Leadership and Management in Nursing

Mary Ellen Grohar-Murray, RN, PhD
Associate Professor of Nursing
St. Louis University School of Nursing

Helen R. DiCroce, RN, MSN
Associate Professor of Nursing
St. Louis University School of Nursing

APPLETON & LANGE
Stamford, CT

Copyright © 1997 by Appleton & Lange
A Simon & Schuster Company

97 98 99 00 01 / 10 9 8 7 6 5 4 3 2 1

Prentice Hall International (UK) Limited, *London*
Prentice Hall of Australia Pty. Limited, *Sydney*
Prentice Hall Canada, Inc., *Toronto*
Prentice Hall Hispanoamericana, S.A., *Mexico*
Prentice Hall of India Private Limited, *New Delhi*
Prentice Hall of Japan, Inc., *Tokyo*
Simon & Schuster Asia Pte. Ltd., *Singapore*
Editora Pentice Hall do Brasil Ltda., *Rio de Janeiro*
Prentice Hall, *Englewood Cliffs, New Jersey*

Library of Congress Cataloging-in-Publication Data
Grohar-Murray, Mary Ellen.
   Leadership and management in nursing/Mary Ellen Grohar-Murray, Helen R. DiCroce. —2nd ed.
      p. cm.
   Includes bibliographical references and index.
   ISBN 0-8385-5646-9 (pbk. : alk. paper)
   1. Nursing services—Administration. 2. Leadership. 3. Nurse administrators. I. DiCroce, Helen R. II. Title.
   [DNLM: 1. Nurse Administrators. 2. Leadership—nurses' instruction. 3. Nursing—organization & administration. WY 105G974L 1997]
   RT89.G76 1997
   362.1' 73' 068—dc20
   DNLM/DLC
   for Library of Congress   96-31743
                                                                               CIP

Acquisitions Editor: Kathleen L. Riedell
Production Editor: Maria T. Vlasak
Designer: Mary Skudlarek

ISBN 0-8385-5646-9

9 780838 556467

90000

PRINTED IN THE UNITED STATES OF AMERICA

Contributors

Judith A. Roos, RN, MSN
Doctoral Candidate, University of Illinois, Chicago
Faculty, Jewish Hospital College of Nursing, St. Louis

Joan H. Carter, RN, PhD
Associate Dean
Associate Professor, St. Louis University School of Nursing, St. Louis

Carroll Ann Quinn, RN, DNS
Associate Professor of Nursing
Fellow, Scripps Gerontology Center
Miami University, Oxford, Ohio

Hugh V. Murray, MBA
Forsyth Securities
Editor, Forsyth Securities Newsletter

Table of Contents

Foreword xix

Preface xxi

Acknowledgments xxiii

UNIT 1: LEADERSHIP. 1

1 The New Health Care System:
   Challenge to Nursing Leadership

   Introduction 3
   Key Concepts. 4
   Health Care Reform 5
   Managed Care 7
   Managed Care Organizations 9
   Characteristics of the Health Care System 10
   Forecast for Health Care 13
   Nursing Leadership's Heritage 14
   Challenge to Nursing. 14
   Leadership Framework. 16
   Differentiating Leadership and Management. 16
   Case Study: Employment in a New Health Care System 17
   Case Study: Leadership or Management?. 18

Summary 18

Student Exercises 19

References 19

2 Leadership Theory

Introduction 21

Key Concepts. 22

Definition of Leadership. 23

Progressive Study of Leadership. 24

Trait Approach. 24

Behavioral School. 25

Leadership Style 25

Leadership Behaviors 26

Situational Theory 29

Contingency Model 29

Situational Leadership Model 30

A New Concept of Leadership 32

Transformational Leadership 33

Connective Leadership. 34

Process Model of Leadership 35

Stage 1—Analysis and Problem Identification 36

The Event. 36

Organizational Factors. 36

Interpersonal Processes between Participants. 37

Controlling Forces 37

Stage 2—Determination of Action 38

Action Plan 38

Stage 3—Evaluation of Action 38

Conclusions on Use of Process 38

Case Study: Laissez-Faire Leadership 39

Case Study: Autocratic Leadership 40

Case Study: Need for Democratic Leadership 40

Summary 41

Student Exercises 41

References 41

3   Interactive Processes of Leadership:
     Communication and Group Process

Introduction 45

Key Concepts. 46

Communication 46

The Message 47

Communication Process. 47

Ten Basics for Good Communication 49

Blocks to Communication 55

Communication with the Health Team. 56

Communication with Difficult People. 57

Communication Networks 60

Group Dynamics 60

Primary and Secondary Groups 61

Characteristics of a Group. 62

Group Processes 63

Leader's Impact on a Group 63

Insight 64

The Group Approach. 65

Understanding 65

Diagnose a Sick Group 66

Flexibility. 66

Evaluation of Group Effectiveness. 67

Case Study: Hostile Aggressive Behavior 68

Case Study: Need for Assertive Communication 68

Case Study: Communication Patterns. 69

Summary 69

Student Exercises 69

References 70

4   Decision Making and Conflict Management

Introduction 73

Key Concepts 74

Decision Making 74

Analysis 74

Prediction of Outcomes 76

Challenge to Nursing 77

Impact of Decisions 79

Systems of Decision Making 80

The Decision-Making Process 81

Identifying Participants 81

Gather Pertinent Facts 82

Generate Alternatives 83

Predict Outcomes 83

Select Best Alternative 83

Plan for Managing Consequences 85

Management of Conflict 86

Nature of Conflict 86

Basis of Conflict 87

Examples of Common Conflicts in Nursing 89

Approaches to Managing Conflict 91

Process Model of Conflict Management 93

Case Study: Coverage by Outside PRN Nurses 95

Case Study: Nurse/Patient Conflict 95

Summary 96

Student Exercises 96

References 98

5   The Ethical Responsibility of the Nurse Leader

Introduction 99

Key Concepts 100

Ethics 100

Ethical Theories 103

Ethical Principles 104

Barriers to Ethical Decision Making 105

Strategies for Enhancing Ethical Decisions in Nursing Practice . . . 106

The Role of Institutional Ethics Committees 107

The Employer-Employee Relationship 108

Peer Relationships 110

Case Study: Ethical Decision Making 112

The Nurse-Patient Relationship 112

Summary 116

Student Exercises 116

References 117

Suggested Readings 119

UNIT 2: AN OVERVIEW OF ORGANIZATIONS
         AND MANAGEMENT 121

6   Organization and Management Theory

Introduction 123

Key Concepts 124

Overview: Organizational Dynamics 124

Classical Theory 125

Scientific Management 126

Administrative Management 126

The Bureaucratic Model 129

Contribution of Classical Theory 130

Modern Theory 130

Behavioral Science 130

General Systems/Social Systems Theory 131

Modern Systems Theory Models 134

Interactional Phenomena 134

    Power 135

    Authority 136

    Responsibility 138

    Status 138

    Process of Delegation 138

Organizational Concepts 138

Organizational Chart 138

Organization Structure 138

Contingency Structure 142

Integrated Health Care System 143

Organizational Model 145

Organization and Management Link 147

Properties of an Organization 147

Case Study: Head Nurse Power 148

Case Study: Authority and Responsibility 148

Case Study: Organizational Structure 149

Summary 150

Student Exercises 150

References 150

7   **Overview of Nursing Management**

Introduction 153

Key Concepts 154

Management Process 154

Levels of Management 155

Management Science 156

Management in Nursing 158

Evolution of Nursing's Management Role 159

Objectives of Nursing Management 159

Management Functions 160

Planning 161

    Types of Planning 162

Organizing 163

Staffing 163

Directing. 164

Coordinating 165

Controlling. 165

Standards 165

Policies 166

Systems of Nursing Care Delivery 167

Case Method 168

Functional Method 168

Team Nursing. 168

Primary Nursing 169

Modular Nursing 171

Case Management 171

Transition to Manager 173

Case Study: The New Manager 174

Management Assessment Guide 175

Summary 176

Student Exercises 176

References 177

8   Delegation: The Manager's Tool

Introduction 179

Key Concepts. 179

Delegation 180

Assignment of Work. 181

The Scalar Chain 182

Decentralization 183

The Purpose of Delegation 183

   Cost Savings. 183

   Time Savings 184

   Professional Growth for Employees 184

   Professional Growth of the Manager. 184

Case Study: Delegation of Staff. 184

Case Study: Improper Delegation 185

The Process of Delegation. 186

Guidelines for Effective Delegation 186

Barriers to Delegation 187

Summary 190

Student Exercises 190

References 190

Suggested Reading. 190

UNIT 3: SPECIAL RESPONSIBILITIES OF THE MANAGER 191

9   Maintaining Standards

Introduction 193

Key Concepts. 194

The Climate for Nursing Practice 195

Professional Basis for Quality Assurance. 196

Practice Framework 198

Legal Basis of Nursing. 198

Ethical and Societal Concerns 200

Governmental Regulations 200

Risk Management 202

Model of Risk Management 203

  Financial Management 203

  Risk Identification 203

  Risk Analysis 203

  Risk Treatment 204

  Risk Evaluation. 204

Impact on Nursing Management 205

Case Study: An Incident Report 205

Summary 206

Student Exercises 206

References 207

10   Motivation in the Work Setting

Introduction 209

Key Concepts. 210

Theories of Motivation 211

Needs Theorists. 211

Personality Type and Motivation. 212

Motivation as Rational Decision Making. 214

Organizational Climate and Motivation. 215

Micromotivation and Macromotivation 218

Motivational Problems. 219

A Situational Approach. 220

Issues Central to Nursing. 221

Case Study: Motivation 221

Case Study: Two Different Worlds 222

Summary 223

Student Exercises 223

References 224

11   Monitoring and Improving Performance

Introduction 227

Key Concepts. 228

Purpose of a Performance Appraisal System. 229

Criteria for Nursing Performance 230

Active Participation in Performance Appraisal 232

Essential Elements 233

Philosophy, Mission, and Objectives 233

Well-Defined Purpose 234

Evaluations that Produce Desired Outcomes. 235

Performance Appraisal Process 237

Planning for the Interview. 238

Participating in the Evaluation Interview 238

Using Evaluation Results 240

Rewards 241

Obstacles to Performance Improvement 245

Case Study: The First Evaluation 247

Case Study: Change in Performance Level 247

Case Study: Evaluations and Morale 248

Summary 249

Student Exercises 249

References 250

12   Legal Issues in the Workplace

Introduction 251

Key Concepts 252

Equal Employment Opportunity (EEO) Laws 253

The Civil Rights Act of 1964 253

Age Discrimination Act 254

Pregnancy Discrimination Act 254

Americans with Disabilities Act (ADA) 254

Sexual Harassment: A Special Case of Discrimination 254

Case Study: Sexual Harassment 256

Case Study: Physical Abuse 257

Case Study: Hostile Environment 257

Labor-Management Laws 257

Unions and Collective Bargaining 257

Strikes 260

Family and Medical Leave Act (FMLA) of 1993 261

Summary 262

Student Exercises 263

References 263

13   Managing Change

Introduction 267

Key Concepts 268

A Theoretical Perspective 269

Basis of Change in Nursing 270
External Forces 270
Internal Forces 271
The Change Process 273
Problem Identification 274
Gaining Support for Change 274
How Changes Are Made 275
Planned Change 276
Radical Intervention 276
Change through Nonintervention 277
Stages of Change 277
Unfreezing 278
Moving 279
Refreezing 279
Change Agents 280
Characteristics of Change Agents 280
Responsibilities of Change Agents 280
Strategies for Change Agents 281
Response to Change 281
Resistance to Change 282
Evaluating Change 284
Case Study: Planned Change Backfires 285
Case Study: Transition from Student to Graduate Nurse 286
Case Study: Parking Lot 287
Summary 287
Student Exercises 288
References 289

UNIT 4: MANAGING RESOURCES 291

14 Managing Resources: The Staff

Introduction 293
Key Concepts 294
Staffing 294

Process and Staffing Plan 294

Staffing Methodologies 296

Case Study: An Understaffed Unit 298

Scheduling Patterns. 299

Work Schedules 299

Management's Role: Planning for Staff. 301

Summary 303

Student Exercises 303

References 303

15   Managing Resources: Time

Introduction 305

Key Concepts. 305

Time Management. 306

Principles of Time Management. 306

Communication. 306

Planning 307

Delegation 307

Prioritizing Goals. 307

Time Management Strategies 308

Time Analysis. 309

Daily Planning. 310

Crisis Control. 310

Problem Analysis 311

Task Analysis 311

Time Control 311

Time Evaluation 311

Barriers to Effective Time Management. 312

Habit. 312

Work Expansion. 312

Case Study: Time Management and the Need to Prioritize. 312

Case Study: Delegation and Communication Problems 313

Oversupervision 314

Underdelegation 314

Losing Sight of Objectives 314

Summary 314

Student Exercises 315

References 315

Suggested Readings 315

16   Managing Resources: The Budget

Introduction 317

Key Concepts 317

Managing Financial Resources 319

Financial Structure 319

The Budgeting Process 320

A Policy Statement 321

Goals and Financial Projections 321

Related Budgeting Concepts 321

Accounting 321

Category One: Income Statements 322

Category Two: The Balance Sheet 322

Category Three: Cash-Flow Statements 323

Cost Accounting 323

Double-entry Accounting 324

Long-range Financial Plans 324

Budget Terms 325

Preparation of the Budget 329

Step One: Review Past Performance 329

Step Two: Review the Organization's Goals and Projections 330

Step Three: Review the Variance 330

Step Four: Actual Preparation of the Budget 331

Case Study: The Budget 331

Case Study: The Lobsterville Clinic: A Study in Financial
         Resource Management 334

Summary 339

Student Exercises 340

Suggested Readings 340

Index 341

Foreword

The health care environment of today is complex, uncertain, and turbulent—there has been a major paradigm shift. The diagnosis, treatment, and management of one patient at a time using the best resources and knowledge available has become managing the care of groups of patients using fewer resources to achieve value-added outcomes.

Registered nurses comprise the largest professional discipline in health care and have a profound influence on all aspects of the health care system. Likewise, the health care system impacts the discipline of nursing. Downsizing, layoffs, hospital closures, and mergers have dramatically impacted the who, when, where, and how of professional nursing care. In the past, change was from one major way of doing things to another major way. Now, we face a plurality of ways of doing things, and must become masters of change to survive—and hopefully thrive—in today's environment. It is at times of radical change such as this that leadership and decision-making skills are of critical importance.

Nurses prepared at the baccalaureate level must, as never before, be prepared to assume leadership and decision-making roles. These roles will not be the traditional roles of supervising segments of a nursing service department. Increasingly, health care organizations have no defined nursing service department. Management titles change or disappear, jobs are transformed, and responsibilities shift as large organizational structures are formed and reformed. Established professions, including nursing, are confronting a potential loss of power as health care organizations create their own multi-skilled assistive workers.

The work of management is evolving into the responsibility of all nurses. The professional nurse is uniquely qualified as the manager of patient care—

individual patients, groups of patients, and communities. In order to enact this role, however, nurses must be able to articulate the **value** of service they provide. They must understand value as a quantity with measurable outcomes in the numerator and cost in the denominator.

This undergraduate textbook provides a framework for the principles of leadership and management for professional nurses to enact their roles in the "brave new world" of health care. Furthermore, it becomes a "jumping-off place" to advanced formal education and higher level responsibilities.

Sandra Blaesing, Ph.D., R.N.
Coordinator, Nursing Service
Administration Specialty
St. Louis University

Preface

The second edition of this text again focuses on undergraduate, senior nursing students. A new feature is a foreword in which the importance of leadership concepts in the undergraduate curriculum is brought to the fore, and curricular articulation from baccalaureate to masters education on the subject is addressed. Comments and suggestions by reviewers of the book served as one source of revisions, along with our own recognition of time-related changes that have occurred in health care delivery and how nursing is practiced since the book was first published in 1992. It became evident that the reorganization of some content was necessary to avoid too-early obsolescence of a new edition. Unit 5 does not appear as such in the new edition. The chapter on ethics has been moved to Unit 1, and the chapter on future directions has been eliminated because the volatility and uncertainty of direction in health care delivery make predictions tenuous. The application of legal considerations to many nursing situations prompted us to include a new chapter on this topic in Unit 3. More case studies from students' experiences have been added to each chapter as they provide a realistic basis for discussion. We feel the students' real experiences expressed in written case studies continue to provide us with an ongoing appreciation of beginners' perceptions of practice today. They provide the student with a safe, comfortable, and confidential way to comment on nursing practice. Students are encouraged to become familiar with the key concepts presented in each chapter and to consider the questions and situations presented in the section entitled "Student Exercises." They are designed to give a sense of the broadness of issues involved in nursing. References for each chapter have been updated, but we have retained many from the past that are classic and timeless.

This second edition is organized into four units. Unit 1 has five chapters that cover the new health care system, leadership theory, the interactive processes of leadership (divided into two chapters), and ethics. The reader will find the same approach to leadership and management as separate entities, as was found in the original publication. Emphasis is on development of leadership skills to be exercised from the beginning of one's practice and as a hallmark of baccalaureate education.

Unit 2 is devoted to an overview of organization and management. In this unit, the reader will find organization and management theory, application of management principles and process to nursing, and a discussion of delegation as a managers' tool.

Unit 3 covers managers' responsibilities. It is divided into five chapters on the topics of standards, motivation, performance, legal issues, and change. The reader will find how students, who are not in formal management positions, can use information in this unit to further their careers in nursing, and to play a role in the advancement of nursing.

Unit 4 is designed to introduce undergraduate students to the management of resources. Effective use of staff and time leads into coverage of budget issues. Care has been given to present all topics in a way that is meaningful to undergraduate students.

In our estimation, our text remains one of the few designed exclusively for undergraduate nursing students in the area of leadership and management. It is our hope that changes that appear in the new edition will benefit student learning and thereby foster greater professionalism among practitioners. A teachers' manual will accompany the new edition, with suggestions on use of the text.

Acknowledgments

We wish to express our continuing appreciation to all those individuals recognized at the time of original publication of our book *Leadership and Management*. We are grateful to the publishers at Appleton & Lange for approaching us about their interest in a second edition. Of particular value to us is Kathleen L. Riedell, Associate Editor, Nursing, for her direction and assistance in the preparation of the manuscript and for keeping us on track in meeting deadlines.

We are fortunate in having the continuing assistance of Hugh Murray for his review and revision of the chapter on financial management, and Judith A. Roos as the author of the chapter on legal issues. We are saddened by the death of Sister Kathleen Krekeler, who added so much to the textbook through the chapter on the ethical responsibility of nurse leaders. We were, however, ably assisted by a colleague, Dr. Carol Quinn, in replacing Sister Kathleen as a chapter contributor. Dr. Joan Carter, who pioneered publication of works on nursing standards, also joined us as a chapter contributor for the second edition. Dr. Sandra Blaesing, Coordinator of the Nursing Service Administration Specialty of the Masters in Nursing Program at St. Louis University, kindly agreed to write a foreword for the second edition. John DiCroce assisted us in preparation of graphics, and we are grateful to him.

We wish to underscore the support we again received from our families, especially our husbands Joseph DiCroce and Hugh Murray. Time in writing for publication takes considerably from valued family activities. Our students continue to teach us and encourage our efforts to assist in their professional education.

Mary Ellen Grohar-Murray
Helen R. DiCroce

UNIT 1

Leadership

The New Health Care System
Challenge to Nursing Leadership

Introduction

Health care is undergoing today what is tantamount to the Industrial Revolution. Under the pressure of government reform, market demand, and internal system reorganization, a dynamic tension has been produced between the health care delivery system and the financing of that care. The nursing profession has long supported our nation's efforts to create a health care system that assures access, quality, and services at affordable costs.[1] The current changes in health care will and are affecting the role of the nurse. Likewise, a real opportunity exists for nursing to help redesign health care delivery. In order to formulate a framework in which the nursing role will be used appropriately, leadership skills will be needed. The goal of this textbook is to introduce the undergraduate student to comprehensive leadership and management theory and to give suggestions for the development of the necessary skills. The objective of this chapter is to describe the dynamic and complex health care system in which future leaders will practice.

KEY CONCEPTS

Ambulatory Care refers to the health care services provided on an outpatient basis; no overnight stay is required. The services provided by ambulatory care centers, hospital outpatient services, physician's offices, and home health care fall under this category.

Capitation refers to a preset amount of money allocated to provide a set of services for a population over a stated period of time, regardless of services used.

DRGs (Diagnosis Related Groups) are one of the first systems that categorized patient and disease information based on averages leading to uniform cost for each category. The following variables determine the category: primary and secondary diagnosis, primary and secondary procedures, age, and length of stay.

Health Care Dynamics is the term used to identify the priorities of the new health care system that form a social structure nurses must practice within.

Leadership is a concept and process that is capable, through interactional phenomena, of influencing a group toward goal achievement.

Management is a concept and a process that uses resources (human, technical, financial, time, etc.) to meet specific goals efficiently and effectively.

Behavioral/Situational Framework is a theoretic foundation that suggests appropriate behavior results from a detailed framework analysis of a situation. The variables that define the situation include the greater society, the organization, a particular event, and leader and follower characteristics. The appropriate behavior refers to leader/manager behavior that provides guidance, inspiration, or direction toward accomplishing an end.

Managed Care refers to the assumption of responsibility and accountability for the health of a defined population and the simultaneous acceptance of financial risk.

Managed Competition refers to the future goal of health care delivery to allow patients and payers to choose among available integrated systems that would best meet their needs. Service, price, quality, and availability would be among the issues to consider.

Primary Care is a term used to describe the basic health care all persons require. It is also the entry point of care in the managed care environment.

HMO (Health Maintenance Organization) is an alternative health care delivery agency and financing mechanism (prepaid comprehensive health coverage for hospital and physician services) which provides primary care services and refers specialty needs to appropriate sources (contracted partners).

PPO (Preferred Provider Organization) is a term used to describe an arrangement between purchasers of care (employers and insurance companies) and a group of practitioners who provide services to patients for a designated network at a discounted rate to encourage use of the available services.

Integrated Health Care System is an organized system that provides a full array of services from primary to tertiary care, with each service representing an independent cost center.

Fee for Service refers to the traditional payment method whereby patients pay doctors, hospitals, and other providers for service rendered and then bill private insurers or the government.

■ HEALTH CARE REFORM

The current health care system is characterized by dramatic shifts in providers, financing, and how and where care will be provided. Because medical spending continues to escalate to a degree our society can no longer support, structural change in the health care system was inevitable.[2] Thus, needed change is occurring to provide access, quality, and affordable care (Fig. 1-1). This movement is in stark contrast to the health care system of the past.

In the mid-1950s, there was a vast expansion of the health care system in terms of volume, intensity, dollars, and personnel. This unrestrained investment in the health care industry led to a rapid escalation of health care cost. All payers (those who reimburse care), especially the federal government, were greatly affected. As a result, in 1983, Congress deliberately enacted what has become known as the Social Security Amendments of 1983 Law HR-1900 (PL 98-21). This legislation included the establishment of a prospective payment system based on 467 **diagnosis-related groups (DRGs)** that allowed pretreatment diagnosis billing categories for almost all U.S. hospitals reimbursed by Medicare. This amounted to a set of maximum fees that would be paid for Medicare patients. Hospitals would make a profit

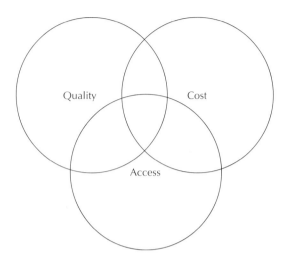

Figure 1-1. The dominant elements of nursing's values for health care reform.

only if the cost of hospitalization was less than agreed upon by the corresponding DRG category. For the first time there was an incentive to keep costs down. This was the major event that started a revolution within the entire medical care industry and that dramatically altered the nature of health care delivery. Soon major insurance companies followed suit by establishing price ceilings as reimbursement for hospital care received. Because health care was accountable for cost containment nursing departments were also expected to account for the cost of direct and indirect care. In the process, nursing service departments reorganized the delivery of nursing care, and in some cases nurses were laid off and several hospitals were no longer operative. Corporate planning groups offered to manage the resources of many existing hospitals to facilitate survival of organizations in a highly competitive environment.

These activities, while substantial, were not sufficient to harness the increasing rise of health care cost. In 1992, 838.5 billion dollars were spent on health care, taking more than 14 percent from the gross national product.[3] In addition, between 35 to 40 million Americans, or 14 percent of the population, were uninsured.[4] In response, the Clinton administration actively attempted to overhaul the health care system and stop the rate of growth. President Clinton formed the President's Task Force on National Health Care Reform. The task force, led by Hillary Clinton, the first lady, was controversial from its inception. Nevertheless, in September 1993, amid considerable public interest and continuing political controversy, the task force proposed fundamental principles. As expressed by Ira Magaziner, senior White House advisor, and Donna Shalala, Health and Human Services secretary, these principals included guaranteed access to primary and preventive care for both children and adults, continued quality of care, and cost containment. In addition, the plan proposed global budgeting, a strategy for providing universal coverage while containing national health costs by setting an annual health budget, and an overall cap on costs. Lastly, preventive and primary care, as well as mental health were emphasized in the plan.[5] Immediately, obstacles to the reform agenda were voiced. These obstacles included the timetable for universal coverage, the future of the employment mandate, the nature of and authority over the basic benefit package, and most importantly, the financing mechanism.[6] Reaching no consensus, the proposed plan was not implemented. Despite the failure of major health care reform led by government initiative, dramatic changes in the marketplace, insurance company financing, and mix of health care providers were initiated. In essence, health care reform had begun, and not surprisingly, the opportunities and challenge to professional nursing have never been greater.

■ MANAGED CARE

The decade has seen unprecedented change in the delivery, organization, and financing of health care, and **managed care** is emerging as a dominant management strategy. There is no universal agreement on how best to define and implement managed care. As such, managed care represents a transitional process.[7] By definition, managed care refers to the assumption of responsibility and accountability for the health of a defined population and the simultaneous acceptance of financial risk inherent in assuming that responsibility.[8] Managed care promotes the effective, responsible and cost-efficient care of the individual within a given population. This management of care is a cooperative process between the managed care organization and the patient.[9] In essence, managed care is a system that integrates the financing and delivery of appropriate medical care by means of the following mechanisms:

- **Care is population based.**
  Population-based care encompasses the concepts and methods of epidemiology and public health. It is comprehensive care that recognizes not only the individual but also the community and environment with special emphasis on healthy practices that promote health. Thus, the

health care professional's role of delivering care to the individual has expanded to considering other factors that impact that care. The overarching goal is to improve the health status of the population.

- **All participants are held accountable.**
Joint accountability is expected on the part of all parties involved for the cost and quality of health care. This includes the patient, practitioner, and administrators of the managed care system. This may be accomplished through coinsurance or a cost-sharing requirement under a health care policy, which provides the insured (patient) will assume a portion of the cost (usually 20 percent) of covered services. The cost, quality, and value of care are evaluated to insure quality of care and efficient use of resources through monitoring, controlling cost, and judiciously using medical services.

- **Information to assess value will be necessary.**
All relevant information is collected about the delivery of care, including patient data, population information, cost data, and technologic information, in order to insure that patients receive the most appropriate care. Quality controls are in place to evaluate care. Reliance on information management will increase as a methodology to insure the most appropriate and cost-effective care.

- **Primary care is of central importance.**
Primary care is considered the chief mechanism by which preventive, therapeutic, and restorative care is provided in the least expensive cost center. Primary care is the entry point to access care, serves as a partner for a long-term caregiving relationship, provides coordination of specialty care, and all other services needed. Typically, this care is provided in **ambulatory care** settings.

- **Interdependence is very important.**
The complexity of today's care requires numerous caregivers and specialists. This demands coordinated care that is not fragmented. Interdisciplinary care has long been used with specific populations (psychiatric and elderly, to mention a few). The concept of the interdisciplinary team takes on more importance in managed care. The ultimate aim is to provide a mechanism for a seamless health care delivery system through a variety of interconnected services.

- **Contracts are used to detail finances and delivery of care.**
Currently, managed care exists on a continuum between the **fee-for-service** method and total population-based care, which will eventually

lead to managed competition. To support this kind of caregiving process, explicit contracts are provided. This informs all involved parties exactly what they will receive and at what financial risk each party will assume. This means all participants—patient, practitioner, and provider—have a responsibility for financing care and incentives to keep cost down.[10,11]

Managed Care Organizations

Managed care represents a new way of approaching health care delivery. It requires restructuring and reengineering of existing structures. There are a wide variety of organizational arrangements that provide managed care. Some of the more common arrangements are referred to as **health maintenance organizations (HMOs), preferred provider organizations (PPOs),** or an integrated system that provides a full array of services for a defined population for a fixed price. These organizations provide a wide range of services from prevention to designated acute care. Participants are encouraged to use services frequently by being charged low monthly premiums and having convenient, accessible medical centers. Managed care is a methodology of providing care when it is least expensive, and providing a financing mechanism that utilizes preset fees with constraints on provider practice.

In a managed care system, the hospital is no longer the center of care. Rather, primary care (ambulatory care service) is the focus. Managed care will place more emphasis on education, self-help, preventive services, and will limit access to tertiary care or hospitals. Because the patient or enrollee is treated in the lowest cost setting, it is not desirable or cost effective to keep every hospital bed filled. In this system, the primary care practitioner is emerging as the central figure in controlling and managing health care delivery.

Managed care represents a first step toward a competitive market-dominated system known as **managed competition.** Managed competition occurs when **integrated health care systems** compete to provide services to defined capitated groups. Because this system is integrally involved with finances, the language used is that of business and the insurance industry. For instance, **capitation** is a term that refers to a given amount of money allocated for a set of services for a particular population over a stated period of time.[12] Prepaid medical groups are given a monthly fee regardless of the services used. With total capitation, the integrated health system is responsible for its enrollees. Patients who are paid enrollees are called covered lives.[13] The system receives payment based on a negotiated single price per covered life, and is paid upfront. The objective of this system then becomes to keep people healthy and out of the hospital, delivering quality care at affordable prices.

■ CHARACTERISTICS OF THE HEALTH CARE SYSTEM

In the managed care environment, health care priorities have been redefined. The following characteristics represent the **health care dynamics,** or the new social structure nurses must now practice within. Each will be discussed independently, and the implications for professional nursing will be addressed.

1. **The changing emphasis from treatment of disease to health promotion and disease prevention.**
   The managed care environment is part of a profound change in the culture of health care whose emphasis is moving away from the treatment of illness and toward wellness and health. Health promotion and disease prevention are long-held values of the nursing profession. Nursing organizations and the nursing press advocate preventive health services, quality of care, and accountability for health care outcomes.[14] Underlying this precept is a major cultural transformation, with patients expecting a very different response from practitioners.[15] Today, an information-rich middle class culture and a population no longer content with emphasis on illness, dominates society. In essence, these attitudes provide a positive environment for nurses, who are uniquely suited to provide this desired style of health care.

2. **An increased need for primary care providers/a decreased need for specialists.**
   Primary care is the routine care needed by most people. It includes an annual physical, treatment for minor illness, periodic immunizations, and health screening. Within the new health care system, primary care is becoming the entry point to receive more complex medical treatment. Currently, there is a shortage of primary care physicians and an abundance of specialists. There are complex reasons for this distribution. Traditionally, specialist care has been rewarded through remuneration for technical procedures by third-party payers, as opposed to the cognitive and interpersonal skills required of primary care practitioners. This ratio will be reversed because of a changing health care culture, the prominent role of primary care, and the government's increased incentive to support primary care education.

Interestingly, it has been recommended that advanced practice nurses (APNs) or nurse practitioners (NPs) be deployed to provide primary care. APNs are registered nurses whose formal education and clinical preparation extend beyond the basic requirements for licensure, resulting in a certificate or master's degree. Specialties of APNs include (1) certified nurse midwives (CNMs), (2) certified registered nurse anesthetists (CRNAs), (3) clinical nurse specialists (CNSs), and (4) nurse practitioners (NPs). Within these specialties are subspecialties for which APNs assume high levels of responsibility.

In particular, NPs are educationally prepared to perform a wide range of professional nursing functions, including obtaining a medical history; performing a physical examination; providing prenatal care and family planning; providing well child care, (screening and immunizations); providing health maintenance care for adults; and collaborating with other health professionals as needed.[16] In addition, NPs are prepared to perform some functions traditionally performed by MDs, such as diagnosing and treating common acute and chronic health problems and minor injuries.[17] NPs have a proven ability to offer quality, cost-effective primary care. Two decades of research summarized in the Yale Journal on Regulation give clear evidence that APNs provide care of comparable quality and at a lower cost than do doctors.[18] Yet, many legislative barriers frustrate their potential. The extent to which NPs are able to perform traditional physician functions [for example prescriptive license (the right to prescribe some medications)] is limited by individual state regulations, although nearly all states have acknowledged in varying degrees the expanded role of the APN.[19] The issue of legislative approval, which changes and expands the scope of APN practice, involves complex public policy, specific legislative actions, and overcoming political obstacles with other health practitioners.[20]

While the president's task force on health care reform recognized the role nursing could play in managing health care delivery, a collaborative system must be in place. That is a system that supports the appropriate use of all levels of health care professions, who deliver care in accord with their education. In this system, nurses could be used to improve access to affordable health care. This is particularly true of patients who are at high risk for serious problems that might have been prevented. In particular, the elderly, mothers, and children are of noteworthy concern. Persons over 65 years of age will be 20 percent of the total population by the year 2030 and will represent a major block of patients requiring health care. In addition, President Clinton's primary and preventive care initiatives for mothers and children (of whom many are minorities, immigrants, and children living in single-parent families) have been targeted for care. This group is traditionally undeserved and exhibits problems that would benefit from preventive care. Examples of some interventions to prevent problems are immunizations and prenatal care. Opportunities for nursing to provide care to these groups is worthwhile and meaningful.

3. More than half the nursing care will be provided outside the hospital, while the hospital will provide only critical care.

Because of health care reform, the acute care hospital has been the most dramatically affected. In a consolidation effort, hospitals have closed, merged, decreased their bed capacity, reorganized their services, and developed integrated health care systems.[21] This massive reorganization resulting in corporatization of the health care industry is one of the largest reorganization efforts since the nineteenth century.[22] This has had a dramatic effect on nursing employment. Prior to reorganization, 66 percent of practicing nurses were employed in a hospital setting.[23] Following reorganization, hospital occupancy rate and patient length of stay decreased, resulting in nurses being laid off.

During this chaotic period as health care seeks equilibrium, nursing employment is erratic. However, as emphasis continues to grow regarding ambulatory and home health care, as well as an expansion of preventive and primary care services, nurses will be required.[24] Findings from studies in which the nursing factor often makes the critical difference in cost can be the basis for a convincing argument in favor of retaining the professional nurse as caregiver. Administrators can be shown that dollars spent on salaries for professional nurses are highly beneficial to the organization.

In addition, new and expanded practice sites, other than the hospital, are emerging. These sites include schools, ambulatory and day surgery centers, clinics, and group practices. Some practice sites are integrated with an acute care system and some are stand-alone. In essence, the hospital is no longer the center of care. Patients who are sick will be cared for everywhere. Patients and the health care team are going to be challenged in dealing with this new environment.

4. Clinical nursing knowledge will be challenged to include new skills.

The new practice environment requires from the nurse a different set of professional skills. In addition to the clinical knowledge necessary for hospital-based care, community and family/group relationships assessment will be necessary. Because the care will be delivered to ambulatory patients, nurses should possess health educator, provider of preventive and primary care skills. In addition, nurses need to be prepared in shared decision making with patients and evaluating treatment effectiveness. The ability to understand the total organizational perspective in the delivery of care will require leadership/management knowledge. The demands of this new system will require lifelong learning of the workforce.

5. **Scientific knowledge and technology will continue to increase.**
Modern times have given us computers and advanced technology whose full capability is yet to be determined. This can only be viewed as a positive step forward for the science of health care. However, modern technology challenges the profession to incorporate these advancements into the holistic philosophy of nursing, which is concerned with the total patient. The expense of modern technology makes cost containment a challenge for the oncoming decade.

6. **Ethical issues will continue to grow in complexity.**
Ethical problems will continue to exist on two levels: (1) those problems that have direct bearing on a patient's life and (2) policies that impact the health care system. Access to health care is emerging as a major ethical and political issue for the health care system. The ability to provide access to proper care is organized around two major issues. The first concerns the available mechanisms to finance health care, and the second concerns the allocation of scarce resources. Both these critical issues are forces that will help shape the debate that ultimately will structure the health care system.

■ FORECAST FOR HEALTH CARE

Nursing as a vital participant in health care delivery is both affected by and capable of influencing the system. Thus, being a leader/manager in an unsettled environment demands that the nurse be prepared with the appropriate knowledge and skills. The nurse manager's preparation should include the analytic ability to identify problems and the skills to effectively lead and manage people through difficult and changing times. This makes the need for nursing leadership even more important to provide creative solutions to facilitate quality nursing and health care. The innovative nurse leader/manager of the future will be expected to use creative problem solving and interpersonal techniques, such as collaboration and negotiation. The future environment for health care delivery for which the nurse leader and manager must be prepared includes recognizing the values held by the nursing profession, supporting and empowering nurses, and marketing the work of nursing not only in the delivery of health care, but also health promotion, disease and accident prevention, research, and education.[25] See Figure 1-2.

■ NURSING LEADERSHIP'S HERITAGE

Throughout history, there have been great nurse leaders. Explanation of their accomplishments has been studied through case study analysis, revealing personal characteristics of greatness. Several studies by Christy reviewed the characteristics and contribution of Lavina Dock, Annie Warbuton Goodrich, M. Adelaide Nutting, Sophia F. Palmer, Isabel Hampton Robb, Isabel Maitland Stewart, and Lillian Wald.[26] These nurse leaders became effective change agents and influenced legislation, nursing practice, and nursing education. Through their efforts, valuable contributions were made in areas of nursing education, nursing literature, and professional organizations, all of which proved to be substantial aids in the development of the profession.

Challenge to Nursing

While changes are required to meet the demands of the managed care environment, some essential elements of the past must be retained to preserve

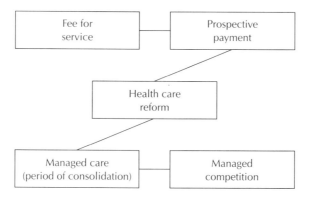

Figure 1-2. A depiction of the evolution of health care from the traditional fee for service to the future of managed competition.

the nature of holistic care, which is central to the very philosophy of nursing. Specific changes in nursing education have been advocated. The National League for Nursing (NLN) called for reform of nursing education to realign programs to be more congruent with the changing landscape of health care. Specifically, NLN says "in a consumer-driven, community-based, primary care–focused based system, nursing education will have to concentrate on increasing the number of primary and tertiary care practitioners."[27] Curriculum changes are needed that encompass a broader knowledge base without extending program length. The increase in the number and diversity of interdisciplinary groups involved in the comprehensive delivery of health care requires sharpening the communication and group process skills of nurses who coordinate the activities of primary care practitioners and specialists. Clinical learning experiences must continue to prepare practitioners with skills needed for quality patient care in the community. Creative educators working with creative practitioners are needed to make the critical difference in redesigning learning opportunities. See Figure 1-3.

The nursing profession has the unique power to influence both health care delivery and health care policy. This demands leadership skill at the national and local policy-making levels. The introduction of health-related policy-making and implementation concepts in baccalaureate nursing curricula, combined with that of leadership, management, and research theory, maximize nursing's service to society.

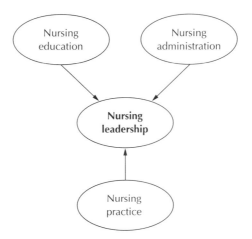

Figure 1-3. Factions of the nursing profession that define and guide the nursing profession and nursing leadership.

Leadership Framework

This is one of the most challenging and potentially rewarding times to be involved in the nursing profession. Never before has leadership been a more important concept to the practice and the profession of nursing. The transition from student to leader and manager is a process that involves knowledge, skill, experience, and time. By reviewing the essential forces that affect a situation, appropriate decisions can be made. For this text the leadership/management process will be grounded in a **behavioral/situational framework,** which refers to the necessary behavior the nurse leader should use to achieve a goal. Appropriate leader behavior is dependent on conditions found in the situation and those affected by the situation. Consistently, the future nursing leader will be exposed to a way of analyzing situations from a broad base. From this perspective, decisions may be formulated from critical factors found in the environment, in a situation, within the leader, and within the group.

New leaders must consider formulating new and efficient methods of nursing care, review factors that renew an interest in the nursing profession, and allow the appropriate use of nurses in new structures. A theoretic basis for leadership and management, as well as work experience, provides a good foundation for the nurse leader during these exciting times. The importance of experience in the development of leaders has been well described in the experiences of executives from the public domain. Successful leaders provide evidence for the need of both knowledge and seasoning. This is particularly important in times of organizational and industrial stress similar to the current health care system. The conclusion suggests that it is unwise to rely on on-the-job training for newly appointed nurse managers. Neither is it wise to promote unqualified individuals just because they are willing to accept the challenge. Identifying potential leadership and management capabilities of individuals is critical in the selection of candidates for important roles. Stress in the work place, staff morale, and general upheaval in the work setting prove to be quite costly when poor leaders and managers are in place. Identifying valuable traditions and practices through the efforts of nurse managers, nurse researchers, nurse educators, and nurse clinicians who work in concert with each other is sensible and brings unity to the profession.

Differentiating Leadership and Management

The terms **leadership** and **management** have been used several times throughout this chapter. It is appropriate to point out the way in which these key terms will be used in this textbook. Leadership and management are viewed as separate entities. Leadership is viewed as being a more fundamental and creative coordinating process than management, which selects actions that use resources effectively and efficiently. Leadership is the process of influencing people to accomplish goals, whereas management is moving an organization toward achievement of its goals. Anyone in a setting can serve as a leader by generating and proposing creative, innovative ideas and by applying predictive principles to apparent problems. To be a leader, one does not have to occupy a formal managerial position. Managers, on the other hand, occupy formal positions in an organization and are accountable for effective use of available resources. The boss expects managers to "make the place run" according to a design. Skills of both managers and leaders are needed for successful operation of any organization. The skills of both might be embodied in one individual, but this is not necessarily true. Some who excel as leaders are poor managers, whereas others excel at managing an established situation while seldom generating ideas for needed redesign. Bennis, a management scientist, points out the differences between a manager and a leader.[28] He says a leader inspires and a manager administrates; a leader develops and a manager maintains; a leader relies on people and a manager relies on the system; and, lastly, a leader requires trust, a manager control.

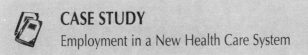

CASE STUDY
Employment in a New Health Care System

Jane Jones just graduated from college with a baccalaureate degree in nursing. Jane entered the profession because she had an interest in serving people and because she believed the job opportunities and security were great. However, when she graduated, she found jobs to be scarce and the immediate future looking bleak. Jane decided to study what was happening in health care. She reviewed the agencies, hospitals, clinics, and same-day surgery centers in her area. She prepared her resumé and prepared for interviews. She was determined. After one month of tireless effort, she was offered two positions. One position was as a staff nurse in the acute care hospital on a surgical division, and the other was a beginning position in adult ambulatory care.

- How would you go about advising Jane as to which position to take?
- What criteria would you use in making a job selection?
- What skills are necessary for each position?

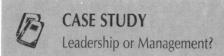

CASE STUDY
Leadership or Management?

In the managed care environment, St. Joseph's Hospital was forced to down-size. The nurses on 4 South, a general surgery division, were becoming increasingly anxious about the future. Were their jobs in jeopardy? Were patients receiving quality care? The nurses felt there was too much emphasis on cost containment and most of the nurses felt they had no control over their jobs in the current situation. Mrs. Smith, the head nurse, recognized the turmoil and called a staff meeting to discuss issues.

- Is Mrs. Smith practicing leadership or management? What is the difference?

■ SUMMARY

This chapter has described the evolution of events that have led to the current conditions in health care today. These characteristics represent the dynamic priorities of health care reform. Future nurse leaders/managers will practice in a managed care environment where emphasis will be on health promotion, prevention, and primary care. Sick people will be cared for everywhere, not just at the hospital, thus nurses must have new professional skills that deal with assessment of individuals and families in a complex integrated health care system. Because cost containment will be a dominant theme, most patients will be provided care in managed care organizations. Technology and scientific advancements will continue. The ethical issue of access to health care will dominate the debate about health care policy. These characteristics represent the forces that will influence the work environment and ultimately the decisions about patient care. The challenge and opportunities available to nursing have never been greater. Fortunately, there is a heritage of past leaders to inspire present efforts. The value of leadership theory is an important tool to influence health care and policy as well as the future role of professional nursing. The transition from students to leaders and managers is a process that requires knowledge, skills, experience, and time. Throughout this textbook, process will be emphasized and structured according to models. Practice takes place in a dynamic environment in which varying degrees of control and structure are possible. It is in a behavioral and situational context that students are challenged to contribute to nursing early in their careers by thinking and acting like leaders.

 STUDENT EXERCISES

1. Name two forces that led to health care reform. In the current climate of health care change, have these forces been addressed? Discuss both the positive and negative effects health care reform may produce on professional nursing.

2. Define managed care. What implications does it have for professional nursing? What would you tell someone interested in entering the nursing profession today?

3. A patient enters the community HMO with a serious respiratory problem. The patient needs immediate medical attention. What will be the likely process of care the patient will receive?

4. What are the chief differences between the old fee-for-service method and the new system of managed care. What are the differences in priorities?

5. As a student in a baccalaureate program, what skills do you require in order to function best in the managed care environment? How would you justify the cost of a college degree for nurses?

■ REFERENCES

1. National League for Nursing, "Nursing's Agenda for Health Care Reform," *American Nurse* Kansas City, MO, 1991, p. 2.
2. Pew Health Professions Commission, *Health Professions Education and Managed Care: Challenges and Necessary Responses*, Pew Health Profession Commission, 1st ed, August 1995, p. 6.

3. Inglis AD, Kjiervik DK, "Empowerment of Advanced Practice Nurses: Regulation on Reform Needed to Increase Access to Care, *Journal of Law, Medicine, and Ethics*, 21:2, 1993, p. 194.

4. Ibid., p. 194.

5. Minarik PA, "Legislative and Regulatory Update: Health Care Reform and Managed Competition: Implications for the CNS," *Clinical Nurse Specialist*, 17:3, 1993, p. 105.

6. Donley R, "Nursing After Health Care Reform," *Nursing Economics*, 13:2, March–April 1995, p. 84.

7. Pew Health Professions Commission, p. 10.

8. Ibid., p. 12.

9. Inglehart JH, "Health Policy Report: The American Health Care System, Managed Care," *New England Journal of Medicine*, Sept. 3, 1992, p. 742.

10. Ibid.

11. Pew Health Professions Commission, p. 12–19.

12. Sovie M, "Tailoring Hospitals for Managed Care and Integrated Health Care Systems," *Nursing Economics*, 13:2, March–April 1995, p. 72.

13. Ibid.

14. Donley R, p. 85.

15. Pew Health Professions Commission, p. 2.

16. Inglis AD, Kjiervik DK, p. 195.

17. Ibid., p. 196.

18. Safriet BJ, "Health Care Dollars and Regulatory Sense: The Role of the Advanced Practice Nurse," *Issue Bulletin*, March 1993, p. 3.

19. Inglis AD, Kjiervik DK, p. 196.

20. Aiken L, Fagin C, "More Nurses, Better Medicine," *New York Times*, March 11, 1994.

21. Sim TW, "Health Care Reform, Window of Opportunity: An Interview with Connie Curran," *ANNA Journal*, 21:3, May 1994, p. 250.

22. Pew Health Professions Commission, p. 5.

23. Donley R, p. 85.

24. Ibid.

25. O'Donnel M, "A Positive Environment," *Nursing Standard*, 5:36, May 1991, p. 36.

26. Christy TE, "Leadership in Nursing." In McCloskey JC, Molen MT (editors), *Research on the Profession of Nursing*, New York: Springer Publishing, 1987, 8:230.

27. National League for Nursing, *A Vision for Nursing Education*, New York: N.Y.U. Press, 1993, p. 3.

28. Bennis W, Manus B, "Leaders," *The Strategies for Taking Charge*, New York: Harper & Row, 1985, 218–222

2

Leadership Theory

Introduction

The health care industry is immersed in a period of scrutiny and rapid change. There is an urgent need for empowered visionary leaders to direct the health care industry into the twenty-first century.[1] Because the work force of nurses is estimated to be 2 million, the largest of the health care discipline, nurses have inherent power to influence the direction health care will take.[2] Therefore, the profession has been challenged to change its education and practice. Nurses must be prepared as leaders who are competent, flexible, and able to energize others to adapt to change. This book will lead the reader to the realization that leadership involves a process that encourages each individual in the work setting to contribute to effectively meeting organizational goals. In addition, it will become evident that the usefulness of a leadership position is in relation to broad situational factors. The objective of this chapter is to describe leadership theory as it progresses from a simple concept to a complex process.

KEY CONCEPTS

Leadership Style refers to the underlying motivation of a leader who directs goal-oriented behavior. These styles are commonly referred to as autocratic, democratic, laissez-faire, or eclectic.

Leadership Behavior refers to the actual choice of the decision-making style the leader uses toward meeting a specific goal. These behaviors are commonly thought to be telling, selling, testing, consulting, and joining.

Great Man Theory defines leaders as those who are born with abilities to lead others.

Trait Approach is a way of explaining leadership in light of a set of traits an individual possesses. These traits include instrumental and interactional characteristics.

Behavioral School is a way of explaining leadership by virtue of decision-making style used by the individual, ranging from autocratic to laissez-faire.

Autocratic is a decision-making style used by a leader in which the leader does not consider the group's input.

Democratic is a decision-making style used by the leader that equally considers the group's input as well as the leader's.

Laissez-faire is a decision-making style used by a leader that is group centered.

Situational Theory is a way of explaining leadership through taking into account forces that occur in the situation, the leader, and the followers. Leaders are determined by the situation.

Contingency Model is a way of explaining leadership on the basis of specific contingencies or variables. They include leader-member relationships, the structure of the task, and the position, or role, of power.

Life-cycle Theory of leadership is a way of explaining leadership based on the following assumptions: (1) the follower's readiness for task completion is based on his or her motivation and competence, and (2) leadership behavior is adaptable based on the follower's task maturity.

New Theory of Leadership is a way of explaining leadership, as offered by Warren Bennis and Burt Manus, through four human handling skills that suggest that leaders are those who have vision, can communicate, are steadfast, and demonstrate a positive self-regard.

Process Model of Leadership is a conceptualization of the essential factors and activities that comprise appropriate leadership decisions and behaviors.

Transformational Leadership is a process of influencing followers through creating relationships that focus on vision and values. This method relies on a climate of trust and mutuality.

Transactional Leadership is the traditional leadership process that emphasizes the leaders influencing process over followers.

Connective Leadership is a process that connects individuals with their tasks and visions to one another, to the group, and to the larger network.

■ DEFINITION OF LEADERSHIP

Leadership has been studied by many disciplines and has been given many definitions with various insights, dimensions, and meanings. Most definitions reflect the discipline's perspective. Thus, the following comprehensive definition, compatible with nursing's values, is offered.

Leadership may be considered as:

> A collective function in the sense that it is the integrated synergized expression of a group's efforts; it is not the sum of individual dominance and contributions, it is their interrelationships. Ultimate authority and true sanction for leadership, where it is exercised, resides not in the individual, however dominant, but in the total situation and in the demands of the situation. It is the situation that creates the imperative, whereas the leader is able to make others aware of it, is able to make them willing to serve it, and is able to release collective capacities and emotional attitudes that may be related fruitfully to the solution of the group's problems; to that extent one is exercising leadership.[3]

Leadership is a complex and multidimensional concept. It includes intrapersonal, interpersonal, intergroup, and situational variables. As a result, it is not easily defined or measured. However, leadership may be analyzed as a process that includes social, ethical, and theoretical components. The social nature of leadership entails the interpersonal skills necessary to be effective in a variety of situations. The ethical nature of leadership involves the inherent power of a leadership position that when exercised should benefit the common good. All components of the leadership process will be discussed throughout the text. The following discussion focuses on the theoretical nature of leadership. This review includes tradition, theory, and research.

Progressive Study of Leadership

The oldest view of leadership considered it a birthright. Kings and queens ascended to thrones because of custom. Kings begot kings and became the leader. Individuals in formal leadership roles were accepted without question. This is similar to the **great man theory,** which states that great leaders are born with the ability to lead, influence, and direct others. As such, only those in possession of these qualities are leaders. Under this perspective, leaders may not be developed. Fortunately, the study of leadership was pursued.

Trait Approach

The serious study of leadership began when the following question was asked: Who is a leader? Early theorists recognized that leadership was by nature elusive, but might be explained by virtue of a leader's traits. The **trait approach** states that leadership exists as an attribute of a personality. If certain traits are exhibited, an individual is a leader. However, because the traits necessary for successful leadership varied from situation to situation, no exhaustive list of traits was offered.

Even though no one leader type was described, certain personality traits have been identified through early psychologic studies to correspond to effective leadership behavior. Among these are intelligence, social sensitivity, social participation, and communication skills.[4] This particular group of traits identifies the leader as the one who has the capability to influence a group through innate intelligence and well-developed interpersonal skills.

Nurse researchers have also conducted studies to determine the characteristics of nursing leaders. Two different studies were conducted independently by Dunham & Fisher and Murphy & DeBack, who sought the characteristics and behaviors of hospital nurse executives.[5,6] Both studies reached comparable conclusions. Nurse executives display similar characteristics, such as being visionary, credible, enabling, willing to serve as role models, and having the ability to master change. Interestingly, Meighan, another nurse researcher, conducted a similar study, only this time using staff nurses with the same leadership characteristics identified.[7] Findings from these studies reveal characteristics that facilitate effective leadership behavior. However, common agreement about strength and priority of the suggested traits, as well as conformity to a single personality profile is lacking.[8] Nonetheless, identified leadership traits serve as adjunct knowledge to explain what makes an effective leader.

Behavioral School

Because traits were insufficient to explain leadership, the study of what leaders do was a predictable next step. This change in perspective examined specific leadership behaviors in the workplace.[9] The early work of Lewin and colleagues explained leadership in terms of decision-making behaviors.[10] Their classic work and terminology is foundational to the study of leadership style.

Leadership Style Leaders have been described in terms of their decision-making styles in one or more of the following ways. **Autocratic,** or dictatorial, means that the leader makes all decisions and allows subordinates no influence in the decision-making process. Such supervisors are often indifferent to subordinates' personal needs. The second system of decision making is entitled participative, or **democratic.** In this case the supervisor consults with the subordinates on appropriate matters, giving them some influence in the decision-making process. This type of supervisor is not punitive and treats subordinates with fairness and dignity. The third system is called **laissez-faire,** or free rein, which means that supervisors allow their group to have complete autonomy. Because they rarely supervise the group directly, the group makes its own decisions. These decision-making styles have become synonymous with the concept of **leadership styles,** which by definition refers to the underlying needs of the leader that motivate behavior. There exists more agreement among authorities on the classification of leadership styles than on a definition of leadership. The **behavioral school** (because of its emphasis on style) has led other authors to expand on its usefulness. For example, styles of leadership can be depicted on a continuum developed by Schmitt and Tannenbaum, ranging from autocratic, or leader-centered, to abdicate, or group-centered, supervision.[11] This continuum is depicted in Figure 2-1.

To make a decision regarding a leader's placement on the continuum, it is necessary to analyze what constitutes a leadership style. This examination includes consideration of one's personality and intelligence, the characteristics of the task to be performed, the roles of the leader and group members who will complete the task, and the characteristics of the group. In essence, this comprehensive analysis will help the leader to understand what is necessary to complete the task and will ultimately lead to the appropriate leadership behavior in a given situation. For a comparison of leadership style and its relationship with the leader, follower, and situation, see Table 2-1.

Leader Centered   **Group Centered**

Use of Authority by Leader

Freedom of the group

Autocrat _____   _____   Democrat   Laissez-Faire

_____ Tells   Sells   Tests   Consults   Joins

Figure 2-1. The relationship between leadership style and leadership behavior. Leadership styles exist on a continuum and are characterized by particular behaviors. *(Adapted from Schmitt, W and Tannenbaum, R.)*

Leadership Behaviors   Leadership behavior refers to a variety of behaviors a leader may enact to meet a goal or to complete a task. These behaviors range from being highly leader-centered to highly group-centered. The leadership behaviors are telling, selling, testing, consulting, and joining (Fig. 2-1); these correspond with the different leadership styles. When a leader identifies a problem, considers alternative solutions, decides on the best course of action without consulting the group, and then informs the group of what is to be done, the leader is using *telling* as a mode of behavior. The group

TABLE 2-1. COMPARISON OF LEADERSHIP STYLE AND LIMITING CONDITIONS

	Autocratic	**Democratic**	**Laissez-Faire**
Leader			
Holds:	Absolute power	Limited power	No power
Knowledge:	Unique	Shared	Same or less
Behavior:	Dominates	Participates	Joins
Position:	Inflexible	Flexible	Neutral
Followers			
Relates:	Dependent	Expects involvement	Independent
Knowledge:	Less	Different	More
Behavior:	Submissive	Involved	Independent
Situation			
Appropriate:	Crisis, emergency, or great skill required of leader only	General goals, controls, and time pressure understood	No clear purpose, control, or time pressure
Inappropriate:	Misuse of employees talents	Cannot influence	Need answer

members clearly do not participate in the decision-making process. This is a most appropriate behavior in an emergency or crisis situation, such as a cardiac arrest. Certainly it would be an inappropriate leadership behavior for decisions affecting professional responsibilities.

Selling, or persuading, is another behavior the leader may use. It involves, as in telling, a leader making a decision without consulting the group. For example, rather than just informing the group members, the leader tries to appeal to the group's sense of logic by identifying the positive aspects of the decision. This might involve pointing out the decision's benefit because of its congruence with organizational goals or the fact that the group's interests have been considered in the decision. An appropriate use of this behavior is when the leader conveys a new policy to the staff, a policy that could otherwise be interpreted in a negative way, by giving the reason for the policy. An inappropriate use of this behavior will occur if the leader only deals with the positive side of a new policy without sharing all relevant reasons for its necessity. The group may resent the leader's positive explanation of a policy or decision that will be very difficult for the staff to follow.

Testing is a behavior available to the leader that begins to involve the group members. In this case the leader identifies a problem and proposes a tentative solution, but before finalizing the decision, the group is consulted for helpful information and input. For example, the leader will discuss the problem with the group and say, "I'd like to have an honest reaction to this proposal." After hearing what the group has to say, the leader will then—and only then—make a decision. It is possible that the leader may change what had been proposed as a solution and follow the recommendations from the group. The proper use of this behavior occurs when the group has the legitimate right to be involved in decision making about policies that they will implement. There is no reason to involve the group if they cannot influence the decision. Indeed, using testing might be harmful to leader-member relationships if the position of the group is ignored.

Consulting is a leader behavior that allows the group to be involved with the decision from the very beginning. The leader presents a problem to the group with its relevant background and asks the group to propose a solution. In effect, the group increases the number of alternative actions to be considered. The leader then selects the decision that best meets the needs of the problem and the group. This is an excellent behavior to use in an interdisciplinary team conference. Another case may be the leader who has a very important yet complicated problem to present to the staff, requiring their input to achieve more commitment to the solution, since they will implement the decision. It would be inappropriate to use this behavior in a highly structured situation in which there simply is only one course of action.

Joining is a leadership behavior that also allows the group to be involved from the very beginning. The leader functions more like a member than a formal leader and agrees in advance to carry out whatever decision the group chooses. The leader does, however, provide the limits within which the decision may be made. This leadership behavior is applicable under special circumstances, such as a problem that requires a solution from a group of people who have comparable positions with equal authority. An example might be the vice president of nursing meeting with other administrators to determine a policy that will influence expansion of the hospital services. An inappropriate use of this behavior would be relinquishing decision-making authority to a group that does not have adequate experience or knowledge to solve the problem.

The aim of leadership development is to produce an effective leader capable of using the proper leadership behavior according to the situation, no matter what the leader's personal inclinations. Leadership style and behaviors are the means by which leadership is exercised. Learning to use these behaviors in the right set of circumstances determines one's personal success as a leader.

Following the classic work of decision-making styles, others in the behavioral school studied leadership effectiveness. For instance, The Ohio State Studies in the late 1940s attempted to (1) develop instruments to measure leadership, such as the Leader Behavior Description Questionnaire (LBDQ) and (2) evaluate factors that influence group effectiveness. Two of the major characteristics that define group effectiveness discovered by these studies were (1) consideration—the extent to which the leader is likely to have a group relationship characterized by mutual trust, respect for subordinates' ideas, and consideration of their feelings and (2) initiating structure—the extent to which a leader is likely to define and structure the roles of subordinates toward goal attainment.[12] The most effective leaders scored high on both of these measures. This kind of research marked the beginning of empiric work to demonstrate the complex interactional nature of leadership.

Later, another study was conducted at the University of Michigan, which concluded that there were four major leader behaviors: (1) supportive behavior—behavior that enhances someone else's feelings of personal worth and importance, (2) interaction facilitation—behavior that encourages members of the group to develop close, mutually satisfying relationships, (3) goal emphasis—behavior that stimulates an enthusiasm for meeting the group's goals or achieving excellent performance, and (4) work facilitation—behavior that helps achieve goal attainment through such activities as scheduling, coordinating, and planning and by providing resources such as tools, materials, and knowledge. To a great extent, the Michigan studies can be credited with being foundational to the situational theories of leadership by expanding the notion of effective leadership action.[13]

Situational Theory

The next stage of leadership theory development was **situational theory.** Researchers suggested that traits required of a leader differ according to varying situations. In 1948, Stogdill conducted a comprehensive review of the literature and concluded that leadership traits differ in varying situations.[14] No single personality typifies a leader; rather, leadership is a relationship that exists among people in a social situation. Thus, a person may be a leader in one situation and not in another. There are three main factors to consider for the leadership process: (1) a leader, (2) a situation, and (3) followers. The group of factors that determine leadership effectiveness are referred to as forces within the managers, subordinates, and situations.

Forces in the supervisor include (1) the supervisor's view of people, performance, and status, (2) the degree of confidence held for the subordinates, (3) leadership inclinations, and (4) feelings of security in an uncertain situation. Forces in subordinates include their (1) need for independence, (2) readiness to assume responsibility, (3) expectations to share in decision making, (4) tolerance for ambiguity, and (5) level of knowledge and experience to deal with situations. Forces in the situation include (1) the organization's values and traditions, (2) the organization's reaction to change (e.g., is it slow to change or volatile?), (3) whether the organization is dominated by physicians, administrators, or nurses, and (4) to what extent the group is effective, cohesive, and able to assume responsibility in different situations.[15]

Situational theories suggest that, based on an analysis of all these critical forces, an individual may be a leader in one situation and a follower in another. Some of the more recent developments in leadership theory are strongly based on the assumptions represented by situational theory.

Contingency Model

One example of leadership effectiveness based on situational theory is Fiedler et al's **contingency model** developed in 1965 (Table 2-2).[16] This very complex theory consists of a three-dimensional model of a given situation. Components of the model are (1) leader-member relations, (2) a task structure, and (3) a position of power. Leader-member relations represent the

TABLE 2-2. FIEDLER'S CONTINGENCY THEORY

Group Situation

Leader-Member Relations	Task Structure	Leader's Position of Power	Leadership Style of the Leader
Good			
—	Structured	Strong	Directive
Moderately poor	—	—	—
—	Unstructured	Weak	Permissive
Poor			

Note: Different sets of conditions predict proper leadership behavior.

amount of confidence and loyalty followers have in their leader. Task structure refers to the number of correct solutions to a given situational dilemma. Position of power means the amount of organizational support available to the leader. Based on this theory, it is possible to predict the most productive leadership style through a complicated analysis of these components and their relationship to a critical situation. For example, if a head nurse who is well-liked has an ambiguous task to request of the staff, a considerate, accepting leadership style is most appropriate. If the head nurse is disliked and asks the same ambiguous task to be completed, a very direct leadership style would be considered best. This theory requires a great deal of study and creates a matrix for the user so that one can change leadership approach after an appropriate analysis of a situation.

Situational Leadership Model

One of the most interesting and useful theoretic perspectives of leadership is the **life-cycle theory** of Hersey.[17] This practical theory suggests that leadership behavior may be predicted on the basis of the follower's readiness. Illustration of the model in Figure 2-2 shows four quadrants, each representing the degree of emphasis on relationship behavior and task behavior. The leader will alter the style of leadership based on an analysis of the follower's readiness. Readiness refers to the level of motivation and competence an individual has for an assigned task. The leader assesses the follower's capacity to complete the assigned task and provides the appropriate leadership behavior that best meets the needs of the follower in the given situation. The leader behaviors are telling, selling, participating, and delegating. The leader behavior conforms to the followers requirements of needing (1) guidance and (2) relationship or emotional support. This is a tool that may be used with individuals or groups.

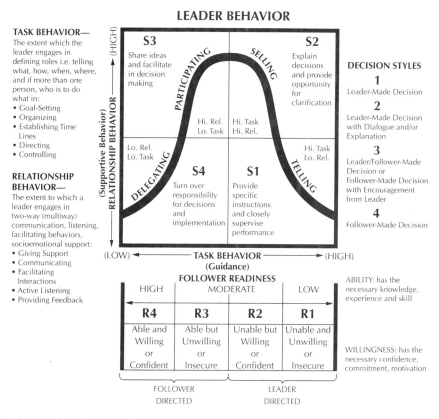

LEADER BEHAVIOR

TASK BEHAVIOR—
The extent which the leader engages in defining roles i.e. telling what, how, when, where, and if more than one person, who is to do what in:
• Goal-Setting
• Organizing
• Establishing Time Lines
• Directing
• Controlling

RELATIONSHIP BEHAVIOR—
The extent to which a leader engages in two-way (multiway) communication, listening, facilitating behaviors, socioemotional support:
• Giving Support
• Communicating
• Facilitating Interactions
• Active Listening
• Providing Feedback

(Supportive Behavior)
RELATIONSHIP BEHAVIOR
(HIGH)

S3 PARTICIPATING
Share ideas and facilitate in decision making
Hi. Rel. Lo. Task

S2 SELLING
Explain decisions and provide opportunity for clarification
Hi. Task Hi. Rel.

S4 DELEGATING
Lo. Rel. Lo. Task
Turn over responsibility for decisions and implementation

S1 TELLING
Hi. Task Lo. Rel.
Provide specific instructions and closely supervise performance

(LOW) ◄——— **TASK BEHAVIOR** ———► (HIGH)
(Guidance)

DECISION STYLES

1
Leader-Made Decision

2
Leader-Made Decision with Dialogue and/or Explanation

3
Leader/Follower-Made Decision or Follower-Made Decision with Encouragement from Leader

4
Follower-Made Decision

FOLLOWER READINESS

HIGH	MODERATE		LOW
R4	**R3**	**R2**	**R1**
Able and Willing or Confident	Able but Unwilling or Insecure	Unable but Willing or Confident	Unable and Unwilling or Insecure

FOLLOWER DIRECTED   LEADER DIRECTED

ABILITY: has the necessary knowledge, experience and skill

WILLINGNESS: has the necessary confidence, commitment, motivation

When a Leader Behavior is used appropriately with its corresponding level of readiness, it is termed a High Probability Match. The following are descriptors that can be useful when using Situational Leadership for specific applications:

S1	**S2**	**S3**	**S4**
Telling	Selling	Participating	Delegating
Guiding	Explaining	Encouraging	Observing
Directing	Clarifying	Collaborating	Monitoring
Establishing	Persuading	Committing	Fulfilling

Figure 2-2. Leader behavior. *(Management of Organizational Behavior. 6th Ed 1993 p. 197.)*

This model's original categories have been refined, and published work demonstrates its success in a variety of arenas besides leadership.[18] The underlying assumptions, however, remain the same:

1. The followers' ability and willingness for task completion based on their task readiness is assessed by the leader.

2. The leader adapts behavior to best guide and/or support the followers to meet the specified objectives.

A New Concept of Leadership

Modern theorists are continuing to struggle with the elusive quality of leadership. One of the most dynamic approaches to leadership is that offered by Bennis and Manus, published in 1985.[19] These authors stated that leadership is the most studied and least understood of the social sciences, and these changing and turbulent times require uniquely effective leaders. They suggest a **new theory of leadership** based on an extensive study of 90 leaders who participated in interviews for the purpose of discovering what is common to leadership and leaders.

The findings of this study concluded that there are four types of "human handling skills" common to leaders. The authors elaborate in great detail the specifics of these skills and refer to them as strategies:

- *Strategy I*—attention through vision
- *Strategy II*—meaning through communication
- *Strategy III*—trust through positioning
- *Strategy IV*—the deployment of self through positive self-regard and the Wallenda factor

Strategy I, or the management of attention through vision, refers to the leader's ability to create a focus or a clear picture of an outcome. The leaders who were interviewed were all results oriented. The ideas they held were very clear in their own minds, making it easy for people to see where they were going.

Strategy II, or the meaning through communication, means that this group of leaders was able to turn its vision into images that others could understand. These leaders had the ability to translate their ideas into symbols with real meaning. From this ability, referred to as the management of meaning and the mastery of communication, leaders are able to inspire by capturing the imagination of others.

Strategy III, or trust through positioning, refers to the leaders' ability to inspire trust in others by contributing to the organization's integrity. This means the leader never loses sight of why the organization exists. The leader knows what the organization stands for and what it has to do. A second component of a leader's contribution to the management of trust is the facilitation of constancy, or staying the course. Like a pilot and an airplane, the leader takes the organization in the right direction. In this way a leader, through positioning, maintains the organization's harmony and purpose but also recognizes the need for change and incongruities and provides for innovations. In essence the leader provides stability for the organization but also allows for the necessary changes that provide for organizational growth.

Strategy IV, or the deployment of self through positive self-regard, means that the leader leads in a very personal way. The leader will display a positive self-image and especially self-respect. This is achieved by the leader recognizing his or her strengths and compensating for weaknesses while nurturing the talents and skills that he or she possesses.

Another aspect of the management of self is the deployment of self through the Wallenda factor. This is best explained through a story about Karl Wallenda, a tightrope aerialist. For three months prior to his fatal fall, Wallenda talked about falling and not succeeding, rather than walking the tightrope. It was as though he were destined to fail. The conclusion is: attitudes influence outcome. Positive attitudes that concentrate on success are what this special group of leaders shared. The ground-breaking work of Bennis and Manus provides much that can be applied to beginning students of leadership. Lee expanded on the new leadership proposed by Bennis and Manus.[20] Lee states that professional performance is highly compatible with the new leadership, provided the leader be open to a new way of thinking. Consider the following to be an application of the new leadership:

- Leadership can be learned and cultivated.
- Leaders are not necessarily charismatic (an inspirational personality). In fact, leadership is more than a characteristic, and charisma just may be the result of effective leadership.[21]
- Leadership is not limited to those who reside at the top of the organization. Rather, leadership opportunities exist at all levels of the organization. It is not so much the exercise of power but the empowerment of others.[22,23]

Transformational Leadership

The work of Bennis and Manus opened the door to others to explore and expand new ways of viewing nursing leadership, such as **transformational leadership.** Burns, an early formulator of transformational leadership, proposes there are two kinds of leadership, transactional and transformational.[24] Traditional or **transactional leadership** occurs when one person takes the initiative for the exchange. Both leader and follower have separate but related purposes, and their differences are the focus of the system. In transformational leadership, both the leader and followers have the same purpose,

and they raise one another to higher levels of performance. This new paradigm relies on mutuality, affiliation, acknowledgement of complexity, ambiguity, cooperation versus competition, an emphasis on human relations,
process versus task, acceptance of feelings, networking versus hierarchy,
valuing intuition, and empowerment of all employees.[25]

The transformational leader mobilizes others and grows and develops
with the followers. Emphasis is on the outcome because the process of
achieving the outcome changes. The right actions may change from day to
day because the focus remains on the goals and end product. The result is
both leader and follower develop a love of the work. The central task of the
transformational leader is to create a vision and build a social architecture that
provides meaning for employees. This leader tries to develop self-esteem
and pride among the followers by being less rule-bound, while maintaining a
clear vision. The measure of a transformational leader's effectiveness is the
success of the followers.[26] Transformational leadership is a values-oriented
relationship, which can only occur within a climate of trust and mutuality. In
practice, establishing and maintaining both organizational and personal trust
with others represents the fundamental strategy of the transformational
leader. Only in an environment of trust can people truly be and act their best.
This form of leadership has been endorsed by many leadership scholars.

A research study by McDaniel and Wolf examined the effects of transformational leadership on work satisfaction and retention on staff nurses.[27]
Among the results were "positive work satisfaction and low turnover" among
registered nurses where transformational leadership was in place.[28] Despite
limitations of the study, such as a small sample from one institution, transformational leadership produced a positive work environment. Another study
conducted by Dunham and Klafehn asked the question, Are nurse executives transformational leaders from their own perception and from immediate
staff members' perceptions?[29] The results revealed the sample of executives
were very much seen as transformational leaders. In addition, the researchers'
data were compared to a study conducted by Bass of world leaders, administrators, and managers.[30] Results revealed the nurse executives' transformational leadership scores were higher than those surveyed in the Bass study.[31]
Transformational leadership is a process that encourages the use of all capabilities among leaders and subordinates.

Connective Leadership

In contrast to transformational leadership, which focuses on cooperation and
conflict, another multidimensional leadership model has been proposed that
focuses on caring. **Connective leadership,** developed by Jean Lipman-
Blumer and based on extensive research with her Achieving Styles Model,

connects individuals creatively to their tasks and visions, to one another, to the immediate group, and the larger network.[32] It empowers others and instills confidence. These strategies produce success, not only in the workplace, but in the interdependent world community. Since health care is moving from fragmentation to a seamless continuum of services, interconnectedness is increasing. Thus, leaders are called upon to exceed their given authority and bridge the gaps and divisions of the organization. It emphasizes the need for a leader to cope with the requirements of multiple constituencies. Health care organizations exist within diverse communities that impact mission and purpose. Connective leadership is seen as an integrative model of leadership that will be appropriate for the twenty-first century.[33]

From this overview of leadership theories, many possible explanations for leadership have been postulated that identify its complex nature. A modern perspective suggests the leader is in a position to use appropriate methods to empower the group.

■ PROCESS MODEL OF LEADERSHIP

For the beginning student, a **process model of leadership** is offered, which summarizes essential factors and activities that comprise a leadership decision or behavior. This model identifies those elements a leader should consider to produce an appropriate, group-oriented, and measurable leadership action. The concepts introduced in the model will be explained more fully throughout the text. See Table 2-3 for a depiction of the process model of

TABLE 2-3. PROCESS MODEL OF LEADERSHIP

Stage One	Stage Two	Stage Three
Analysis of Events	*Determination of Action*	*Evaluation of Action Plan*
1. Describe the nursing event and state the desired outcome.	6a. Generate ideas for action to accomplish desired outcome.	8. Monitor.
2. Identify the participants and how they see the problem and solution.	b. Weigh each alternative.	9. Correct errors.
	c. Select the best alternative.	10. Provide feedback.
3. Describe the organizational factors—structure and climate.	7. Identify barriers associated with selected action and plan for managing the conflicts.	
4. Describe the quality of interaction between the participants—locus of power.		
5. Describe the controlling factors that influence the situation.		

leadership. The model is composed of three stages. Stage 1 involves the analysis of the problem, stage 2 includes the determination of an action plan, and stage 3 involves the evaluation of the selected action.

Stage 1—Analysis and Problem Identification

The analysis stage categorizes elements of the problem or event. This categorization provides a framework to select the critical aspects from the broad organizational influences, as well as the actual (problem/conflict) event. The analysis stage is composed of the following variables: (1) the event (problem), (2) the participants and their perceptions, (3) the organization factors (organizational structure and climate), (4) interpersonal processes (locus of power), and (5) controlling forces or limiting factors. The following discussion explains these terms.

The Event. The event can range from an obvious problem to a feeling of dissatisfaction with the status quo. The *problem* begins the analytic process. A simple question (e.g., Is this an isolated event or does it occur frequently?) will suggest a simple or complex decision-making process. Isolated problems should be treated differently than problems that occur regularly. Eliminating the cause of problems often includes assistance from more than one department. For example, what is the effect on patients when no effort is made to solve the problem of dietary trays always being late? Certainly the effect on diabetic patients goes beyond inconvenience.

Next, the *participants* of the event should be identified. All persons from each department who have a direct impact on a particular activity should be involved in the solution. People perceive their own behavior from their very unique *perceptions*. It is essential that those involved in the event express their point of view and objectively state "what happened" so that the elements of the event can be commonly understood and an acceptable solution can be reached.

Organizational Factors. Events that occur in organizational settings vary in the scope of how broadly they affect others. Organizations form *structures* composed of division of labor, authority, and responsibility, which require coordination through the processes of leadership and management. The manner in which the organizational structure connects work, people, and managers impacts how a problem may be solved. The event occurs as people try to work together in an organization that by its very nature separates people so that communication and ultimately understanding are more difficult. Thus, impact of a problem should be considered on the work area as well as on the total organization. For example, does the problem have a time pattern? Do problems occur only during peak vacation months? If so, what is the policy regulating vacations, and can it be modified as part of the solution? In a complex organization, can a policy modification affect only one or two groups, or must the modification include personnel in all departments? What kinds of morale problems might result from such changes? Organization theory offers a variety of theoretic rationales that will be discussed elsewhere in the text for the purpose of explaining the complexities modern organizations hold for incumbents.

The other factor to consider is the *climate* of the total organization and its influences on the work area. Climate, by definition, is a characterization of the socioemotional effect produced by the emphasis placed on human relationships and work. Problem-solving activities have to consider the existing structure, with its programmed demands, and the climate to produce a solution, that is consistent with organizational goals and psychologically satisfying.

Interpersonal Processes between Participants. The interaction between the leader and the subordinates affects the means by which decisions are made. The combination of these processes defines the degree of compatibility seen in the work group. The length of time and effort to arrive at a decision is partially determined by this compatibility, as well as the respect shared by the leader and group. When a group member emerges as a strong, opposing leader with little regard for the formal leader, effort and time are diverted from the main problem and instead focus on the group's internal relationships. Incompatible working relationships develop when people do not recognize the leader's broader organizational responsibilities. The ability to manage conflict situations is an important skill for the nurse leader/manager. (The skills of communication, conflict resolution, and decision making will be addressed in Chapters 3 and 4 of the text.) The concept of power, both an individual characteristic and force, impacts decision making. A position of *power* refers to the variety of transactional and legitimate forces that produce the ability to influence others. Power may well be the most critical force in determining an outcome.

Controlling Forces. There must be a basic understanding and agreement to certain rules and regulations that allow the organization to run with efficiency. Controlling factors, such as protocols, procedures, and standards of professional and personal behavior, dictate norms that reduce ambiguity in the work place.

Stage 2—Determination of Action

Action Plan. After taking into consideration the myriad of factors that contribute to the situation, a course of action must be determined. The activities of stage 2 necessitate the use of decision making as discussed in detail in a later chapter. The process, in brief, considers the defined problem and categorizes information about it based on specific information of *what, who,* and *how* best to solve the problem. To arrive at the best action, many *alternative solutions* must be considered, and prediction of the outcome should be attached to each alternative solution. The predictive effort should include consideration of both *positive and negative outcomes* of each solution proposed. Selecting the solution offering the greatest overall advantages and least disadvantages is part of the ongoing process. Leadership and management theory offer concepts that make this a selective process. The leader then clearly describes relationships between the desired outcome and each possible alternative.

Stage 3—Evaluation of Action

The last stage of the process model is evaluation of action. *Evaluation* as an activity makes a judgment that determines worth and value. The major aim is to reduce subjectivity and to increase objectivity through measurable criteria.

Following implementation of the selected action, the results should be evaluated in terms of actual outcome, even if it is an unexpected outcome based on the established criteria. These criteria should judge the immediate effect of the management decision. In addition, criteria should be included that are sensitive to the total system. The long-range effect of any decision has to be considered to reduce the sources of new problems.

The *evaluation criteria* should be compared to a variety of issues, such as (1) the *acceptability of action* for a particular organization or setting, (2) the *psychologic-social acceptance* of the selected action, (3) the *effect,* direct and indirect, on the quality of nursing care, (4) the possible *growth* for the group implementing the plan, and, finally, (5) the *solution's* ability to maintain order.

Conclusions on Use of Process

Nurse leaders are expected to meet professional standards and organizational goals. Using a process model of leadership is one mechanism that highlights the necessary forces in a situation, leader, and followers that influence decisions to achieve successful outcomes. A process leadership model in all its stages requires application of theory to determine the best possible leadership action. The knowledge and skill level of the duly appointed leader directly and indirectly influence the short- and long-range goals of the organization. Interpersonal relationships significantly influence the possible alternatives that might be generated to solve a problem or to make a decision. The creative leader who possesses innate intelligence, resourcefulness, dominance, and self-sufficiency will be able to facilitate a course of action.

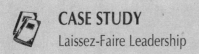

CASE STUDY
Laissez-Faire Leadership

You are a new staff nurse in a sizable ambulatory care setting where 150 to 200 patients are seen each day in 25 specialty clinics. Your reason for joining the staff in ambulatory care is your interest in the nursing functions you believe are essential to the setting (e.g., patient teaching, being an advocate to patients/families in maintaining health and in adapting to changes in their lives imposed by illness, and serving as a liaison and coordinator between patients/families and members of the health care team).

Shortly after your orientation period it becomes apparent to you that these are not consistent functions of the nursing staff in the department. You become frustrated when assigned to *receptionist functions,* such as logging patients in and assigning them to examining rooms, and to *task functions,* such as taking and recording vital signs and weights on patients. When you attempt to become more involved in *total care functions,* you sense the alienation of the other nurses. In addition, it becomes apparent that the organizational structure necessary to carry out giving and documenting total care does not exist. It is difficult to identify a person as the leader. An ineffective, free-rein style seems to be in operation. The lack of visible structure in the department leads you to higher level nursing administration for assistance in dealing with your professional role conflict.

You make an appointment to see the director of outpatient clinics. Although the director listens to you, she admits this is a new area and is in the process of forming a workable structure. The director asks you to submit ideas for change in the setting.

- What changes do you think would facilitate the work flow?
- What style of leadership would be most effective in this situation?
- What attributes should the leader display in this situation?

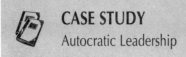

CASE STUDY
Autocratic Leadership

Mrs. Meyers is the head nurse on 3 South, a very busy general surgery division. Mrs. Meyers is known for "running a tight ship." For instance, Mrs. Meyers makes out all the assignments on the division in a very detailed manner. She prefers to call physicians for new orders and to report problems. Mrs. Meyers consistently provides more structure than the task requires.

Many of the professional nurses have tried to discuss the problem with Mrs. Meyers, but the conversation goes nowhere. Mrs. Meyers insists that the responsibility of a head nurse is great and that without her vigilance, errors would occur. Of late, RNs are asking to transfer from 3 South almost as fast as they are hired. The associate director for surgical divisions suspects that the problem may be Mrs. Meyers' leadership style.

As a result of inquiry and observation, the associate director concludes that Mrs. Meyers is a major factor in the turnover. She offers some alternatives to Mrs. Meyers, including a leadership development mini course.

- What should such a course offer to an experienced head nurse who must learn to use leadership behavior in a more acceptable manner?
- Is it possible for a person to understand the needs of subordinates and to become more flexible in her leadership style?

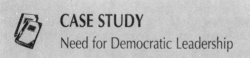

CASE STUDY
Need for Democratic Leadership

You are a new nurse in an Emergency department. You observe a very busy area where rooms are filled with patients awaiting attention. The charge nurse is responsible for prioritizing who is seen first. This often necessitates certain patients are not seen for long periods of time, so that more seriously ill patients may be treated or admitted. You notice that on a regular basis, waiting patients and families become very angry. Often, nurses repeat blood work for patients, and there is general disorganization. You are convinced the head nurse is too laissez-faire. You believe the work place needs order.

You believe if the group was called together, solutions could be found that would enhance the work flow.

- What type of leadership style would be effective in this situation?
- What leadership behaviors would be necessary to bring more structure to the flow and treatment of emergency patients?

■ SUMMARY

This chapter has provided a progressive discussion of leadership from a birthright to a complex process. The various perspectives have provided sequential insights for modern theorists who highlight the need for effective leaders in these unpredictable times. The conceptual basis for leadership is still not fully understood. However, each succeeding theory adds more understanding to the process. Leaders in nursing are suggesting the thoughtful study and implementation of transformational leadership as a congruent method with nursing's values and organization requirements. A process model of leadership was offered to highlight the multiple concepts that need to be understood for a leader to be truly effective.

 ## STUDENT EXERCISES

1. In your own words, describe leadership.

2. From your personal clinical experience which leaders do you admire? Why?

3. What is your evaluation of transformational and connectional leadership?

■ REFERENCES

1. The Missouri Nurse, "National Commission Urges Dramatic Reductions in New Doctors," *Registered Nurses*, ANA publication, 65:2, 1996, p. 4.
2. Ibid., p. 18.
3. Brown JAC, *The Social Psychology of Industry*. Baltimore, MD: Penguin Books,1954: 129–130.

4. Peterson A, "The Changing Management Role: Autocratic Doer to Team Facilitator," *Nursing Management,* 2:4, December 1994, p. 209–212.

5. Dunham D, Fischer E, "Nurse Executive Profile of Excellent Nursing Leadership," *Journal of Nursing Administration Quarterly,* vol. 15, 1990, p. 1–8.

6. Murphy MM, DeBack V, "Today's Nursing Leaders Creating the Vision," *Nursing Administration Quarterly,* vol. 16, 1991, p. 78–80.

7. Meighan MM, "The Most Important Characteristics of Nursing Leaders," *Nursing Administration Quarterly,* vol. 15, 1990, p. 63–69.

8. Stevens-Barnum B, "Leadership: Can It Be Holistic?" *Holistic Nursing Practice,* October 1994, p. 9–15.

9. Ibid., p. 10.

10. Lewin K, Lippitt R, White RK, "Studies in group decisions," In Cartwright D, Zander A, *Group Dynamics,* New York: Harper & Row, 1953.

11. Schmitt W, Tannenbaum R, "How to Choose a Leadership Pattern: Skills that Build Executive Success," *Harvard Business Review,* 6:116, 1964.

12. Korman AK, "Consideration, Initiating Structure, and Organizational Criteria—A Review." In Sorenson PF Jr., Baum Hill (editors), *Perspectives in Organizational Behavior,* Champagne, IL: Stripes, 1973.

13. Fleishman EA, *Leadership Climate and Supervisory Behavior,* Ohio State University Press: Columbus, OH, 1951.

14. Stogdill RM, "Personal Factors Associated with Leadership in a Survey of the Literature," *J Psychol,* vol. 25, January 1948, p. 35–71.

15. Schmitt W, Tannenbaum R, p. 118–121.

16. Fiedler FE, Chermers MM, Mahar LC, *Improving Leadership Effectiveness: The Leader Match Concept,* New York: Wiley, 1976.

17. Hersey P, Blanchard K, LaMonica EL, "A Situational Approach to Supervision: Leadership Theory and the Supervising Nurse," *Super Nurse,* 7:17, May 1978, p. 20–22.

18. Hersey P, Blanchard KH, *Management of Organizational Behavior: Utilizing Human Resources,* 6th ed, Englewood Cliffs, NJ, Prentice Hall, 1993.

19. Bennis W, Manus B. *Leadership: The Strategies for Taking Charge,* New York: Harper & Row, 1985.

20. Lee JL. "Leadership in Practice." In Ismeurt RL, Arnold EN, Carson VB (editors), *Concepts Fundamental to Nursing,* Springhouse, PA: Springhouse Corporation, 1990, p. 438.

21. Lee JL, p. 438.

22. Ibid.

23. Bennis W, Manus B, p. 224–225.

24. Burns JM, *Leadership,* New York: Harper and Row, 1978.

25. Klakovich MD, "Connective Leadership for the 21st Century: A Historical Perspective and Future Directions," *Advanced Nursing Science,* 16:4, 1994, p. 42–54.

26. Ibid., p. 43.

27. McDaniel C, Wolf GA, "Transformational Leadership and the Nurse Executive," *JONA*, 22:2, 1992, p. 60–65.
28. Ibid., p. 63.
29. Dunham J, Klafehn KA, "Transformational Leadership and the Nurse Executive," *JONA*, April 1990, p. 18–31.
30. Bass BM, *Leadership and Performance beyond Expectations*, New York: The Free Press, 1985.
31. Dunham J, p. 32.
32. Lipman-Blumer J, "Connective Leadership: Female Leadership Styles in the 21st Century Workplace," *Sociology Perspective*, 35:1, 1992, p. 183–203.
33. Klakovich MD, p. 52.

Interactive Processes of Leadership
Communication and Group Process

Introduction

Leadership theory discusses the process of leadership from a variety of perspectives. Emphasis on vision, values, and motivation is stressed, but how does one enact leadership? Can anyone become a leader? The importance of identifying nurses with leadership potential early in their careers and helping them to further their ability has been recognized as a critical activity. Traditionally, leaders have been developed in the hospital, but in this era of rapid change, opportunities for leadership development need to be incorporated into the new landscape of health care organizations. Leadership development remains of continuing interest to nurses. Especially now with organizational reorganization, insuring a succession of competent leaders and managers is necessary for professional advancement and stability of patient care delivery.[1] In a review of the nursing leadership literature, nurse scholars advocate the use of mentorship, networking, and continuing education as valuable methods to develop leadership behavior.[2,3] Fundamentally,

45

leadership skills consist of communication skills and knowledge of group processes. The objective of this next chapter is to discuss leadership development, focusing on communication and group process skills.

KEY CONCEPTS

Communication is the transfer of understanding from one person to another.

Communication Process is the means by which ideas are transferred through ideation, encoding, transmission, receiving, decoding, and response.

Group Dynamics is the variety of behaviors and characteristics that are demonstrated in a group and that allow a group to meet a goal.

Nonverbal Behavior is the behavior, expressions, and accompanying gestures that oppose or support the communicated message.

Message represents that which one individual wishes to convey to others.

Communication Climate is a general socioemotional feeling (positive or negative) that results from the interplay between leader and followers.

Assertive Communication is a confident pattern of speaking and dealing with others.

Passive Communication is a seemingly uninvolved, shy, or withdrawn communication pattern of speaking and dealing with others.

Aggressive Communication is a bold, forthright confronting pattern of speaking and dealing with others.

Lateral Communication refers to a pattern of communication among those of equal rank.

■ COMMUNICATION

Leadership is an interactive process, whereby a leader influences a group. The nature of the leader's influencing process remains an ambiguous topic among leadership scholars. Through research efforts, it has been established that leadership consists of personal, functional, and situational variables. Formal educational and training programs have provided a foundation to the belief leadership skills may be developed.[4] Nonetheless, **communication** is the medium by which leadership is conveyed to the group (Fig. 3-1).

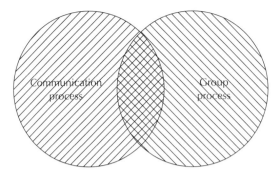

Figure 3-1. The main components of leadership: communication and the group process.

Communication, by definition, is the transfer of information and understanding from one person to another. This occurs by means of the communication process, consisting of a sender, message, and receiver, which are influenced by an environment. Each of the components of the communication process is capable of enhancing or inhibiting the understanding of the message.

The Message

The **message** is the idea to be conveyed. A leader should keep in mind that the meaning of words resides not in the message but rather in people who interpret the message. Words do mean different things to different people; thus, individuals assign their own meaning and it may be different from what was intended. The message is composed not only of symbols (words), but also a tone and **nonverbal behavior.** The tone of the message reflects an emotional level whereas nonverbal behavior, consisting of facial expressions, pauses, gestures, posture, and guarded remarks, reinforce or contradict the primary message. The relative importance of each aspect of the message has suggested that words are far less important than the tone of the message and the accompanying body language.[5] Subsequently, the message is conveyed by means of the communication process (Fig. 3-2).

Communication Process

The **communication process** consists of six steps: ideation, encoding, transmission, receiving, decoding, and response (Fig. 3-3). *Ideation* refers to the message, the idea, or the thought to be communicated to the individual or a group. *Encoding* is the manner in which the message is conveyed. The manner may be something other than verbal, such as a written message, a visual

THE MESSAGE

1. *Verbal*
   What you talk about

2. *Nonverbal*
   How it is communicated
   Facial expression
   Guarded remarks
   Pauses
   Gestures
   Posture
   Tone of voice
     Accepting
     Rejecting
   Body language

COMMUNICATION CLIMATE

Positive—enhances the message
or
Negative—detracts from understanding the message

Figure 3-2. The essential elements of the communication components: the message and the communication climate in which the message is delivered.

or spoken cue. Encoding also takes into account the nonverbal behaviors that accompany the message, such as a gesture or an expression. *Transmission* is the transmittal of the message. For the listener or reader to receive the message, intact senses and appropriate ability are required. *Decoding* refers to the mental mechanisms used to receive and, consequently, interpret the message. The *response* or feedback should, in turn, tell the leader if the individual or the group understood the message. The communication process will now reverse for the leader's understanding. Both the leader and followers share responsibility to understand each other.

The nurse leader/manager uses communication skills in all aspects of organizational life. Today, the nursing student is well grounded in therapeutic communication skills. However, different skills are required to communicate effectively with groups of professional workers. The ability to communicate effectively is particularity important today, with the growing emphasis on interdependence in health care. Experts agree: success in the workplace is directly related to human relations skills. Effective communication among professionals is one way to establish and maintain the desired atmosphere of professional competence which insures quality patient care.

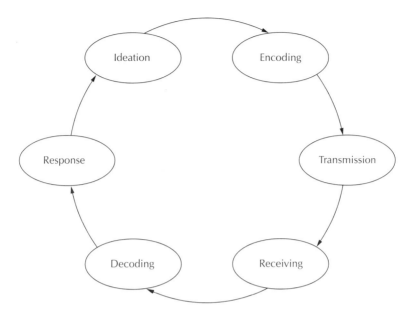

Figure 3-3. The conceptual components of the communication process. The circle is used to denote the dynamic and reciprocal properties of the communication process.

■ TEN BASICS FOR GOOD COMMUNICATION

Skillful communication is an integral process for successful leadership. The following suggestions are offered to enhance communication in the workplace.

1. Clarify your ideas before communicating to others.

Before speaking to an individual or a group, plan and organize what it is you are going to say. Analyze your thoughts carefully, and keep in mind the objective you wish to meet as well as the unique characteristics of those to whom you are speaking. Provide an opportunity for questions and answers to enhance the clarity of the message. If necessary, return to the objective to increase the likelihood of mutual understanding. The steps to take to assure your message is clear are as follows:

- Tell them.
- Have them tell you.
- Have them write it down.
- Schedule follow up meetings or reports.[6]

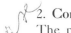

2. Consider the physical setting.

The physical setting can be either conducive or a serious block to communication. Environmental distractions interfere with the communication process. People may be trying to have a serious conversation when a sudden, distracting noise occurs that directs attention away from the message and toward the environmental stimuli. Consider the following situation: a head nurse is explaining the medication error policy to a new staff nurse, and the phone rings or there is a knock at the door. This is distracting, and both parties will have to compensate for the interruption before they are ready to continue their conversation. The physical environment should support the opportunity to have a meaningful two-way conversation. This means insuring a quiet, private, comfortable setting in which all parties will be able to concentrate on communicating.

3. Consider the psychological environment.

The psychological environment is also referred to as the communication, or social, climate. A **communication climate** is defined as the general socioemotional feeling that is produced between the leader and group as a result of the emphasis placed on productivity and human concerns. A psychological and emotional contract results within the work group, producing either a supportive or defensive climate. If you as a leader have created a supportive and open (positive) environment, you will have less difficulty communicating with your staff than you would within a defensive and hostile (negative) environment (Fig. 3-4). A supportive communication climate is characterized by a leader who listens; is empathetic; offers acceptance of individuals; exhibits a shared, problem-solving attitude; is open; and values equality in the workplace. The group members exhibit the same attitudes and behaviors. In a supportive environment, a bond between leader and follower insures safe, consistent, and meaningful communication. Conversely, a defensive climate is characterized by a leader who may be controlling, punishing, evaluating, advice giving, and insists on being right. The followers, on the other hand, are submissive or hostile, and communication is usually nonproductive and may be unpleasant.

The value of a positive communication climate is that it fosters behaviors among the leader and followers that lead to trustful and cooperative working relationships. To a great extent, following the 10 basics of good communication will contribute to a positive communication climate. It is much easier to problem solve when working relationships are good.

Positive climate behavioral characteristics

Listening
Empathy
Acceptance
Shared problem-solving attitude
Openness
Equality

Negative climate behavioral characteristics

Controlling
Punishing
Evaluating
Advice giving
Superiority
Certainty

Figure 3-4. The characteristics of both a negative and positive communication climate. These behaviors are exhibited by the leader or the followers or both.

4. Consult with others when necessary to be sure your information is accurate.

A major mistake for a leader is to communicate incorrect information to the members of the group. If misinformation is given to an individual or to the group, the leader should acknowledge the error and correct the situation as soon as possible. This demonstrates to subordinates and to superiors that the leader deals with mistakes in a direct, honest, and forthright manner.

5. Be mindful of the tone as well as, the words of the message.

Tone refers to the emotional level of the message. It may be interpreted as angry, friendly, dictatorial, fair, or a number of other emotional reactions. The tone may be opposite from the words that are being spoken. If you say something of a very serious nature and smile and laugh, you are giving mixed messages, making it very difficult for the listeners to know what you are trying to convey. The tone of your voice or written memo should support your message, not detract from it.

6. Take the opportunity to convey something of help, value, or praise to the receiver.

People need to know that their contributions are useful and respected. This is not just limited to subordinates; you also might wish to acknowledge the helpful contributions of superiors. Give credit for the contributions of others when genuinely deserved. It is amazing how powerful praise can be in establishing positive feelings in other people. By giving praise, the leader is actively involved in the development of the followers as well as a good work environment.

7. Follow up your communication.

Feedback is necessary to make sure that the message was understood as you intended it to be understood. To encourage feedback, watch for nonverbal signs of confusion. Encourage and reward questions from the group. Ask open-ended questions such as, "What do you think about the plan?" Avoid closed-ended questions like, "Is that clear?" Take the initiative by assuming responsibility for any potential misunderstandings by saying, "Sometimes I am not clear. Would you repeat your understanding of what I have just said, so that I can check myself?" Depending on the nature of the communication, you may require serial contacts or meetings. This is all a part of leadership, and you, the beginning leader, are showing your serious and committed effort to help people understand the message.

8. Nonverbal behavior should support communication.

For the most part, nonverbal behavior is unconscious, and since most individuals don't control these reactions, they tend to be extremely revealing. Thus, be sure your actions support your communication in two ways. The first is in the delivery of the message. Facial expressions and body posture should be consistent with the message. Demonstrating self-confidence and erect posture evokes confidence in what you are saying. The second component of nonverbal behavior is with follow-through of the message. If the leader makes a request of the group, the leader should also comply with the request. This promotes trust. If actions and attitude are in conflict, there will be confusion, and people will tend to deny what has been said. For example, if the leader tells the staff that they must be on time for work and then the leader is consistently late, the message will not be taken seriously.

9. Be an active listener.

To improve your listening skills, certain behaviors should be learned and practiced as you interact with people. Active listening begins as you give full attention to the person speaking. This means that you listen carefully with your mind as well as with your gestures and facial expressions. Look directly at the person to whom you are speaking. Direct eye contact conveys your undivided attention to the speaker. It is also a good idea to indicate your desire for understanding by asking for clarification, paraphrasing, summarizing, and requesting information as necessary. The most important aspect of active listening, and also the most difficult, is keeping silent, which shows respect for the other person. Active listening will enhance understanding of messages by facilitating communication through appropriate feedback. Listen to what the person has said as well as the way it was said. Listening takes discipline, effort, and time to develop. Discipline requires emotional, intellectual, and behavioral control. A leader will have to develop the self-mastery to be silent when someone else is speaking. This means putting another's ideas before your own. Active listening implies a good faith effort on the part of the leader to understand the message.

Developing active listening skills includes the following suggestions:

- **Stop talking.** To be able to listen to another person, stop what you are doing, eliminate distraction, and give full attention to the speaker.
- **Put the other person at ease.** Try to be relaxed yourself, and open the conversation with a nonthreatening comment, such as, "Anything I can help you with?"
- **Don't interrupt.** This is particularity important if the person is upset. It is important for people to believe that they have been heard.
- **Empathize.** Indicate by your response that you are concerned. You might ask for help by saying, "I would like to understand your problem. Will you help me?"
- **Paraphrase.** Try to summarize what you have heard and restate it to the satisfaction of the person.
- **Ask open-ended questions.** This form of questioning is indirect and provides for more clarification of points of view. A question such as, "What do you suggest we do?" engages the other individual in a meaningful way.
- **Use silence.** Silence in a conversation may produce tension. This tension may be necessary to insist that the other individual respond. Using discriminant periods of silence may enhance the ability to problem solve.
- **Allow reflection.** In many cases, the leader's role may be to be a sounding board for the group member. This also is called passive listening. The leader will gain a better understanding of the other's views, which enhances the potential for a positive solution.[7]

10. Be assertive when expressing your view.

Communication patterns exist on a continuum from passive to aggressive. Assertiveness is the desirable style for the nurse leader and manager. **Assertive communication** and behavior maintains a balance between aggressive and passive styles. The assertive style considers the rights of all persons involved in the communication process. The Nurse's Bill of Rights, identified by Hermann, states very clearly what these rights are:

- The right to be treated with respect
- The right to be listened to
- The right to have and to express thoughts, feelings, and opinions
- The right to ask questions and to challenge
- The right to understand job expectations as well as have them written
- The right to say no and not feel guilty
- The right to be treated as an equal member of the health team
- The right to ask for change in the system
- The right to have a reasonable workload
- The right to make a mistake
- The right to make decisions regarding health and nursing care
- The right to initiate health teaching
- The right to be a patient advocate or to help a patient speak for himself or herself
- The right to change one's mind[8]

The assertive style is demonstrated by communication that says directly and clearly what is on your mind. It is also demonstrated by listening to what others say. The leader uses objective words, uses "I" messages, and makes honest statements about the leader's ideas and feelings. Part of an assertive style is the use of direct eye contact, spontaneous verbal expressions, and appropriate gestures and facial expressions while speaking in a well-modulated voice. Assertiveness is also a process that comes with maturing in a role and gaining self-confidence in one's own knowledge and experience. An assertive style is appropriate and is based on self-respect and consideration for other people.

Aggressive communication, on the other hand, is concerned only with the rights of one position and is very goal oriented. This style may be characterized as being forceful, and may be inappropriate, or confronting. It may or may not be overtly hostile.[9] This style uses subjective words, makes accusations, and sends "you" messages. It may be confronting, sarcastic, or rude. This individual often belittles others while seeming to take charge of the situation. The rights of all individuals have not been considered.

A **passive communication** style, on the other hand, is uninvolved. This style may be withdrawn and shy or purposefully withholding. Women in particular may tend to be silent in group situations, and beginning leaders may have to overcome some hesitation about speaking to groups. Some suggestions that can help include recognizing your value and rights in a professional situation. Try to make one contribution in each group situation. Gradually you will feel more comfortable speaking in groups. Plan in advance what you wish to say, and if possible speak from a prepared text.

Communication among professionals is an essential hallmark of health care. Keep in mind that the leader and followers have a basic right to give and to receive information in a professional manner. Communication skills grow and develop over time and are the means by which leadership is exercised. It is important to remember that communication does not mean agreement or harmony concerning every issue but rather an understanding of the message between leader and followers.

■ BLOCKS TO COMMUNICATION

Blocks to communication refer to obstacles that prevent the message from being delivered or understood. Some of the more common reasons for blocks to communication are *poor listening habits, time and work demands, semantics,* and *frame of reference.*[10] Blocks to communication are the reasons why people leave meetings with half messages and incomplete or inaccurate information.

Poor listening skills, or the inability to listen attentively to people, result from a variety of sources. Among the reasons are that the leader prejudges the conversation with prior expectations and assumes to know what the speaker is about to say. Some leaders may assume hearing and listening are the same activity. Other reasons for inattention are disinterest in the conversation and allowing the mind to wander. We hear faster than people can speak; thus, active listening will facilitate focusing on the speaker.

Time and work demands also may interfere with our ability to communicate effectively. The stress of the work environment with all its constraints minimizes the ability to concentrate. Stress produces an intense reaction and likely will produce a temporary block to communication. The individual stops listening, or may hear part of the message, and the mind is closed to other ideas. Stress is a powerful force that interferes with concentration. Before constructive communication can continue, time has to be set aside and work responsibilities met.

Semantic barriers can also pose problems for communication. Semantics refers to the study of words. In day-to-day conversations, people may use the same words but ascribe different meanings. Since words are symbolic, their meaning is subject to multiple interpretations. The leader should try to be aware of the choice of words or phrases used in conveying a message to avoid misinterpretation or sending the wrong message to the group. In addition, the leader should consider the context of words and their relationship to a particular idea. Using messages in the proper context will enhance communication. For example, a head nurse wishes to praise the staff because of their outstanding efforts during an extremely hectic period. The head nurse tells the group, "You are all guilty of doing an unbelievable job!" Unfortunately, it is really not clear what the head nurse is trying to say or for what period of time or particular activity. In this case, there is a great deal of room for misunderstanding the message.

People speak and think from their personal frame of reference and experience. Eliciting feedback allows the leader to judge the listener's understanding. This can be accomplished by asking the right questions, phrasing questions within a frame of reference, and requesting that questions asked of you be also placed in a frame of reference. As always, acknowledge the message and affirm that both you and the speaker have the same understanding. If it is appropriate, thank the other person for being honest and expressing feelings. Listening is a skill for which you as a leader will be rewarded because it will lead to effective behavior.

For the beginning leader it is important to be aware of the powerful role communication plays in the organization. Those aspects of the situation and within the leader and followers that contribute to an understanding of the communicated message should help you to refine your ability to communicate with the health team. Avoiding blocks to communication will contribute to successful interaction.

■ COMMUNICATION WITH THE HEALTH TEAM

The future leader will be in a position to communicate with subordinates, other leaders/managers, and superiors. Communication with other managers or leaders holding comparable positions is referred to as **lateral communication.** Because of the structural arrangement of the organization, it is highly probable that a great deal of a manager's time is spent with other managers of equal rank to examine or to create policy. The same recommendations for good communication exist with lateral communication. It is extremely important, in fact, that this group communicate well because of the significant influence the decisions they make have on the organization as a whole. See Figure 3-5.

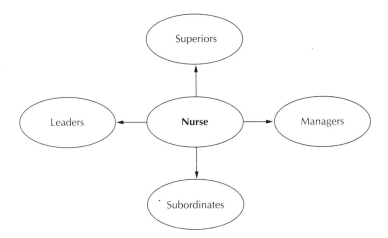

Figure 3-5. The members of the health team with whom the nurse communicates on a regular basis.

Superiors are those individuals with more legitimate authority, or those people who possess more power and status. For the beginning leader or manager, communication with superiors can be threatening and intimidating, due to the social differential between the two. Dealing with those more powerful is a fact of organizational life. For a formal or previously arranged meeting, the new leader will have an opportunity to be prepared for the topic to be discussed. In this case, reviewing the fundamentals of good communication will be helpful in facilitating participation in the meeting. Spontaneous meetings with superiors may be difficult for the beginning leader. However, the same communication rules apply, to facilitate the communication process: stay focused on the topic, make sure your message is understood, and listen actively to understand (Fig. 3-6). Despite the different roles played by the various team members and their accompanying levels of status, communication is the critical process that focuses the work of the organization.

Communication with Difficult People

Positive communication is a desirable goal, but problems may arise with certain individuals. In any organization, there may be a few people who deal with others in an unreasonable way. They may be overtly hostile or unwilling to speak at all. Difficult people who consistently interact in an unproductive way cause problems for those who must interact with them.

What are the reasons for impossible behavior? People learn and use behavior that gets results for them. If bullying others gives one power and

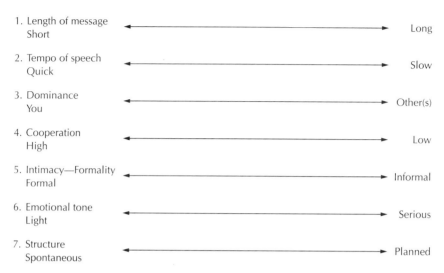

Figure 3-6. The factors that need to be considered for the most effective communicated message.

control, goes unchallenged, and is reinforced, a behavioral pattern develops. While human behavior is a complex phenomenon, responsibility for that behavior belongs to each person. Individuals who continually cause havoc with other's sense of equilibrium may be termed "difficult." Dr. Robert Branson has made a study of personality types that cause the most disruption in the workplace.[11] He has identified them to be hostile aggressive, complainers and negativists, silent and unresponsives, super agreeables, know-it-alls, and indecisives. He has proposed particular coping mechanisms for those who must deal with these individuals. Difficult people make up less than 10 percent of any organization.[12] However, they cause untold problems in morale, turnover, and productivity. The usual ways of dealing with these people include explaining and excusing their behavior or reacting in a defensive and frustrated manner. Dr. Branson offers another response: coping in highly specific ways to the different personalities.

The new leader should consider the underlying coping strategies which include the following presumptions:

1. One individual cannot change another's behavior.
The behavioral reactions of difficult people are long-standing and well-developed. These reactions are a result of stress, and are used to gain control of the situation even if other people are affected.

2. Behavior that is not confronted will not change.

Individuals who display problem behavior don't use conventional methods of problem solving. Thus, if dealing with these people, leaders must facilitate problem-solving skills.

3. Coping skills with difficult behavior may be learned.

It is more appropriate and less taxing to learn techniques that deal effectively with problem behavior. It empowers the leader to be in charge of potentially emotionally charged situations.

Specific coping strategies that deal with individual personalities follows.

Hostile aggressive people behave as they do when under stress. They typically blame other people for their situation and for triggering their angry, demeaning reaction. The way to cope with this behavior is twofold. The first is to stand up for yourself, and the second is not to engage in an argument. Your statement might include, "I don't agree," or "I see things differently. Let's discuss this further." Do not engage in an argument; it will only make the situation worse. It is very important that you keep an emotional distance from hostile aggressive attackers. This is done by remembering that there is an issue that needs to be addressed, besides the overwhelming behavior. The behavior is the responsibility of the hostile aggressive person. You have a responsibility as a coworker to try to deal with the issue, not the behavior. If at all possible, remove the hostile aggressive person from public view. Suggest that you converse in a private setting or at later time so that emotions can calm down.

Complainers and negativists are individuals who criticize or are unsatisfied with given situations or decisions. These individuals feel powerless in the face of a problem, as though they have no control over events. Coping strategies include not agreeing with them, and asking for their view on how to (1) structure the problem, (2) analyze the negative consequences of the final decision, and (3) help them solve or accept the negative aspects of the best solution while reminding them of their role in constructing the solution.

Silent unresponsive people have learned that, by simply never speaking, they don't have to participate in problem solving. This way they don't have to take responsibility for decisions. Coping with this behavior includes, after posing your concern, keeping silent until the person speaks. If the individual refuses to speak, repeat your concern and remain silent. If all attempts to engage the person in communication fail, conclude and state that because there is no response, you will make the final decision.

Super agreeable people are those who want to please everyone, even if they can't. It is highly stressful for them to explain they are unable to do something because it might displease the leader. When they fail to do what they said they would do, it becomes a problem. Coping with this behavior requires the leader to assure the persons that it is all right to say if they are currently unable to complete their work. Follow-up and encouragement are also helpful activities for the leader.

Know-it-alls are people who are only impressed with their own views and facts, even if they aren't always correct. To cope with this behavior, the leader must use their own words and facts to dissuade them. The leader should suggest that they review the facts of the situation, and point out discrepancies in those facts. In this way, know-it-alls convince themselves of their error.

Indecisive people have a difficult time making decisions. There is a great deal of stress for them to choose a course of action because they see impediments to any given course of action. To cope with this behavior when a decision must be made, the leader should say, "In any plan there are problems. What gets in the way of this one? Please tell us even if you feel it is insignificant." Be assured, what they tell the leader is not insignificant; it is a major block to the decision-making process, and it is up to the leader to offer a compromise.

If leaders can learn to use different communication and behavior patterns that facilitate group members to make responsible decision, working relationships will be highly productive.[13]

Communication Networks

Communication patterns, or networks, form within the organization and among the health team, allowing information to be circulated. These same networks also affect the ways groups solve problems. The actual pattern of the communication network may be as varied as the number of groups in existence. However, common patterns are downward, upward, downward and upward, circular, or multichanneled. Figure 3-7 illustrates the communication networks. In essence, the leader either talks in a downward pattern to the group or there is a sharing both up and down with the participants of the group as well as communication that is shared among the participants. The real issue is not whether every participant shares a two-way communication channel with every other member but whether the communication is effective. Open communication patterns are preferable to restricted networks.

■ GROUP DYNAMICS

Communication skills are one aspect of leadership development, equally important is the knowledge of group dynamics. **Group dynamics** include

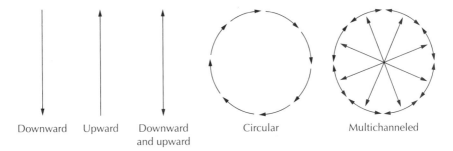

| Downward | Upward | Downward and upward | Circular | Multichanneled |

Figure 3-7. Some of the ways communication networks can form.

the study of how people form and function within a group structure. The group becomes a unit when it shares a common goal and acts in union to meet that goal. Particular problems in organizations can only be studied through group behavior; for example, a labor and management dispute represents different points of a collective view.

Primary and Secondary Groups

A group may be defined as a collection of individuals who interact with each other on a regular basis, are psychologically aware of each other, and see themselves as a group. Groups are categorized as primary or secondary. *Primary groups* are composed of individuals who interact on a "face-to-face" basis, and the relationships are personal. In addition, there are no written, formal rules or regulations because they are unwarranted. Examples of primary groups are families or groups of friends. In the workplace, primary groups also exist in the form of those who affiliate because of something held in common. Similarity distinguishes this group. For instance, the group members may be all women in the administrative field, all graduates from the same institution, or all of the same ethnic background. *Secondary groups* are larger and more impersonal. These groups are organized around formal rules, procedures, policies, and other regulations. The workplace is composed of secondary groups that are found in departments and levels forming the work group.[14]

The leader deals with secondary groups in the workplace. Secondary groups may also be categorized as formal and informal groups. *Formal groups* are the official or legitimate work group, whereas *informal groups* form for a variety of reasons. The leader must be able to influence both groups and thus move the work group toward meeting its objectives. Most research on effective leadership behavior focuses on formal leaders in positions of authority. However, there is a growing interest in the role and influence of the informal leader.[15]

An effective work group, composed of formal and informal groups, is characterized by the ability to meet its goals through a high degree of appropriate communication and understanding among its members. This group makes good decisions based on respect for all members' viewpoints. Another characteristic is the ability to arrive at a balance between group productivity and individual need satisfaction. This group is not dominated by the leader; instead, there is a flexibility among the leader and members to use individual talents appropriately. This group is cohesive and can objectively review its work and face problems in a way that balances emotional and rational behavior for a productive group effort. The leader who enhances cohesion and cooperation will be moving the group toward completion of its goals.

Characteristics of a Group

Group affiliation is a source of need satisfaction. Membership in primary and secondary groups meet social and psychological needs. To a great extent, people choose groups that are in keeping with their values. This can be explained on the basis of group characteristics, consisting of values, norms, and conformity. Groups share a value structure that comes about through the influence members have on one another. For example, some groups value their expertise, friendship, or higher wages. The ability to influence one another may be positive or negative.

Another characteristic of a group is conformity to norms (without some degree of conformity, there is no group or group identity). Norms refer to the expected behaviors within a group. If an individual violates these norms, he or she is at risk of becoming an outcast. Take for instance the new staff nurse from fictional University Hospital who has worked with every conceivable medical and nursing advancement. As this individual works with patients in a highly competent way, it is likely the new nurse will be discussed by coworkers who feel threatened. Their discomfort springs from a threat to their knowledge and skill level. The new nurse is a stimulus for a different norm and the group has several ways of dealing with this challenge. The first may be to say, "Look at Super Nurse," and then to exclude her from the group until the productivity level becomes comparable. Norms of a group are powerful enforcers for human behavior. Compliance to the norm means group membership.

While most group members conform, all individuals, however, do not. The single, most important, individual characteristic that leads to group conformity is the degree to which the individual finds the group attractive psychologically. For the individual who feels that membership in this group gives status, participation will follow. For those who don't perceive membership as a positive activity, participation will be more doubtful. The leader who understands each member's potential contribution will be able to encourage both conformists' and nonconformists' strengths and orchestrate the diversity. This is accomplished through the different roles and positions available to group members.

Group Processes

How to work more effectively with group situations has been summarized by Lippitt as a result of his extensive work with small groups.[16] He contends that leadership skills can be learned and practiced within a group context, and skill with groups can be developed. Some individuals have a very natural and easy ability to work with individuals on a one-to-one basis, but the idea of dealing with a group needs special attention. Lippitt contends that to work more effectively with groups, a leader needs to develop the following:

- An awareness of the leader's impact on a group
- Insight into other's needs, abilities, and reactions
- A sincere belief in group decision making
- An understanding of what makes a group tick
- Ability to diagnose a sick group
- Flexibility as a leader or member of the group.[17]

Each of the necessary skills to become an effective leader will be discussed below.

■ LEADER'S IMPACT ON A GROUP

A leader's impact on a group refers to the leader's affect on other people. *use*
When dealing with a group, ask yourself some questions. Are you comfortable in group situations, or do you feel a bit insecure? Some individuals enjoy groups while others find working with groups difficult. If you find yourself in the latter group, make a conscious effort to objectively evaluate how your behavior, regardless of your feelings, affects the group. Pay attention to (1) how you act, (2) how much or how little you speak, and (3) what the group's reaction is to you. Does the group listen to you, or do they overlook your silence? Does the group really appreciate your attempts at humor, or do they find such comments irritating and distracting? By developing a sensitivity to the reaction of others, you will become aware of the group members' reactions to you, either in what they say or in what they do (e.g., the subtle expression on someone's face, the tone of a person's voice, or how relaxed or

tense the atmosphere of the meeting becomes when you introduce a thought). The consistent reaction of the group to your presentations will be a gauge of your effectiveness. Conversely, you should also consider the reaction other people and their behavior have on you. As a leader, it is helpful to focus on communication as opposed to reacting to the individual.

Insight

Insight into the needs and abilities of others is an important leadership group function. It recognizes that people belong to groups for different reasons. Individuals participate in groups to meet their needs. If needs are not being met, the individual will become hostile or apathetic. The wise leader understands that individuals bring different capabilities to group productivity, and the most important activity the leader can engage in is to look for unexpected talent in individuals. The leader allows the member to participate in different ways that broaden the individual and build the participant's ego. This is accomplished by allowing members to participate broadly so that capabilities may emerge.

Some of the available behaviors that participants in the group may exhibit are broadly grouped as *task* or *maintenance functions*. Task functions serve to facilitate and to coordinate group effort in the selection and definition of a common problem and in the solution of that problem. Behaviors that fall in this category are:

- *Initiating*—suggests new ideas or a different way of looking at an old problem; proposes new activities.
- *Information seeking*—asks for relevant facts and feelings about the situation at hand.
- *Information giving*—provides the necessary and relevant information.
- *Clarifying*—probes for meaning and understanding in whatever the group is considering.
- *Elaborating*—builds on previous comments and thoughts and thus enlarges the concept under consideration.
- *Coordinating*—clarifies the relationships among the various ideas and attempts to pull things together.
- *Orienting*—defines the progress of the discussion in terms of goals to keep the discussion in the right direction.
- *Testing*—checks periodically to see if the group is ready to make a decision or to recommend some action.
- *Summarizing*—reviews the content of past discussion.

Maintenance functions are carried out through behavior that maintains or changes the way in which the group is working together. These behaviors seek to allow the group to develop loyalty to one another and to the group as a whole. These behaviors include:

- *Encouraging*—the giving of friendly advice and help. Praising and agreeing with others also define this behavior.
- *Mediating*, or *harmonizing*—helps others to compromise or to resolve differences in a positive way.
- *Gatekeeping*—allows the fair and equal participation of all members of the group by such comments as, "We haven't heard from Jane."
- *Standard setting*—the action that determines the yardstick the group will use in choosing its subject matter, procedures, rules of conduct, and, most important, its values.
- *Following*—going along with the group either passively or actively during a discussion or in response to the group's decision.
- *Relieving tension*—diverts attention from unpleasant to pleasant matters. Often this behavior smooths the way for constructive communication.[18]

The Group Approach

Fundamental to a successful group is a sincere belief that a group can be effective and productive. Not every one works well in group situations, and some individuals seek ways to be alone and independent no matter what the circumstances. A group approach enables you to bring a wide variety of experiences, backgrounds, viewpoints, and technical competencies to deal with a problem. Good decisions rely on informed participants, and the leader's attitude has much to do with successful interaction.

Understanding

An understanding of what makes a group work will enable you to maximize a group's effectiveness. This requires the group to have clear objectives and purposes. Groups exist for specific purposes (e.g., to provide quality patient care, to solve a budgetary problem), and the formal boundaries of the group's jurisdiction should be clear. Group members need to know if their decision is binding or advisory. In addition, the leader should make clear that all members are expected to participate with honesty and candor. Allow the group to do its own best thinking and withhold your own solution to a problem until all members have shared their point of view. The leader should try to elicit as many ideas as possible before beginning the evaluation process; otherwise, alternative solutions will not be considered, and the first few ideas will be the only ideas discussed. To make the group more important than individual members, disassociate ideas from the person who put forward the idea. Keep personalities and personal rivalries out of the discussion. This can be accomplished by giving each idea an impartial title, such as plan A or B.

It is wise to not make decisions until all information is available; try not to guess or to make premature decisions that may have to be changed. As a leader, try to gain consensus rather than take a vote. It is very important that all persons, particularly the more negative members of the group, voice their view.

Diagnose a Sick Group

Sometimes a group just does not work. On the surface, the group may be composed of highly competent people, but for some reason productivity suffers. As the leader, you must try to understand why the group is not operating as it should. The usual reason for a nonproductive group consisting of competent people is that individuals have unexpressed feelings and motivations that cause them to fight among themselves or even to withdraw from a constructive solution. This is often referred to as a hidden agenda, or the real reason that a group member is not participating with the group to solve the immediate problem at hand. There will be no constructive group effort if hidden agendas remain concealed. The leader must try to bring some of these agendas out in the open so that they can be dealt with and not distract from the immediate situation. Without resolve, there is no hope for constructive and effective group action. One very interesting technique to deal with this problem is to enlist the aid of the group to diagnose the difficulty. This can be accomplished through asking for postmeeting evaluations of the process of the meeting, such as an anonymous postmeeting report and suggestions for the next meeting. What you as the leader are trying to do is to make the group conscious of its own procedures and of its own responsibility to criticize and to correct its inadequacies. Without accomplishing this, the group may not succeed and will have to disband. It is a myth to think that every group automatically will succeed; however, much can be done to help it succeed.

Flexibility

Finally, the leader must be flexible. Within a group, members assume a variety of roles. For the most part, people take certain roles and maintain them as they participate in group meetings. It is advisable for the leader to vary roles from time to time. Versatility should energize you and stimulate the group to creativity. In addition, different roles are necessary to elicit alternative actions.

Group processes are the means by which individuals deal with the social interactive component of organizational life. A leader will be in a position to better influence a group if there is some understanding of these dynamics. Today, it is a highly desirable skill to be able to communicate with groups and to influence the outcome of the group effort.[19]

Evaluation of Group Effectiveness

An effective group leader is able to evaluate how well the group performed. To facilitate this process, a tool is provided to evaluate group behavior (Fig. 3-8). In addition, problems will be more obvious through the use of an objective measure.

	1	2	3	
ACTIVE PARTICIPATION was lacking. We served our own needs. We watched from outside the group.	1	2	3	ACTIVE PARTICIPATION was present. we were sensitive to the needs of our group. Everyone was "on the inside."
LEADERSHIP was dominated by one or more persons.	1	2	3	LEADERSHIP was shared among the members according to their abilities and insights.
COMMUNICATION OF IDEAS was poor; we did not listen. No one cared about ideas.	1	2	3	COMMUNICATION OF IDEAS was good. We listened and understood one another's ideas.
COMMUNICATION OF FEELINGS was poor. No one cared about feelings.	1	2	3	SINCERITY was present. We were revealing our honest selves.
SINCERITY was missing. We were just acting parts.	1	2	3	
REACTION among GROUP MEMBERS was a problem. Persons were rejected, ignored, or criticized.	1	2	3	REACTION among GROUP MEMBERS was active give-and-take.
FREEDOM OF PERSONS' IDEAS was stifled. Persons were not free to express their individuality. They were manipulated.	1	2	3	FREEDOM OF PERSONS' IDEAS was enhanced and encouraged. The creativity and individuality of persons was respected.
CLIMATE OF RELATIONSHIP was one of hostility, suspicion, anxiety, or superficiality.	1	2	3	CLIMATE OF RELATIONSHIP was one of mutual trust. The atmosphere was friendly and relaxed.
GOALS were fuzzy, contradictory, or just plain missing.	1	2	3	GOALS were clear to all. We had a definite sense of direction.
PRODUCTIVITY was low. Our group was irrelevant; there was no apparent agreement.	1	2	3	PRODUCTIVITY was high. We were digging hard and were earnestly at work on a task. We created and achieved something.

1 = problem
2 = neutral
3 = productive

Figure 3-8. Summary of those characteristics of group life that allow a group to either be effective or not. As they are listed, they form an evaluation tool of group effectiveness. The student can categorize the various aspects of the group's behavior as a problem, neutral, or productive.

CASE STUDY
Hostile Aggressive Behavior

Dr. Adams is a well-known and experienced surgeon. However, at the very least, he is known to be a difficult individual. He has gained this reputation because he shouts before he thinks, blames before he knows the facts, and generally has a short fuse. Sally Hainer, RN, didn't know Dr. Adams and inadvertently walked onto the unit to transfer a patient. In typical fashion, Dr. Adams couldn't find the laboratory work on the chart and began a temper tantrum aimed at Sally. She looked him in the eye, told him to stop shouting, and, when he could be reasonable, to restate his request. The spectators to this event were speechless.

- What kind of communication technique did Ms. Hainer use?
- What would you have done?

CASE STUDY
Need for Assertive Communication

Miss Jones, RN, has been invited to represent the nurse's view of case management in an interdisciplinary group composed of physicians, administrators, physical therapists, and the financial officer. At the first meeting the group members assembled, and Dr. Incharge presided over the group, and called the meeting to order. Miss Jones happened to notice she was the only nurse and female in attendance. Shortly after the meeting was brought to order, Dr. Incharge asked Miss Jones if she would take the minutes at the meeting.

- What should she say and do?
- Why was Miss Jones chosen for this task?

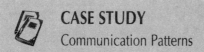

CASE STUDY
Communication Patterns

Mary Mitchen is a new staff nurse on a general medicine pediatric division. She had completed her senior practicum on this particular unit and was also working as a student nurse. Her first week of work was relatively uneventful, and she was feeling confident about her new position. One day, at the end of her shift, she was about to tape her change of shift report, when the head nurse stopped her and asked her some questions about one of her patients. Mary began to answer when the head nurse interrupted her, so Mary tried to continue to answer her questions when it happened again. Every time Mary tried to talk, the head nurse cut her off. Finally, Mary said, "Please let me finish my thoughts, I am new here and want to learn, and would be interested in how to improve."

- What type of communication patterns were being expressed?
- Analyze Mary's reaction to the interaction. Do you agree with her response?
- What should Mary do if this happens again?

■ SUMMARY

This chapter discussed leadership development from the standpoint of the interactional, or social, components of communication and group process. These are the fundamental concepts that the leader should understand and then practice. Since leadership has been defined to be a process, time and experience will facilitate leadership development, as well as following the examples of the leaders in your own organization.

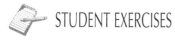

STUDENT EXERCISES

1. Explain to your class of nursing students how to do CPR. Would you teach the class in the same way to a group of Girl Scouts? What is involved in making your decision?

2. Use the various communication networks suggested in the chapter and circulate a message. Which network produced the least distortion in the message?

3. Based on your own individual experiences, compare positive and negative communication climates. Discuss the characteristics in each.

4. Observe the group dynamics in one of your classes or groups. What do you see in terms of roles played by the different participants? What is your role?

5. Try to influence the outcome of your next group meeting by using the fundamentals of communication and by being aware of how groups function. Share with the class your experience.

6. Try to find people in your experience who fit the various roles played by group members. Do they consistently use the same behaviors, or do they alter as the situation requires? Share with the class your observations, and discuss the relative effectiveness of the different behaviors in influencing the group.

■ REFERENCES

1. Johnson J, Costa L, Marshall S, Moran MJ, Henderson CS, "Succession Management: A Model for Developing Nursing Leaders," *Nursing Management*, 25:6, 1994, p. 50–55.
2. Manning G, "Invest: A Plan for Developing New Managers," *Nursing Management*, December, 1991, p. 26–28.
3. Bruderle ER, "The Arts and Humanities: A Creative Approach to Developing Nurse Leaders," *Holistic Nursing Practice*, October 1994, p. 68–74.
4. Bass BM, *Bass and Stodgill's Handbook of Leadership*, 3rd ed., New York: New York Free Press, 1990.
5. Osborne WL, Covits NF, "Better Communication Makes More Compassionate Hospitals." *Nursing Management*, 22:8, August 1991, p. 31–38.
6. Kreitner R, *Management*, 6th ed., Boston, Toronto: Houghton Mifflin Co., 1995, p. 370.
7. Van Fleet JK, *Conversational Power*, Nightengale Conant Corporation, Chicago: Prentice Hall Inc. Audio, 1990.
8. Hermann SJ, *Becoming Assertive, A Guide for Nurses*, New York: D. Van Nostrand, Co., 1978, p. 27.

9. Johnson JR, "The Communication Training Needs of Registered Nurses," *The Journal of Continuing Education*, 25:5, 1994, p. 213–218.
10. Newbauer S, "The Learning Network: Leadership Development for the Next Millennium," *Journal of Nursing Administration*, 25:2, 1995, p. 25–32.
11. Branson RM, *Coping with Difficult People*, New York: Dell (Doubleday), 1988, p. 2.
12. Ibid., p. 1
13. Ibid., p. 4
14. Kreitner R, p. 436–437.
15. Altieri L, Elgin PA, "Decade of Nursing Leadership Research," *Holistic Nursing Practice*, 9:1, p. 75–82.
16. Lippit G, Seashore E. *The Professional Nurse Looks at Groups Effectiveness*, Washington, DC: Leadership Resources, 1966, p. 4.
17. Ibid., p. 4–5.
18. Ibid., p. 14–15.
19. Newbauer S, p. 26.

4

Decision Making and Conflict Management

Introduction

A leader is in a position to facilitate the group's progress toward sound decision making and conflict resolution. The objective of this chapter is to continue discussion of leadership development through decision making and management of conflict. Decision making and conflict management were introduced in Chapter 2 during discussion of the process model of leadership. They are activities people engage in frequently throughout the course of everyday activities. They range from unimportant to critical and have consequences that affect others, sometimes seriously. In the following sections of this chapter, aspects of both decision making and conflict resolution will be explored. The two topics are presented in the same chapter because of their relationship—decisions cause or prevent conflicts, and conflicts are solved through the decision-making process.

✦ KEY CONCEPTS

Analysis is a critical function essential to sound decision making.

Conflict is an unsettling condition that causes a clash of ideas about what is expected or established. Conflict can be friendly or hostile.

Creativity is a human quality needed for generation of ideas in decision making.

Decision is a complex conclusion derived from a set of premises that relate to a situation.

Decision-Making Process is a process of arriving at a conclusion after analysis of units of related information. It is purposeful and goal directed.

Internal Climate is the dynamic socioemotional milieu that establishes the harmony/conflict ratio among people.

Power in group dynamics, is a force within people that shapes the way in which others can function. Two types of power are described in this chapter: (1) *directive power*—a negative force that exploits others by advancing the power wielder's interest and (2) *synergic power*—a positive force that cherishes others by incorporating their values.

Prediction is identification of likely outcomes of a decision given consideration of all known facts about a given situation. It is a critical part of selecting a decision.

Premise is a proposition about something that serves as a basis for decisions. A premise can be correct or incorrect and serves as the unit of analysis when evaluating decisions.

■ DECISION MAKING

In nursing, the quality of **decisions** are measured in relation to professional standards that emanate from contemporary societal forces. The focus of the discussion of the **decision-making process** is on **analysis** of situations that require action and **prediction** of possible outcomes of the action of choice.

Analysis

From the outset, decisions must be viewed as highly complex conclusions drawn from multiple **premises.** From such a view it is understood that the

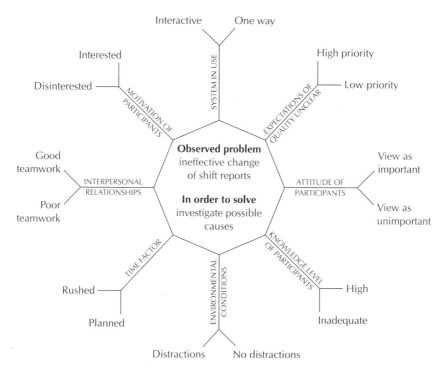

Figure 4-1. Illustration of an observed problem with an array of possible causes. In the center of the figure the observed problem is stated, and the reader is directed to investigate possible causes described in the eight spokes that extend out from the center. Each possible cause forks into two possible responses. The choice of responses at the forks provides information unique to a situation that provides direction for decision making about possible solutions to the problem.

decision itself cannot be analyzed but rather that the units of analysis are the premises from which decisions are formulated. Units are all factors that influence a total situation. The configuration of factors is what differentiates one situation from all others. Figure 4-1 illustrates a situation in which the quality of change-of-shift reports is being questioned. A variety of possible causes for the problem is shown. Action to be taken to correct the situation depends on which factor, or combination of factors, is identified as contributing to the problem.

According to Simon, there are two classes of premises that make up the basis for decisions in organizations: (1) the *criterion of efficiency* and (2) *identifications.*[1] Simon defines criterion of efficiency as conserving the scarce resources the organization has at its disposal for accomplishing its task. He says identifications mesh the subgoals of components of an organization with the goals of the whole organization. Identifications are intangible, psycho-logic loyalties and values that individuals subscribe to that relate to mission and purpose. Both classes of premises are at play in organizational settings, sometimes as competing forces. Decisions about efficiency issues frequently involve known boundaries. Take for instance a budget that has an absolute ceiling. Making rational decisions about spending can be done with relative ease in light of known limits. No institution, however, operates solely on effi-ciency issues. In the business world, profit is tempered by sensitivity to qual-ity and human values. Companies are satisfied with adequate profits, share of the market, and fair prices in place of monopoly. Nursing, a service profes-sion, is even more affected by concern for values and standards, and there must be a delicate balance between resources and values.

When identifications involve goals and values of several different departments in an organization, *how* spending is distributed becomes an issue. It is at this time that nursing must be prepared to justify, in a measur-able way, the budget for delivery of nursing care. Garre discusses the rela-tionship between decision-making methods and the nature of the problem to be solved.[2] Analysis of cost effectiveness is a helpful approach to decision making when only a few factors are involved in the problem situation. Conversely, when multiattributes must be considered, cost as a basis for a decision becomes problematic because there are too many conflicts that can arise when cost is weighed too heavily. When professional values and stan-dards are compromised, attrition and morale problems are sure to follow and the solution to those problems can be very costly. The expectation of broader and more active involvement of nurses in organizational operations is rela-tively new, and it becomes more important as fundamental professional issues come under scrutiny. Efficiency within the overall organization is increasingly a consideration that calls for new ways of decision making. Analysis of nursing decisions must be considered in light of how they affect the whole organization. Good decisions are the stabilizing force in balancing efficiency and values. Correct premises about both, as they relate to nursing practice, are essential to arrive at good decisions. Figure 4-2 illustrates how decisions affect balance of efficiency and service values in nursing.

Prediction of Outcomes

Improving skill in decision making through study and experience is impor-tant in nursing. In organizational settings, nursing decisions affect others, be it staff, patients, the organization, or even society in general. Few, if any, deci-sions made about nursing issues or events are unimportant. Consider that a

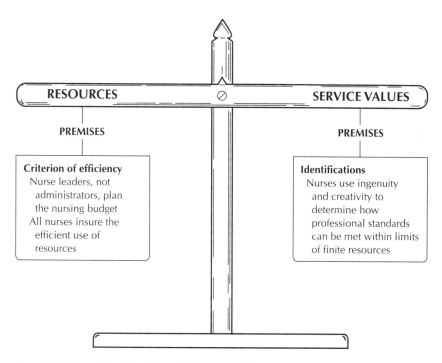

RESOURCES   ⊘   **SERVICE VALUES**

PREMISES   PREMISES

Criterion of efficiency
Nurse leaders, not
administrators, plan
the nursing budget
All nurses insure the
efficient use of
resources

Identifications
Nurses use ingenuity
and creativity to
determine how
professional standards
can be met within limits
of finite resources

Figure 4-2. Illustration of the delicate balance needed to provide quality professional nursing services within the limits of finite resources. Resources should be interpreted to include material supplies, personnel, and time. Nurses' decisions and performance determine balance or imbalance between resources and services.

decision about the time and place for a coffee break can have unwanted effects on the morale of the staff. In his book *Administrative Behavior,* Simon says that in group situations we need to think about decision making as a way of thinking about issues that concern others and that there are good and bad decisions relative to any issue a group might encounter.[3] Understanding what is included in the decision-making process is essential to making good decisions or to improving the quality of decisions to avoid unmanageable, negative consequences that can accompany them.

■ CHALLENGE TO NURSING

Traditionally, nurses were involved almost exclusively with meeting holistic needs of individual patients, leaving budgetary and other business matters to others. Such a position fostered a paternalistic attitude that led to administrative control of the nursing department in much the same way that a head of a household controls spending within the family.

The soul of nursing leadership is to control decisions affecting the practice of nursing in the organization. Taking control will facilitate a shift from a paternalistic attitude to one of a collegial attitude between nursing and agency administration. Nurses at all levels need to be prepared to engage knowledgeably in decision making in matters that affect all aspects of nursing. Improved knowledge of and skill in decision making will enable nurses to contribute more effectively to organizational viability. Opportunities exist daily for nurses to study situations that call for decisive action. Analysis of unique factors in situations improves the quality of decisions.

Just as nurses at every level are directly or indirectly affected by decisions that come down from administration—from parking places to available equipment needed in the delivery of nursing care—so too are patients affected by decisions nurses make relative to delivery of nursing care. An area in which all nurses can engage thoughtfully in decision making is in determining the pattern of patient care assignment in care settings. It is an area that belongs exclusively to nurses.

There are differences in patterns of patient care assignments, and analysis of their makeup relative to patient needs and staff competencies leads to critical selection. The pattern selected—case management, team approach, primary nursing care, or functional task approach—is one element in determining low-, adequate-, or high-quality outcomes for patients. Determining the best pattern for any given situation is based on multiple considerations, such as (1) credentials of available staff, (2) their level of competency, (3) acuity level of patients, and (4) boundaries to be observed. Too frequently there is the tendency to adopt the newest pattern as the best for all situations. It is clear that such a position can be problematic in terms of quality of patient care and staff morale. Analysis of all units of information about a given pattern of patient care delivery in relation to a given set of patient care requirements is needed before a decision can be made to adopt any pattern.

There are situations found in nursing that are stressful and that call for quick decision making. Analysis of all information is not possible. Bourbonnais and Baumann describe the effects of stress on decision making.[4] In a review of literature, they found evidence that stress causes erosion of general cognitive ability to cope with complexity. As a result, the range of cues used in decision making is altered; initially, peripheral cues are missed, and as stress builds, central cues are not perceived. According to Carnevali and Thomas a mild level of anxiety produces broad perceptions and increased learning, moderate anxiety produces narrowing perceptions and decreased learning, severe anxiety produces scattered perceptions and an inability to understand, and panic level of anxiety produces distorted perceptions with new learning being impossible.[5] Decisions made under adverse circumstances must be revisited if possible when the situation allows for more deliberation.

▉ IMPACT OF DECISIONS

Everyone is affected by the manner in which new policies are designed and implemented. Take for example current changing policies on smoking in work settings. When rationale for a change is sound and is presented in such a way as to invite input from everyone affected, the inevitable restriction is accepted differently than if the decision is one-directional, from the top down. In like fashion, in making decisions about patterns of patient care, the impact that a change in the established pattern can have on those who provide the care can be positive or negative, again depending on competent people being informed and having an opportunity to influence the final decision. Many dissatisfactions of nurses spring from having no control over decisions that affect their practice. Being informed, active decision makers can lead to more control over the practice of nursing in an organization and therefore to higher levels of satisfaction.

The goal of health care organizations to provide the best possible care to clients within a given set of circumstances can be served by well-prepared personnel who help formulate and implement decisions. Organizations that have knowledgeable individuals at all levels are better able to accomplish their mission. Understanding decision making as a process is basic to this mission and can be studied theoretically through the use of simulation scenarios. Student exercises included at the end of the chapter are designed to facilitate use of process in decision making and to eliminate bias frequently associated with a single-dimensional approach to problems. Students are encouraged to develop their own scenarios from their first-hand experiences. Good decision making hinges on, among other things, good communication skills and knowledge of group dynamics. Decision making in nursing is teamwork that calls for both cooperation and coordination. It is not sufficient to agree on a common goal, but each participant must also understand the plan. Coordination of group efforts provides stability in the face of differing opinions about an issue. For example, the purpose of signals in football or bidding in bridge is to enable each player to form accurate expectations as to what each teammate is going to do.[6] Group decision making, then, must take place in some structured way with effective communication flow, agreement on a common goal, and coordination of group activities. Further discussion appears later on in the chapter under "Management of Conflict."

■ SYSTEMS OF DECISION MAKING

How individuals or groups set about making decisions might be similar to how leadership is exercised. Style ranges from autocratic or bureaucratic to democratic. An autocratic or bureaucratic approach produces different outcomes than does a democratic approach. Consensus as an outcome is frequently the ideal. The autocratic or bureaucratic system is frequently unattractive to competent groups. Such a system, however, might be best in emergencies such as "man overboard." In a crisis event, one individual must be charged with controlling the situation and be assured of the cooperation of others. Crisis situations are not the only instances in which an autocratic system is effective. For example, a symphony orchestra's performance is the result of an autocratic system, and it is by no means a crisis. Both examples represent events in which the group freely allows one individual total control. In instances when control is taken by one person without the approval of the group, the outcome can prove to be destructive. Use of the autocratic system must be carefully reviewed to avoid serious conflicts.

A democratic system of decision making might be highly satisfying to a group that feels it is important that everyone's input be considered in decisions, especially when all group members have similar professional competencies. It is not, however, necessarily the best system to employ in all situations because within every group are individuals with different strengths. It might be a fact that because of the nature of an issue, some individuals have nothing to offer in choosing between alternative decisions, whereas they might be experts in other areas. To include them simply out of commitment to a democratic style is inefficient and time consuming and potentially damaging to established group cohesiveness. The nature of teamwork is that at sometime everyone "sits on the bench." Any style of decision making can be misused, overused, or used appropriately. The situation dictates which should be chosen.

Some decisions are carved in stone and are based on firmly established criteria that are rooted in doctrine, culture, values, and tradition. Many cannot be modified through reason. Others are modifiable but controlled by economic constraints, such as a salary scale. All organizations are influenced to some extent by this type of bureaucratic decision making. Nurses, as nurses, seldom have active roles in these types of decisions, but they are affected by them and need to know about them and their sources. These decisions are "givens" in a situation and as such do not come under scrutiny in a formal way.

Consensus is a possible outcome of decision making in which all participants satisfy part of their point of view while having to give up some other part. Arriving at consensus is time consuming, but the final product is mutually satisfying and can be of superior quality. Consensus provides a rich source of new knowledge about an issue and fosters regard for others' points of view.

Skillful decision making is highly useful to groups engaged in a common effort. How a group formulates decisions provides valuable information about their effectiveness in an organization. Through their decision-making activities, untapped creativity is released, potential leaders are identified, and areas needing development are identified.

■ THE DECISION-MAKING PROCESS

A group can adopt any of several decision-making models, or a group can design its own model. Symbols used in the construction of a model vary, but essentially they all share the same steps or stages, as follows:

- Identify participants.
- Gather pertinent facts.
- Generate alternative decisions.
- Predict outcomes.
- Plan for managing consequences.
- Select the best alternative.

A brief discussion of each stage follows.

Identifying Participants

The configuration of the group charged with formulating a decision should have adequate representation of all who are going to be directly affected by the decision. Decision makers on a nursing unit should be selected for attributes they possess that can facilitate good decisions. Interest without the other attributes for sound decision making is insufficient during the process. Interest, however, should be encouraged, and those individuals should participate in the capacity of observers until they have sufficient knowledge of related factors and of the decision-making process to be able to contribute constructively. Experiences they gain can be valuable assets to themselves and to the group for future use.

Arbitrary assignment of individuals to decision-making teams should be avoided to ensure quality outcomes. Recognition of individual staff members' assets in some organized way, such as anecdotal notes kept by the head nurse or periodic collection of data from staff as to their development and interests, can help improve utilization of group strengths. The head nurse must take appropriate steps to design opportunities for nonparticipants to improve their decision-making skills so that the unit runs efficiently and effectively. Planning exercises for nurses to gain skill through use of a process model is one way to accomplish this. Expectations of participation and growth in quality of participation must be clear and understood by everyone. Consequences of participation and performance must also be clear and understood by everyone. Nurses beginning their careers should expect to be given opportunities to gain skills needed to participate in the decision-making process.

Gather Pertinent Facts

Gathering of pertinent facts can be compared to great rivers that draw from many tributaries.[7] Ignorance of factors that relate to a problem leads to poor decisions because premises are wrong. Poor decisions have to be reversed, which of and by itself causes loss of confidence in the decision makers. Communication is a critical skill during the stage of gathering data. The possibility of information being withheld for reasons that support individual efforts must be considered and corrected when it exists. Sufficient time should be allowed for this step. When the group is satisfied that important facts that relate to the issue have been thoroughly presented, what follows is the task of prioritizing and arranging the complex bits of information into an effective scheme. Each of these operations calls for analytic and predictive thinking as well as adequate knowledge of the subject matter. This step forces balance between the competing forces efficiency and values. Prioritizing can give rise to serious conflicts as the competing forces collide. In nursing, professional standards must dominate while being tempered by efficiency constraints.

Generate Alternatives

The third step in the process is to generate as many alternative decisions as possible. The emphasis is on quantity, and judgment about alternatives is curtailed temporarily. **Creativity** is a valuable trait in idea generation. Free reign should be given to the imagination during this step, and group participants should agree in advance not to criticize any suggestions. Skill in using techniques such as brainstorming, forced association, self-interrogation checklists, think tanks, and Delphi technique are highly useful. See Table 4-1 for a description of each of these techniques.[8] The more time-consuming and sophisticated techniques can be trimmed to suit a situation and still contribute to better quality decisions in the end.

Brainstorming is the oldest and most common of the creative-thinking techniques. Brainstorming involves four principles:

1. Don't judge ideas.
2. Let your mind wander.
3. Aim for quantity.
4. "Hitchhike" on previous ideas (i.e., look for variations on ideas).[9]

Brainstorming is easily used as a group activity or by individuals. Students are encouraged to use two or three techniques from Table 4-1 as learning experiences to generate ideas about solutions to problems they encounter in their daily, clinical, nursing experiences.

Predict Outcomes

When group members feel adequately satisfied with the list of alternative decisions, they can move onto predicting outcomes of each. Knowledge of groups and how they are affected by changes is useful during this stage. The realm of a group's possible responses to any decision is an important consideration. During this stage, weighing strengths of the desired and undesired outcomes of each alternative leads to the narrowing of the alternative courses of action. Quality dominates as the list is condensed and becomes the source from which the final selection will be made.

Select Best Alternative

A process model of decision making appears in Table 4-2. The nature of process is such that stages are interdependent. There is movement back and forth in an iterative cycle as new information becomes available to be incorporated into the model. Students are encouraged to make use of the model in carrying out activities at the end of the chapter.

TABLE 4-1. TECHNIQUES FOR IDEA GENERATION

Technique	Description
Brainstorming	Used to generate a large quantity of alternatives to solve problems. Anything goes, and participants are completely free to propose any suggestions. They are encouraged to think without constraint—the wilder the better. Ideas can be toned down later. No judgments, criticisms, or negative statements are allowed during the spontaneous brainstorming session. All suggestions are recorded within a time limit. Later, the most promising alternatives are analyzed and evaluated.
Forced association	This deliberately breaks down habitual associations and seeks new relationships. The item needing action or improvement is stated, and then participants use free association to create a list of 10 words usually associated with it. Then an entirely different item is selected and free association used to create a list of 10 associated words. The two lists of 10 words are written in parallel columns. Participants are asked to make their mind work back and forth between columns, seeing relationships between the original item and the work list of the different item. Ideas are then critically analyzed to choose the useful ones in addressing the item needing action.
Self-interrogation checklist	Questions are used to develop new perspectives on a problem. They stir the imagination, and the writer withholds judgment until all ideas are written down. Questions serve to define and to uncover problems, obtain extra facts, make decisions, and generate ideas for change. Questions might be (1) Can we do more? (2) Can we streamline and eliminate excess? (3) Can we get information elsewhere? (4) Can we handle the task ourselves? (5) Does it reduce costs? (6) Is it practical? (7) Does it improve efficiency?
Think tanks	Getting a select group of people together to harness imagination and to encourage creativity is one form of think tank. Members must be carefully selected for specific attributes. Group size should range from five to eight members. The right kind of meeting place is essential: often exotic or different places stimulate innovation, and a relaxed atmosphere generates divergent and unusual ideas. A specific problem or goal must be clearly stated for participants to try to solve. Meetings should occur often enough for germination, pollinations and flowering of ideas. Think tanks are particularly useful for future projections.
Delphi technique	This technique is useful for forecasting, surveying views and attitudes, problem solving, formulating strategies, and airing controversial views. A group of experts in the area being addressed is selected. The experts anonymously react to a questionnaire, expressing their opinions and views. The questionnaires are analyzed, and each expert receives anonymous feedback about all the responses. They are then asked to respond again, taking feedback into consideration. Feedback analysis is again provided. The process is repeated as many times as needed until a consensus is reached about the problem.

TABLE 4-2. PROCESS OF DECISION MAKING

1. Participants	2. Gather Pertinent Facts	3. Generate Alternative Decisions
Determine qualified decision makers. Select based on: —Nature of issue —Experience —Knowledge —Interest —Personal traits that foster group efforts	Employ fact-finding techniques. Survey others. Remember that each fact is a premise and that decisions are a combination of multiple premises.	Employ techniques that cultivate creativity. Don't judge ideas. Aim for quantity. Entertain what seems ridiculous. Look for variations in ideas.

4. Predict Outcomes	5. Select Best Alternative	6. Plan for Managing Consequences
Recognize desired and undesired outcomes of each alternative. Concentrate on quality. From list determine alternatives with undesirable outcomes that cannot be managed. Condense list accordingly.	Weigh the undesirable outcomes against the value of desirable outcomes of remaining alternatives. Select the best alternative.	Secure support of the whole group. —Communicate to all who are affected by the decision. —Be honest about pros and cons. —Show how the pros outweigh the cons. —Suggest ways to handle undesirable outcomes. —Offer to assist where possible.

Improving quality of decision making pays high dividends as groups encounter conflicts in the work setting. Dealing with conflicts can be time consuming. Quality of decisions made relative to a controversial issue can make the difference between managing the conflict or being managed by it.

Plan for Managing Consequences

The group must look at negative consequences with an eye for those that cannot realistically be managed in a way to avoid further and perhaps most serious problems. Because each alternative has both desired and undesired consequences, each eliminated alternative represents a loss in terms of the very best, idealized choice; but the outcome is one that is workable and in the overall interest of everyone.

A final note about decisions based on consideration of all elements in the process: each is uniquely valuable in a specific situation. Skill in use of the process is therefore very important for quality nursing practice.

■ MANAGEMENT OF CONFLICT

Nature of Conflict

Interactive processes of leadership are multifaceted, and the management of conflict might well be the most challenging process of all. Acknowledging the dual nature of conflict as potentially constructive or destructive and recognizing cues that spell blessing or trouble is the goal of managing conflict.

Some conflicts are preventive and reduce hindrances to goal attainment. Effective leaders learn to curtail conflict on one hand and to design or to allow its influence on the other, becoming increasingly astute in determining the need for each. Obsolete practices of entrenched groups can be shaken loose by allowing or imposing conflict events. For example, different expectations that introduce new ideas and ways of doing things can pump new blood into stagnant, but otherwise competent, groups. Members gain new appreciations and readily incorporate changed expectations if the conflict event is managed well. In the case of destructive conflict, early intervention is needed to defuse volatile emotions that threaten attainment of group purpose. Disarming instigators in some way through use of various techniques is one way of handling destructive conflict. Specific strategies for managing both constructive and destructive conflicts are offered in the following section.

To begin, it is necessary to dispel the notion that all conflict is bad. In settings where conflict has been traditionally viewed as something that is only destructive, a new look can broaden perspectives to include potential benefits that come from dealing effectively with conflict. A simple question (Will some change harm or help a situation?) leads to analysis, which is the first stage of conflict management. Analysis reveals the nature of the particular conflict, which must be considered within the context of a given situation and point in time to determine its potential outcome.

Degree of conflict in a setting is an important factor to consider when analyzing its effects. Situational factors influence the point at which a conflict is good or bad. Competent groups handle conflicts differently than weak groups. The collective strength of effective groups accommodates weaknesses among their members. Such accommodation is not found in disjointed groups. The style and strength of leadership operating in a setting influence individuals' and the group's responses to disruptive events. The overall **internal climate,** therefore, is an important determinant of the outcome of any given conflict. It is important to acknowledge the fluid nature of factors that contribute to internal climate so that frequent monitoring of the environment occurs. It cannot be assumed that a cohesive group remains so always.

Conflicts do not fall on a fixed point on a scale from beneficial and growth producing to harmful. Multiple, interactive, situational factors determine the merit of conflict. A conflict event might produce the cutting edge needed for growth at one point in time and cause problems at another. For example, in times of organizational prosperity, an announcement of no raises or of cut back in salaries will have a very different outcome on the workers than at a time of economic constraint and retrenchment that threaten job security. The same announcement with the same individuals, but with different situational factors, produces different consequences. The assumption that dissatisfaction can be expected from the former situation and cooperation from the latter could be quite accurate depending on the degree of shared information, understanding, and fairness. If cuts affect only staff while managers remain completely unaffected, and no explanations are given, a perception of misuse of power is likely, whether or not it is true. Conflicts rooted in misunderstanding, lack of cooperation, misuse of power, and unfairness generally produce detrimental outcomes. They must be terminated as quickly as possible. At times, skilled negotiators are needed to settle disputes when cooperative efforts fail. Differences in perceptions of events occur in nursing from time to time, and it is important that nurses develop an appreciation of conflict as a significant force influencing nursing practice. Failure to understand or handle conflicts appropriately can account for serious, internal, professional problems.

■ BASIS OF CONFLICT

Conflict can be of an intrapsychic (i.e., personal), interpersonal, or intradepartmental nature. Nurses encounter varying degrees of each and need to develop understanding and skill in managing them. Individuals can experience serious internal personal conflicts that temporarily force reordering of their priorities. Personal conflicts can put an individual at variance with work goals. In such instances, collective strength of effective work groups can temporarily compensate for the individual's poor performance, but resolution is ultimately the responsibility of the individual.

Interpersonal influences, such as personality differences and conflicting ideas, produce conflicts that can lead to either positive or negative results. Antagonism between individuals can be good or bad based on the degree of mutual respect shared between them. Outcome of any interpersonal conflict is due to complex, time-related, situational factors surrounding the entire event.

Conflict is frequently associated with felt, unequal distribution of power, status, and resources. It may be real or the result of inaccurate perceptions. In either case, problems arise that must be handled swiftly if complications are to be avoided. Outcome of conflicts is determined by four critical forces: (1) the issue, (2) power base of participants, (3) cooperation between participants, and (4) communication. Selected courses of action can keep issues to manageable proportion or can escalate them. Power can be used to coerce or to compromise. Individuals can hold onto bias or work to dissipate it. Information can be freely shared or withheld as a means of control, and listening can become an integral part of communication.

Clause and Bailey describe the use of **power** in two ways: *directive* and *synergic*.[10] Directive power shapes others for the purpose of advancing the interest of the power wielder and is viewed as a negative force. It is an example of unequal distribution of power. Synergic power, on the other hand, incorporates group values and cherishes other people. Synergic power is an essential element in balancing control in competitive environments. Nursing is in a competitive environment in which bureaucratic goals dominate, putting professional goals and values at risk. A strong, cohesive voice from nursing plus intelligent and articulate nurse representatives are necessary to keep professional values/bureaucratic efficiency conflicts to manageable proportions in complex organizations. In today's climate of health care delivery, ways must be found to conserve resources and to use wisely what is available. Professional nurses must spend their time providing professional services rather than secretarial and hotel services that frequently consume too many professional nurses' hours. An honest look at practices might reveal a degree of purposefully holding onto these activities. Such activities do provide opportunities for closure of a task, which is satisfying, whereas many professional activities leave nurses with some ambiguity about outcomes of their efforts. Experience plus maturity allow nurses to handle the ambiguity more effectively.

Recognition of the basis of conflict can be helpful in managing it. Knowing events that are bound to be problematic can allow for effective interventions to reduce their magnitude or to eliminate them altogether. Decisive action is complex, and analysis of premises from which action was formed is ongoing and interactive.

Examples of Common Conflicts in Nursing

Nobel and Rancourt present evidence of a lack of cohesiveness in perceptions and values among nurses, which causes major intradepartmental conflicts.[11] They discuss different modes of knowing and knowledge accessing style as causes of such conflicts. As a result of the differences, nurses perceive the world of nursing and how they conceptualize legitimate knowledge from opposing viewpoints. Educational preparation was suggested as one factor in accounting for the differences, with university-educated nurses, both staff nurses and nurse managers, being more flexible in applying information in conflict situations. Nurses with broader educational backgrounds were able to appreciate a variety of perceptions about a situation, whereas non-degree nurses tended to hold onto their own perceptions as being correct. Unwillingness to develop greater flexibility can lead to anger and fear as responses to conflict.

Earlier research by Kramer and Schmalenberg has shown that commonly occurring conflicts in nursing can be categorized according to type.[12] Labels given to the types of conflicts are helpful in identifying the source and participants of conflict in nursing and provide clues about interventions. Examples of classic conflicts in nursing include *professional/bureaucratic, nurse/nurse, nurse/doctor, personal competency gap, competing role, expressive/instrumental*, and *patient/nurse* conflicts. Many nurses will be able to see themselves in each one at one time or another. How they are managed and what is learned from them is important. A description of each type follows.

Professional/bureaucratic conflicts are the result of incompatibility of expectations produced by the system and perceived professional standards and responsibilities. Imbalance of power is frequently at the root of such conflicts. As such, they lead to a great deal of frustration for nurses who feel helpless in a situation.

Nurse/nurse conflicts result when differing values toward the philosophy of nursing are held by nurses who work together. The differences interfere with teamwork. There can be ongoing problems between nurses who are consistently task oriented and those who wish to do holistic care. Assignment preferences of task-oriented nurses are based on procedures to be performed, whereas nurses who prefer holistic care choose continuity of patient care from admission to discharge. Both approaches cannot exist on the same unit. Recently, nursing is experiencing the need for sensitivity training in order to manage staff conflicts that arise out of multicultural issues. Martin, Wimberly, and O'Keefe present a new view of multiculturalism's impact on the health care industry.[13] U.S. standards emphasize the individual, competition, and accomplishment. Nurses in our culture strive to assist patients to become more independent in health care matters. Western language is considered to be low context and many words are used to make a point. In contrast, Eastern cultures are group oriented, and the individual is subordinated. Harmony is prized and language is considered to be high context with few words used for necessary communication. Philosophical differences can become sources of misunderstandings that can turn into conflict without planned efforts to improve understanding.

Nurse/doctor conflicts spring from differing expectations of each other in the delivery of care. There are differences in the "medical model" and the "nursing model." Each emphasizes different aspects of health care that complement each other. Conflict comes about because of imbalance of power traditionally found in the system. Development of collegial relationships in which there is mutual respect for each other's complementary roles can prevent the time-consuming and senseless problems that take attention away from shared goals of nurses and doctors.

Personal competency gap conflicts occur when nurses' skill levels interfere with their own expectations of standards of practice for themselves. This type of conflict occurs when nurses are pulled to areas of practice they are unfamiliar with, especially to intensive care units (ICUs) and trauma centers. The practice of reassigning nurses to different units as a means of taking care of shortages is common and expedient in advancing efficiency. It must be noted, however, that efficiency and effectiveness are different entities. If standards of practice are frequently ignored, some elements of professional/bureaucratic conflict are seen through imbalance of power.

Competing role conflicts occur when the same person fills the roles of nurse, student, spouse, and parent, all of which exert a pull on the individual's time, energy, and attention. Demands outside of nursing, as well as demands from within nursing, contribute to this type of conflict. Today, to some extent, such conflicts cannot be avoided. Economic conditions frequently require two incomes to maintain an acceptable life-style. Single-parent families mean a period of day care for children that is not always ideal. Educational level for nurses must be upgraded to meet their career goals.

Expressive/instrumental conflicts occur when nurses are torn between technical care demands and human or expressive needs of patients. Ethical issues, legal issues, patient and family requests and personal values, and the philosophy of the nurse all operate as elements in this type of conflict.

Management of expressive/instrumental conflicts is among the most difficult. They can be a daily source of conflict in ICUs and trauma centers. Nurses in critical care and trauma care settings must work effectively with an expanded professional team and handle sensitive situations with families.

Patient/nurse conflicts result when nurses' goals for care differ from patients' goals for care. When nurses maintain an effective, therapeutic role in caring for patients, this type of conflict can be kept to a minimum. Respecting patients' and families' decisions about their care, especially when their choice is an informed and considered one, is part of holistic care and is an expected standard. It is, however, not easy to accept nontraditional choices, but nurses are sometimes in the position to support them without personal value judgments.

There is another entire category of patient behavior that comes from increasing violence and crime in our society that can bring about serious nurse/patient conflicts. Daum describes the disruptive antisocial patient who is simultaneously perpetrator and victim of drug trafficking, neighborhood violence, and other criminal activity.[14] They are individuals who have limited ego strength, who act impulsively due to limited ability to delay gratification of their needs, and who accept violence as a way of life. They present nurses with challenges formerly not experienced. These situations call for strong leadership and collaboration among all caregivers for firmness and consistency in caring for the patient. At times the presence of security guards or even local police is necessary in order to insure safety of other patients and the staff.

No doubt many nurses, both beginners and veterans, have experienced some or all of the types of conflicts described. These conflicts appear to be timeless and are a reality in nursing practice. Nurses must be prepared to prevent them when possible or to manage them effectively so that their effects are minimized.

Approaches to Managing Conflict

Strategies and techniques for managing conflicts are more easily described than prescribed. At the outset, consider that conceptualizing conflict positively and describing events in positive terms can help produce positive outcome. Conversely, conceptualizing conflict negatively and describing events in negative terms can cause negative outcomes. Some positive terms are suggested in the Conflict Management Module of Teaching Improvement Projects System (TIPS) developed at the University of Kentucky at Lexington.[15] Positive terms are *exciting, creative, helpful, courageous, stimulating, growth-producing, strengthening,* and *clarifying.* In the same reference, Hocks and Wilmot found, however, that more frequently in our society, conflict is depicted in negative terms, such as *destructive, confrontational, disagreement, tension, anger, pain, hostility,* and *anxiety.*[16] It would appear then, that there is much work to do in order to foster a positive attitude about the potential that conflict can have. Various strategies can lead to win-win, win-lose, or lose-lose outcomes. Some can give rise to legal and ethical problems and must be used cautiously. Situational factors surrounding any conflict are numerous and varied in combination, and planning approaches to solve conflicts is based on situational contingencies. Some techniques for managing conflict described by Booth are *confrontation, bargaining, smoothing, avoidance,* and *unilateral action.*[17] Each has its place in conflict management, since situations are uniquely different. A definition of each technique follows.

Confrontation can be difficult and uncomfortable. But its constructive use can be learned. For this approach to be healthy and successful, three prerequisites are necessary: (1) each party must be motivated to resolve the issue, (2) each party must have equal power relative to the issue, and (3) each party must have necessary information about the issue. Successful confrontation brings important issues out in the open, facilitates honest and spontaneous sharing of views, and provides information that improves participants' knowledge about the issue. When successful, it leads to a win-win outcome.

Bargaining, as the term implies, involves giving of something to gain something in return. A negotiator or arbitrator is useful when bargaining is the technique of choice. The arbitrator must be briefed on the position of each party and on the preferred solution of each. The approach is time consuming and expensive but can yield a satisfying win-win outcome. It is more frequently employed in settling major issues where important matters are at stake.

Smoothing minimizes the importance of differences so that they are not acknowledged, and therefore no solution is found. All parties lose, and in time the problem presents itself again. It might be used temporarily as a strategy to gain time while attempting to improve cooperation between rivals.

Avoidance, another no-win technique, sweeps problems under the rug where they are more likely to compound than to go away. It too might be employed temporarily while interactional conditions between parties improve. Avoidance is the technique of choice if the issue itself is too trivial to warrant attention.

Unilateral action implies active involvement by one party while the other is either avoiding action or is helpless in the situation. It might be a power-based conflict and result in a win-lose outcome. This approach can create more problems than it solves and can lead to legal and ethical problems. On the other hand, it can be the technique of choice in certain crisis situations.

Favorable outcomes of conflict situations depend on purposeful selection of the best technique based on the unique circumstances surrounding each issue. It is conceivable that any one of the techniques described could be the approach of choice in a given event. Determining the best choice takes place through use of a structured process. Following is a description of a process for student use.

■ PROCESS MODEL OF CONFLICT MANAGEMENT

The process model of conflict management presented in Figure 4-3 is composed of four stages. Stage 1 has four parts: (1) *issue*, (2) *power*, (3) *cooperation*, and (4) *communication*. Stage 2 is use of *facilitative* techniques. Stage 3 is movement toward *resolution*. Stage 4 is plan for *implementation* of decisions.

In the four parts of stage 1, there are questions to ask about each. Is the issue important, how important and how much time will be needed to arrive at consensus? Is *power* equal enough for negotiation to take place? Can it be equalized? Is the level of *cooperation* such that all sides regard other's point of view? Can it be developed? Is *communication* open and spontaneous and without hidden agendas? If it is determined that the conflict is legitimately nonnegotiable by virtue of policy, resources, or contractual agreement, group effort is inappropriate and individuals must reassess their own situations and proceed accordingly. If, on the other hand, the conflict is one for group resolution, they proceed to stage 2.

Stage 2, *facilitative techniques*, includes the selection of a mutually agreeable neutral setting so that neither side has an advantage because of space. When possible and by choice of those involved, a setting away from the workplace can be helpful. It is important that discussions proceed along depersonalized positions (for example: suggestion A, suggestion B, etc.). Each point is then considered as to its advantages and disadvantages. A realistic time frame should be established in order to insure forward movement of the process while giving it the importance it deserves.

In stage 3 the group moves toward *resolution*. Short, frequent exchanges are important and provide a way to clarify and validate terms, restate positions, and validate perceptions. A final definition ends stage 3.

During the fourth and final stage, a plan for *implementation* is devised. New expectations are described, who will be affected by them is identified, and how a smooth transition can be accomplished is defined. The new practices will be monitored until the new expectations are established. The

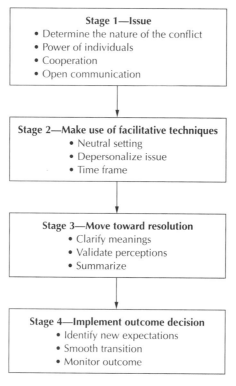

Figure 4-3. Process model of conflict management. Stages occur in one-way sequence. The model is adaptable to a variety of situations involving groups or individuals within groups, or between groups.

resolution of some conflicts can be handled quite successfully by staff nurses, such as those that stem from and are limited to the operation of a nursing unit. Others are better handled by nurse managers, such as those having legal consequences and those that involve several layers of the organizational hierarchy. Managers are recognized as formal leaders, as spokespersons, and as those who have ready access to information not available to others. In either case, it is well to consider Numerof's position that negotiation of conflict is the most difficult aspect of Communication.[18] Communication has been covered extensively in Chapter 3. It is of major importance in organizations, and the need for ongoing refinement of skill cannot be overemphasized.

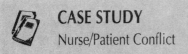

CASE STUDY
Coverage by Outside PRN Nurses

Lately, full-time staff nurses on a busy acute care unit at Hospital X are find-ing themselves working alongside PRN nurses from a rent-a-nurse agency. While the PRNs are highly competent in the actual delivery of patient care, full-time staff nurses must teach the PRNs the physical resources of the unit, procedures for ordering tests and supplies, directions to various depart-ments, physicians' protocols, etc. In short, when staff nurses are the busiest, it is like having new employees to orient.

Compounding the problem is the recent resignation from the unit of some of the staff nurses to go to work for the rent-a-nurse agency. Their move is motivated by the salary and work schedule of PRNs. Nurses at the rent-a-nurse agency decide their own days and hours and earn $6 an hour more than the highest-paid staff nurse at hospital X.

This is certainly a situation in which the grass seems greener on the other side. Analyze the situation and propose alternatives to administration of hospital X that will ensure quality care and improve staff morale. In ana-lyzing this situation, consider the following points:

- Using professional standards, cite conditions that are essential for high-quality patient care.
- Offer cooperation in the form of constructive input from the staff in solving the problem.
- Clearly state the level of dissatisfaction among the nursing staff and the possible consequences if the situation continues as is.

CASE STUDY
Nurse/Patient Conflict

Marcus Butler is a 19-year-old patient recently transferred from the surgical ICU to the open surgical unit. He had suffered gun shot wounds to his abdomen and left leg during a gang confrontation in the early hours of the morning four days ago. His condition is stable, but he is expected to be in the hospital for three to four more days. It isn't long before the nurses realize that his behavior presents a real challenge for them. He is demanding, his language is insulting, and his numerous visitors provide him with food items that are not on his restricted diet. Together they play loud music and/or the television late into the night. Nurses have been threatened when they request any form of cooperation from the patient or his visitors. A security guard is stationed on the unit, but his presence seems to make little difference because he is not recognized as a law enforcement agent by the gang members. It is apparent that Marcus does not share or appreciate any of the nurses' values and concern for his health and well-being. Their best efforts have made no difference in his response to them.

- How would you structure a plan for the care of this patient?
- What is your response to his unconventional behavior?

■ SUMMARY

In this chapter, decision making and management of conflict are discussed. Effective communication improves understanding between parties in complex work settings, and healthy group dynamics facilitate decision making. In turn, quality decision making fosters effective management of conflict. Not all conflict is detrimental, but those that are must be managed and brought under control. Some conflict is growth producing and leads to revitalization of efforts. Experience in decision making and conflict management leads to heightened precision in communication and improved group relations. Outcomes of both are good or bad, depending on the willingness of participants to work toward success and on their skill level. Process models of decision making and conflict resolution are offered.

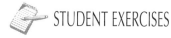 STUDENT EXERCISES

1. With the advent of third-party payment, a large medical center found it feasible to change operating practices in several of its departments. One affected department was the outpatient department, where most clients are Medicare and Medicaid recipients. A complex fee system was devised based on services including consultation, laboratory tests, radiographs, etc. Nurses in the department were accustomed to a sim-

pler fee schedule, depending on whether patients had a prescription filled. They were upset at the thought of patients being charged higher fees. Since nurses were responsible for completing the form indicating the extent of services a patient received, many decided to check the lowest category, "Seen by nurse only." They reasoned that the designers of the new system could not understand poor clients' situations. The agency lost a great deal of revenue it could have collected from Medicare and Medicaid sources as a result. Comment on the nurses' decisions. Comment on the organizational decision.

2. The nursing service department has been asked by administration to select a representative to serve on an ad hoc committee that will decide distribution of widely scattered parking places owned by the hospital. Administration is tired of the bickering about who wants to park where, so they established a system that each department alphabetically selects individuals to serve on the committee. Suggest an alternative method of assignment; give your rationale.

3. Using the description of Delphi technique in this chapter and considering your fellow students to be "experts" in use of learning climates, construct a brief questionnaire concerning library hours (or some other issue). Try to survey at least five students. Do at least two feedback analyses (three if possible). Share a report of findings of the process and findings with fellow students.

4. Administration has deemed it crucial to freeze salaries for the coming year. Groups within the organization respond to the news with wide variation, from "rally round" to "sabotage." Administrative personnel are surprised that so many are not being cooperative, because they thought they had a "familylike" cooperative team. How would you respond to this situation?

5. The head nurse on your unit has received a communication from administration that change-of-shift unit census reports are arriving late in the office more and more frequently. The census and acuity level of patients on the unit have been high. How are unit census reports used in the nursing department? What steps would you suggest to facilitate meeting the needs of everyone?

6. More and more the formation of a hierarchy within the ranks of staff nurses is being observed. There are floor duty nurses, trauma nurses, intensive care nurses, transport nurses, and outpatient nurses all employed in the same institution at the same level. There is an

unmistakable attitude of some being more important than others. List potential conflicts associated with such a hierarchy.

7. The nursing unit is without the services of a ward secretary for a week. The head nurse wants to be fair to her staff and decides to take her turn at filling in. For the full week she serves as the unit secretary. Analyze premises in this decision. Weigh the gains and losses for the unit.

■ REFERENCES

1. Simon HA, *Administrative Behavior: A Study of Decision Making Processes in Administrative Organizations*, 3rd ed, New York: The Free Press, 1976, p. xi.
2. Garre PP, "Multiattribute Utility Theory in Decision Making," *Nursing Management*, May 1992, p. 33–35.
3. Simon HA, p. ix.
4. Bourbonnais FF, Baumann A, "Stress and Rapid Decision Making in Nursing: An Administrative Challenge," *Nursing Administration Quarterly*, Spring 1985, p. 85–91.
5. Carnevali DL, Thomas MD, *Diagnostic Reasoning and Treatment Decision Making in Nursing*, Philadelphia: J.B. Lippincott, 1993.
6. Simon HA, p. 71.
7. Ibid., p. xii.
8. DeBella S, Martin L, Siddall S, *Nurse's Role in Health Care Planning*, Norwalk, CT: Appleton & Lange, 1986, p. 34.
9. Johnson C, "Cultivating Your Creativity," *Toastmaster*, August 1988, p. 8–10.
10. Clause KE, Bailey JT, *Power and Influence in Health Care: A New Approach to Leadership*, St. Louis: Mosby, 1977, p. 9.
11. Nobel KA, Rancourt R, "Administration and Intradisciplinary Conflict Within Nursing," *Nursing Administration Quarterly*, Summer 1991, p. 36–42.
12. Kramer M, Schmalenberg C, "Conflict: The Cutting Edge of Growth," *American Journal of Nursing*, October 1976, p. 19–25.
13. Martin K, Wimberly D, O'Keefe K, "Resolving Conflict in a Multicultural Nursing Department," *Nursing Management*, 25:1, January 1994, p. 49–51.
14. Daum, AL, "The Disruptive Antisocial Patient: Management Strategies," *Nursing Management*, 25:8, August 1994, p. 46–51.
15. Sedlacek, J, *Conflict Management*, University of Kentucky, College of Allied Health Professions: TIPS, 1989, p. 13.
16. Ibid., p. 17.
17. Booth RZ, "Conflict Resolution," *Nursing Outlook*, September/October 1982, p. 447–453.
18. Numerof RE, "The Manager as Conflict Negotiator," *Health Care Supervisor*, April 1985, p. 1–15.

5

The Ethical Responsibility
of the Nurse Leader

Introduction

As early as 1980, Flaherty wrote: "Whenever nurses meet, they express concern about the number and complexity of ethical dilemmas that they face and the effect of these on the quality and quantity of their professional practice."[1] How many more dilemmas present themselves, particularly to the nurse manager, as we approach the twenty-first century?

Special situations, such as the explosion of the acquired immune deficiency syndrome (AIDS) and human immunodeficiency virus (HIV) infections, and the proliferation of organ transplantations, have escalated the number of ethical dilemmas for nursing practice. In addition, nursing leaders and managers are faced with dilemmas associated with a rapidly changing health care system, such as allocation of scarce resources and maintaining quality of care in an era of severe cost cutting. The object of this chapter is to discuss the ethical responsibility of a nurse leader/manager in today's complex health care system.

⚜ KEY CONCEPTS

Ethics is that branch of philosophy that examines ideal human behavior.

Morality is based in values derived from religious precepts, cultural belief systems, or other forms of community expectation or social convention.

Values are the basis for codes of behavior that affect ethical decisions.

Deontology Theories presume that one does the good act and avoids evil.

Consequentialist Theories define good actions as those of utility.

Autonomy provides for the privilege of self-determination in deciding what happens to one's body in health care.

Beneficence requires that care providers contribute to health and welfare and not merely avoid harm to patient or client.

Nonmaleficence prohibits deliberate harm and demands weighing risks with benefits of treatment.

Justice requires that individuals be given what they are entitled to, deserve, or can legitimately claim and that resources are distributed fairly.

Affirmative Action a new ethic, but also written into statutes, provides for employment and promotion opportunities for qualified persons in proportion to the existence of representative ethnic groups in the geographic area.

Ethics Committees are groups designed to educate health care providers in ethical decision making and to provide consultation in resolving ethical dilemmas.

Whistle-Blowing is a cry against wrongdoings, a call for correction of an injustice, abuse, or neglect.

■ ETHICS

The term **ethics** is used to refer to that branch of philosophy that examines ideal human behavior. **Morality** is a term used to refer to general rules of social and personal conduct and the practices or actions that derive from those rules. While "moral" is a term sometimes used as a judgment about whether an action is right or wrong, in the field of ethics, "ethical" and "moral" refer, not to the rightness or wrongness of actions, but to a category or class of actions that pertain to ethics.[2] Morality is based on strongly held or fundamental values derived from religious precepts, cultural belief systems, or other forms of community expectation or social convention. Ethical dilemmas are those situations that present a conflict between two or more fundamental **values,** are complex and have no apparent solution, and for which all possible solutions have equally undesirable outcomes. While ethical dilemmas confront nurses and nurse managers daily, not all difficult situations encountered by nurses are ethical dilemmas. A situation may have ethical aspects but still be primarily an organizational, communication, or legal problem. For instance, a patient may have a valid living will stating that the patient does not want to be resuscitated in the event of cardiac arrest, but that document is not in the patient's chart. While this situation has ethical implications for the patient's treatment, it is primarily an organizational or legal problem. The Patient Self-Determination Act clearly outlines the hospital's responsibility to assure that advance directive documents be put in the patient's chart.[3]

Ethics is a reflective endeavor in which the individual moves beyond the acceptance and internalization of traditional rules of the social group and moves into the realm of reflecting upon those rules.[4] Ethical decision making for the professional nurse is guided by general rules of social conduct, the nurse's personal values, and the values of the nursing profession. The fundamental values of nursing are expressed in the Code for Nurses.[5] They are the values, such as respect for patient autonomy, acting in the patient's best interest and maintaining professional competence, that all nurses commit to uphold when they enter the profession:

1. The nurse provides services with respect for human dignity and the uniqueness of the client, unrestricted by considerations of social or economic status, personal attributes or the nature of health problems.
2. The nurse safeguards the client's right to privacy by judiciously protecting information of a confidential nature.
3. The nurse acts to safeguard the client and the public when health care and safety are affected by the incompetent, unethical, or illegal practice of any person.
4. The nurse assumes responsibility and accountability for individual nursing judgments and actions.
5. The nurse maintains competence in nursing.
6. The nurse exercises informed judgment and uses individual competence and qualifications as criteria in seeking consultation, accepting responsibilities, and delegating nursing activities to others.

7. The nurse participates in activities that contribute to the ongoing development of the profession's body of knowledge.
8. The nurse participates in the profession's efforts to implement and improve standards of nursing.
9. The nurse participates in the profession's efforts to establish and maintain conditions of employment conductive to high-quality nursing care.
10. The nurse participates in the profession's effort to protect the public from misinformation and misrepresentation and to maintain the integrity of nursing.
11. The nurse collaborates with members of the health professions and other citizens in promoting community and national efforts to meet the health needs of the public.

An important part of professional socialization is learning to use these fundamental values to guide one's actions in professional situations. Other professional values are more instrumental, in that they are helpful or necessary to achieve the fundamental values expressed in the Code. For instance, nurses value their professional autonomy and the right to control their own practice, because these activities are necessary to assure that patients' best interests are well-served. Nurses value assertiveness because they may find it necessary to confront other professionals or family members if a patient's right to participate in decision making is being threatened.

In a study of professional values of nursing students and graduate nurses, Schank and Weis discovered that respondents "have not fully developed the value orientation of the profession embodied in the Code" for nurses.[6] The values elicited—caring, interpersonal goals, helping, respect, patience, honesty, loyalty, faith, accountability, self-happiness, and education—refer to the first six code statements, which deal with professional issues. The values related to social issues, reflected in the last five code statements, are not identified as readily as professional values by the respondents in this study.[7] Another way of interpreting these findings is that nurses tend to first internalize those values related to their individual responsibility to the patients directly served. As the nurse more fully develops as a professional, there is a greater understanding of, and commitment to, the profession's collective responsibility to society. The last five statements of the Code for Nurses speak to professional activities that help to implement and improve standards of high-quality nursing care, provide a sound scientific basis for nursing practice, protect the public from misinformation, and collaborate with others to promote health of the public. These more socially oriented goals can only be accomplished when nurses band together in collective activities, such as setting national standards of practice and engaging in political action.

Professional values guide nursing actions and motivate one to continue to function within standards and codes. Professional values are developed through education or by observation of role models and mentors. A very important part of the nurse leader's role is to role-model commitment to the individual and collective values of the nursing profession and to mentor other nurses in their growth as professionals.

Ethical Theories

The two categories of ethical theories prevalent in guiding moral decision making are **deontology theories** and **consequentialist theories.** These theories explain reasoned analysis of ethical dilemmas and account for the moral decision of one person as opposed to the moral decision of a second individual. For example, one person may determine that an action, such as telling the truth or keeping a promise, is good in itself and may perform that action regardless of the consequences. A second person may look at the results of the action and determine not to do it. From their perspective, it may be hurtful to someone to tell the truth or keep a promise.

Consequentialism is the theory that actions are right or wrong according *only* to their consequences. The most common form of consequentialism is utilitarianism. In a somewhat oversimplified form, this theory is expressed as "the end justifies the means" or as promoting "the greatest good for the greatest number of people." Thus, the consequences of a specific action assume a very significant role in the decision-making process. Ethical decisions founded on a utilitarian base may be made from the perspective of "act utilitarianism," which judges the consequences or utility of single acts situationally, or "rule utilitarianism," which judges the utility not of single acts but of adhering to certain moral rules. For an act-utilitarian, deceiving a patient about a diagnosis may be morally acceptable because, in a particular situation, it satisfies the family's needs and may protect the patient from a possible depression. A rule-utilitarian may believe that deceiving the patient is wrong because the greatest good to society comes from adhering to the moral rule "Do not lie."[8,9]

Deontologic theories are based on the premise that judgments about the rightness or wrongness of actions are based on features other than or in addition to the consequences of the action. Deontologic theories presume that one does the good act and avoids evil. Good or right actions honor truth, promises, contracts, and significant relationships, including the nurse-patient and manager-worker relationships. For example, a deontologist may believe that deceiving a patient about a diagnosis is always wrong because deception in and of itself is wrong, regardless of its consequences. Ethical decisions made within a deontological framework are grounded in religious traditions, natural law or "common moral consciousness."[10]

Ethical Principles

Several ethical principles derived from ethical theories are applicable in health care and nursing situations. The principles most often utilized in resolving dilemmas are autonomy, beneficence, nonmaleficence, and justice.[11]

Autonomy provides for the privilege of self-determination in deciding what happens to one's body in health care. Since the late 1960s, society has affirmed the right of the individual to make decisions about medical care. The President's Commission for the Study of Ethical Problems in Medicine emphasized that the competent adult has the right to decline medical treatments even though it would result in death.[12] Several famous court cases, such as the Nancy Cruzan case, established the patient's legal right to refuse treatment, and that right was given additional force with the passage of the Patient Self-Determination Act in 1990.[13] The Code for Nurses speaks directly to the autonomy principle in its first and third statements.[14]

Paternalism, in which the physician or health care provider makes decisions about treatment on the basis of what the provider deems best for the patient, is directly opposed to autonomy. The principle of self-determination, or autonomy, requires that patients have adequate information about treatment options to make an intelligent decision and to give informed consent to a specific form of therapy.

Beneficence requires that care providers contribute to the health and welfare of the patient and not merely avoid harm to the patient or client. Providing for discharge planning early in hospitalization to facilitate rehabilitation or protecting a patient's reputation by maintaining confidentiality of information are examples of following the principle of beneficence.

Nonmaleficence prohibits deliberate harm and demands weighing risks with benefits of treatment. Not using proper precautions in caring for patients with infectious or communicable diseases and thus endangering self and other patients would contradict the principle of nonmaleficence. Physically restraining a patient without carefully weighing the benefits against potential risks of restraint could lead to serious problems for the patient, causing more harm than good and thus violating the principle of non-maleficence. The nurse manager who does not protect the confidentiality of personnel information can do a great deal of harm to a staff member's reputation and professional future.

Justice requires that individuals be given what they are entitled to, deserve, or can legitimately claim. Patients have rights to considerate and respectful care, and nurses are entitled to safe working environments. Generally, physicians deserve to have their orders carried out. Administrators and supervisors can legitimately claim that workers spend their time on the job in productive activity.

The principle of justice has to do with the fair allocation of resources. Decisions about how to allocate become more difficult when resources are limited. As health care reform measures place greater emphasis on containing costs, all health providers struggle to make allocation decisions that will be as fair as possible for all parties concerned, and still maintain an acceptable level of quality of care. Staff nurses making decisions about how to divide their time among several critically ill patients are allocating the scarce resource of their time, and should examine how they make those decisions.

Barriers to Ethical Decision Making

Several factors relating to individual nurses and the social context in which they practice can present barriers to making sound ethical decisions. Some of these factors are a result of contemporary social conditions from which the nurse leader cannot escape. For instance, over the past few decades, an apathy toward the Judeo-Christian doctrine and moral code has emerged. More individuals reach adulthood having had limited opportunity to develop strong moral convictions to guide their personal actions. Violence and abuse have become commonplace in American society and seem to reflect a diminished value for human life. As our country becomes more culturally diverse, individuals from other cultures and religious traditions bring different perspectives on ethical issues such as end-of-life decisions and questions of justice and fairness. Ethical decisions regarding care for such persons require an understanding of their cultural belief systems, an understanding that is often lacking.

Many situations have both ethical and legal ramifications. Current social attitudes place emphasis on individual rights rather than responsibilities, contributing to the tendency to turn to the courts to uphold those rights. Within health care, this tendency contributes to the potential for legal actions that may or may not be justified by the facts of a situation. The result is that professionals are cautious in decision making and fearful of litigation. For example, in questions such as whether or not to continue life-sustaining treatments, the ethically good action may be stifled by fears of litigation.

Advances in technology have resulted in such emotionally explosive practices as intrauterine diagnosis or treatment and gene therapy. New technologies have challenged our beliefs about what constitutes life and death. Cost considerations have created concerns about when and to what extent society can afford to provide available technology, thus raising the question of whether or not the ethically good action is affordable.

Other potential barriers to moral judgments exist in the nursing practice environment. The nurse leader may not be central to ethical decision making but is subject to physicians and to administrators while being accountable to patients according to codes of ethics. Nurses have overlapping responsibilities with other health care professionals, thus making it unclear exactly where accountability rests and making it difficult to trace and correct errors. There is often inadequate staffing and frequent rotation of nurses, which may place nurses in a position of knowing what is the right thing to do for patients but being unable to fulfill those responsibilities because of lack of time and situational support.

■ STRATEGIES FOR ENHANCING ETHICAL DECISIONS IN NURSING PRACTICE

One aspect of ethical decision making over which nurses have control is their own moral development and their perspectives of professional obligations. For example, nurses can determine to what extent they accept traditional male and female roles in health care delivery and understand how these traditional roles affect their ability to advocate for patients. Nurses can make choices that will increase or reduce their risks for experiencing burnout or substance abuse. They can develop understanding of how burnout or substance abuse can impede a nurse's ability to carry out professional ethical responsibilities as outlined in the Code for Nurses.

Nurses and nurse leaders may not have received adequate preparation in moral development theory and ethical decision-making models. Despite this, it is their responsibility to participate in ethical decision making. Nurses need to recognize that without adequate education about systematic ethical analysis, their conclusions about the right action in an ethical dilemma are mostly a reflection of what "feels good" to them. What feels good or right for one person may or may not be the best action for someone else. Systematic analysis of situations, applying the tools of ethical theory and ethical principles, helps to assure that the values and beliefs of one person are not inappropriately imposed on others. To attain the necessary tools of ethical analysis, nurses can attend courses in ethics. Nurse leaders can help provide staff development programs and in-service education to keep staff up-to-date on ethical issues in practice. Professional publications, such as the Code for Nurses with Interpretive Statements or various position statements from the American Nurses Association, can be helpful sources to expand the nurse leader's vision of professional ethical responsibilities.[15] Other activities that facilitate individual development include regularly scheduled nursing ethics rounds or brown bag discussions. These forums provide opportunities for staff to clarify their legal rights and responsibilities and to begin to deal with the ambiguities and limitations inherent in all ethical dilemmas.

Vigilance against unconditionally accepting the health care decisions of administration and the medical staff will help the nurse leader guard the role of patient advocate in ethical dilemmas. The ability to challenge administrative or medical pronouncements comes with self-confidence in the leadership role based on educational preparation in philosophy, ethics, and moral decision making, as well as management and leadership. Other resources to support ethical decision making include the institution's philosophy and mission statements, patient's bill of rights documents, position statements on ethical issues from professional societies, standards of care, chaplain services or pastoral care departments, and risk-management departments. An ethics hot line can provide anonymity for individual employees with problems that cannot be taken directly to immediate supervisors. Perhaps the most important resource for managing ethical dilemmas is the institutional ethics committee.

The Role of Institutional Ethics Committees

The work of **ethics committees** lies in three areas: education (including education of the committee itself), policy and guideline recommendations, and case review.[16,17] Ethics committees are *not* established to serve as a second medical opinion, to assume decision making for the patient, or to function as a peer review or grievance committee.

The educational process for the committee members can include a short course in bioethics, reading materials, and attendance at workshops or seminars on ethical issues. Thereafter, education in ethical decision making for the institution, for individuals, and for the community can be provided.[18]

Some of these educational experiences will lead naturally to the second objective, which is policy making. The need for more effective communication and clearer definition of roles will dictate specific procedures and policies, reflecting the values of the institution.[19,20] The third function, case review, provides opportunities for persons representing a range of professional and patient perspectives to systematically analyze cases and clarify options for action. Nurses' perspectives on ethical issues should be well-represented on institutional ethics committees. Nurse leaders can encourage and identify well-prepared, articulate staff nurses to serve in this capacity. The nurse leader can help caregivers and families understand how the ethics committee referral process works and encourage them to utilize this system.[21]

▪ THE EMPLOYER-EMPLOYEE RELATIONSHIP

Employer-employee relationships are those that exist between the department of nursing (as represented by the vice president of nursing), nurse managers, and the professional nursing staff. Professional nurses should learn the philosophy and goals of the employing agency. A hospital's philosophy is a statement of beliefs that direct the goals and purposes for which the institution exists. It achieves its aim only when the beliefs are operationalized within each department. Knowledge of the philosophy of the hospital can be compared with personal values and ethics. If the hospital's philosophy and the nurse's values and ethics are congruent, then as ethical issues arise, the nurse can act with the assurance that personal values support institutional values, and vice versa. The individual nurse then has the right and responsibility to "live out" the ethical philosophy and goals of the institution as well as practice somewhat autonomously in relation to position and responsibilities.

Because value judgments and ethics influence institutional policy formulation and implementation, the nurse leader keeps communication lines open with administrators, participates as fully as possible in decision making, and remains committed to identifying with and acting on the values of the organization.[22] This kind of loyal commitment to an institution presumes fairness or justice in employment relationships.

Two very specific fairness issues are job security and equitable treatment of employees. Job security necessitates a contract with four requirements: (1) full knowledge by both parties of the nature of the agreement, (2) no intentional misrepresentation of facts by either party, (3) no enforced entrance into the contract with duress or coercion, and (4) no contract binding the parties to an immoral act. Equitable treatment of employees involves respecting the employees' rights to due process and fair dealings and to achievement of personal growth, fulfillment, human dignity, and emotional health.[23]

One way in which organizations express commitment to the values of justice and fairness is through affirmative action programs. **Affirmative action,** a new ethic currently written into many federal and state statutes, provides for employment and promotion opportunities for qualified persons in proportion to the existence of representative ethnic groups in the geographic area. A similar policy applies to employment by sex. Considerable controversy surrounds affirmative action laws and programs, particularly in regard to whether or not such programs are fair for all parties involved. Currently, however, with few exceptions, affirmative action guidelines must be followed when hiring and promoting personnel. The nurse manager must be aware of such policies and work closely with the human resource or other appropriate institutional departments to assure that policies are closely followed.

Sexual harassment policies are another approach to upholding principles of justice and fairness in the workplace. Sexual harassment is morally and legally objectionable; it infringes on human rights and interferes with an individual's privacy and autonomy. Employers have a responsibility to maintain a harassment-free workplace.[24] Nurse leaders can take the lead in formulating sexual harassment policies and educating everyone in the workplace about sexual harassment.

As an employed professional the nurse is in a somewhat unique position. All employees hold a certain amount of loyalty to the institution for which they work. This loyalty stems in part from the fact that, when hired, employees make a commitment to accept and support the philosophy and mission of the institution. Employee loyalty also relates to the more practical fact that supporting the goals of the institution helps to insure the employee's paycheck. However, nurses as professionals also have a loyalty to the patients they have promised to serve. Likewise, nurses hold a certain loyalty to other health professionals, such as nursing peers and physicians. While nurses' roles have become increasingly autonomous, assisting the physician is still an important nursing role. Sometimes nurses find themselves in situations in which these loyalties to employer, patients, and other professionals are in conflict. For example, a nurse may be aware of an incident of possible medical negligence. Loyalty to the patient seems to dictate that the nurse take the necessary steps to inform the patient and/or report the situation through appropriate administrative channels. However, loyalty to the institution and to a physician as a colleague may influence the nurse to remain quiet about the incident. These situations are very difficult for nurses to resolve and can create considerable suffering for the nurse. If the nurse acts out of loyalty to the patient and chooses to report the incident, the nurse may be taking on a role of whistle-blower.

Whistle-blowing is defined as a cry against wrongdoing, a call for correction of an injustice, abuse, or neglect.[25] All possible attempts to solve patient care deficiencies through open communication and confrontation with individuals involved should be exhausted before a nurse goes "outside the unit" to call for correction. While blowing the whistle may be the ethically right action, such action places the nurse in a vulnerable position.[26,27] Whistle-blowers may be fired, demoted, harassed, or shunned.[28] The key to success, in terms of how effective the complaint will be in rectifying the problem, lies in the manner in which the complaint is made.[29] The nurse in a whistle-blowing situation needs to carefully follow the administrative chain of command and thoroughly document all aspects of the situation, keeping personal copies of all documentation.[30] In some states, whistle-blowers are protected by law. In many instances of abuse, neglect or incompetence, professional codes or legislation require the reporting of such injustice. Nurse leaders should know the state laws regarding the reporting of abuse.

■ PEER RELATIONSHIPS

Peer relationships are defined as those that exist between head nurses as colleagues and between staff nurses as colleagues. The informal nurse leader may be either a head nurse or a staff nurse. As a consequence of personal characteristics or knowledge, a staff nurse may be recognized as a leader but not assume a position of authority in the organization.

Mutual respect, collegiality, and cooperative and productive interdependency are essential for effective relationships between nurses and physicians and are equally necessary for healthy and positive relationships with peers.[31] Such working relationships facilitate discussion of the ethical issues that arise from an increasingly complex and technological health care environment. Nurses' daily encounters with critical illness and death, angry and grieving families, and conflicting demands within the workplace can very quickly lead to feelings of burnout. In fact, the burnout phenomenon has been attributed to confronting ethical dilemmas without an arena in which to work through these dilemmas in a reasoned way.[32] Providing opportunities for nurses to ventilate their feelings about difficult patient care situations or their frustrations about heavy workloads, fears of litigation or ethical dilemmas may prevent the burnout so prevalent among nurses in today's acute care settings. However, once this ventilation of feelings has taken place, the role of the nurse leader is to help staff members move beyond the focus on emotions and develop productive problem-solving strategies. In the case of ethical dilemmas, one productive strategy is to seek consultation with the institutional ethics committee.

Unfortunately, a common dilemma that nurses face is the unprofessional or unethical conduct of peers. Since the Code for Nurses includes a commitment to safeguarding the client and public from incompetent, unethical or illegal practice of any person, awareness of any such activity on the part of peers requires some type of action. Policies are established to guide employee behavior. Blatant disregard for policy requires intervention from the nurse leader. Psychologists have attributed employees' dishonesty to emotional exhaustion and depression but such persons are not justified in stealing materials or drugs, damaging property, malingering or wasting time, cheating on time cards, or extending breaks or meal periods.[33] Abusing drugs, falsifying patient records, or acting in ways that compromise patient safety are other examples of unethical or illegal conduct that nurses cannot condone in their peers. A nurse leader as peer could point out these unethical behaviors by approaching the offending party and respectfully confronting him or her with genuineness, honesty, and understanding. Skillful communication of the consequences of such dishonest behavior for the offender as well as for peers and institutions is a mark of professionalism. If resolution of the problem does not result from one-to-one confrontation, the nurse leader should carefully follow the chain of command in reporting the offending behavior.

If a nurse suspects that a peer may have a substance abuse problem, the appropriate response involves carefully following institutional policies to assure patient safety and to get the individual into rehabilitation. Most state nurses' associations have a Peer Assistance Program to help and support nurses who depend on alcohol or mood-altering drugs.[34,35] Impairment due to alcohol and substance abuse creates huge financial, professional, and personal costs.[36] By knowing the policies and procedures of the employing agency as well as the state laws on reporting of substance abuse, and utilizing programs such as peer assistance programs or employee assistance programs that offer counseling for impaired individuals, nurse leaders can help to reduce those costs.

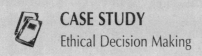

CASE STUDY
Ethical Decision Making

Mary Kay O'Connor has been working in the intensive care unit (ICU) for over six months. Mary Kay loves her work and finds the staff approachable and competent.

One evening, Mary Kay noted that the narcotic count was off. Mary Kay tried to find out what had happened to the missing narcotic. She reviewed the charts and patient requirements and could not locate the missing morphine. She reviewed the hospital policy for such a problem, called the evening supervisor, and filled out the appropriate forms.

Mary Kay did not give the matter another thought. She assumed it was an oversight, and she was happy to learn how to handle such situations for the future.

A month later, the same thing happened, and Mary Kay was working with the same staff personnel. Mary Kay observed the staff and suspected that one of the new registered nurses might have a drug problem.

- What should she do?
- What are the pros and cons for any action she may take?

■ THE NURSE-PATIENT RELATIONSHIP

The nurse-patient relationship is the foundation for all professional nursing activity. The nurse's obligation to the patient has always been a part of the professional code, but it has assumed increasing emphasis over the years. The first official code for nurses, published in 1950, emphasized nurse's primary obligation to the physician. In later versions, the emphasis shifted to loyalty to the employing institution. Starting with the 1976 edition of the Code for Nurses, all 11 principles of the code emphasized the primacy of duties to patients.[37]

In general, nurses' obligations to patients as outlined in the Code involve putting the patient's interests before one's own, respecting the patient's right to exercise personal autonomy by taking part in decision making, respecting the dignity and privacy of patients, maintaining professional competence, and engaging in activities that establish and maintain quality patient care. The Code for Nurses serves as a public statement of nursings' commitment to individual patients and to society at large. It serves as a social contract between nurses and their clients. When new nurses enter the profession, they are making a type of public commitment to uphold the obligations outlined in the Code.[38] Nurses also have certain obligations to the institution that sometimes may seem to be in conflict with promises or loyalties to patients. For example, in the current environment of cost cutting, the nurse leader may be pressured to reduce nursing staff beyond what the nurse leader believes is adequate for good patient care: loyalty and appreciation for the needs of the institution conflict with the nurse's professional promise to provide high-quality care to patients. The leader's responsibility is to clearly document and communicate patient care needs and advocate with administration so that care is not compromised.

Many situations arise in which the nurse leader must advocate to protect patient autonomy. Providing for patient involvement in decision making means taking the time to assure that patients fully understand any consent forms they are signing. It means respecting and facilitating the use of advance directives or helping patients who wish to complete these documents. Respect for autonomy involves respecting the patient's right to refuse treatments, even if nurses, physicians, or families disagree with the competent patient's decision. Nurses in leadership roles often find themselves "caught in the middle" between patients and families and physicians. While this may seem an uncomfortable position to be in, nurses are perhaps the best people for such a role. Nurses should feel confident that their strong communication skills, rapport with patients and families, and good working relationships with physicians are just the skills needed to foster the dialogue needed in these situations.

Referring to specific ethical guidelines can be helpful to the nurse leader in her relationships with patients, families, and other health care professionals. "A Patient's Bill of Rights" (see page 114) and "The Patient's Choice of Treatment Options" are published by the American Hospital Association.[39] Similar Bill of Rights documents are available for nursing home and home care patients. The ANA publishes the "Code for Nurses with Interpretive Statements" and "Ethics in Nursing: Position Statements and Guidelines."[40] The Hastings Center has produced "Guidelines on the Termination of Life-Sustaining Treatment and the Care of the Dying."[41] Addresses for each of these organizations can be found in the end-of-chapter references.

Patients Bill of Rights
A Patient's Bill of Rights
American Hospital Association
1973

On 6 February 1973 the American Hospital Association's House of Delegates approved A Patient's Bill of Rights. Other historically significant documents in the United States, which predated this Bill of Rights, were a document drafted by the National Welfare Rights Organization (1970) and the preamble to the Standards of the Joint Commission on Accreditation of Hospitals. The AHA Patient's Bill of Rights, printed in full below, has been influential in the development of similar documents in other parts of the world.

The American Hospital Association presents a patient's Bill of Rights with the expectation that observance of these rights will contribute to more effective patient care and greater satisfaction for the patient, his physician and the hospital organization. Further, the Association presents these rights in the expectation that they will be supported by the hospital on behalf of its patients, as an integral part of the healing process. It is recognized that a personal relationship between the physician and the patient is essential for the provision of proper medical care. The traditional physician-patient relationship takes on a new dimension when care is rendered within an organizational structure. Legal precedent has established that the institution itself also has a responsibility to the patient. It is in recognition of these factors that these rights are affirmed.

1. The patient has the right to considerate and respectful care.
2. The patient has the right to obtain from his physician complete current information concerning his diagnosis, treatment, and prognosis in terms the patient can be reasonably expected to understand. When it is not medically advisable to give such information to the patient, the information should be made available to an appropriate person in his behalf. He has the right to know by name, the physician responsible for coordinating his care.
3. The patient has the right to receive from his physician information necessary to give informed consent prior to the start of any procedure and/or treatment. Except in emergencies, such information for informed consent, should include but not necessarily be limited to the specific procedure and/or treatment the medically significant risks involved, and the probable

duration of incapacitation. Where medically significant alternatives for care or treatment exist, or when the patient requests information concerning medical alternatives, the patient has the right to such information. The patient also has the right to know the name of the person responsible for the procedures and/or treatment.

4. The patient has the right to refuse treatment to the extent permitted by law, and to be informed of the medical consequences of his action.

5. The patient has the right to every consideration of his privacy concerning his own medical care program. Case discussion, consultation, examination, and treatment are confidential and should be conducted discreetly. Those not directly involved in his care must have the permission of the patient to be present.

6. The patient has the right to expect that all communication and records pertaining to his care should be treated as confidential.

7. The patient has the right to expect that within its capacity a hospital must make reasonable response to the request of a patient for services. The hospital must provide evaluation, service, and/or referral as indicated by the urgency of the case. When medically permissible a patient may be transferred to another facility only after he has received complete information and explanation concerning the needs for and alternatives to such a transfer. The institution to which the patient is to be transferred must first have accepted the patient for transfer.

8. The patient has the right to be advised if the Hospital proposes to engage in or perform human experimentation affecting his care or treatment. The patient has the right to refuse to participate in such research projects.

9. The patient has the right to expect reasonable continuity of care. He has the right to know in advance what appointment times and physicians are available and where. The patient has the right to expect that the hospital will provide a mechanism whereby he is informed by his physician or a delegate of the physician of the patient's continuing health care requirements following discharge.

10. The patient has the right to examine and receive an explanation of his bill regardless of source of payment.

11. The patient has the right to know what hospital rules and regulations apply to his conduct as a patient.

No catalogue of rights can guarantee for the patient the kind of treatment he has a right to expect. A hospital has many functions to perform, including the prevention and treatment of disease, the education of both health professionals and patients, and the conduct of clinical research. All these activities must be conducted with an overriding concern for the patient, and, above all, the recognition of his dignity as a human being. Success is achieving this recognition of his dignity as a human being. Success in achieving this recognition assures success in the defense of the rights of the patient.

■ SUMMARY

This chapter focuses on the multiple and complex ethical issues that face nurses and nurse leaders/managers. It defines the terms *ethics* and *morality*. Values are considered as they affect the nurse personally and professionally.

Two ethical theories, deontology and consequentialism, are contrasted in terms of how they guide thinking and acting in ethical dilemmas. The basic principles derived from these classical theories—autonomy, beneficence, nonmaleficence, and justice—are described and related to the Code for Nurses. Some barriers to the ethical decision-making process are examined and strategies for enhancing good ethical decision making in health care settings are offered.

Specific situations creating ethical dilemmas are explored in the relationship of employer to employee, peer relationships, and the nurse-patient relationship. Examples are included that apply ethics principles as they coincide with the tenets of the Code for Nurses.

To conclude this chapter, student exercises provide opportunities to apply the content to selected ethical dilemmas. A reference list includes up-to-date resources as well as addresses of organizations and associations offering professional and ethical literature.

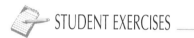 STUDENT EXERCISES

1. A newly admitted patient continues to ask why she was hospitalized. Her primary nurse wants to tell her that her diagnosis is cancer of the lung. The patient's family insists that the diagnosis be kept from her. Indicate the ethical theories or principles that provide direction for the nurse and for the family. How would you solve this ethical dilemma?

2. A fragile man in his eighties has many sensory and motor deficits from a cerebrovascular accident. When his heart stops, he is resuscitated, and he awakens to find himself hooked up to tubes and machines. He begs to be allowed to die but is repeatedly resuscitated. What ethical principle is being violated in this situation? As his nurse, what steps would you take to be his advocate?

3. One of your coworkers refuses to care for suicide patients in the intensive care, saying, "They wanted to die, so let them." As a peer, how could you appeal to this nurse's moral sense? What principles of ethics are in jeopardy?

4. It is not the practice in your institution to issue contracts to nursing service personnel. How would you, as a nurse leader, initiate a change in this practice? Describe how you would use ethical principles in your arguments in favor of contractual agreements.

5. You discover that one of your colleagues is stealing insulin syringes to take to her diabetic grandmother who cannot afford to buy such disposables. List the steps you would take in confronting her and the ethical principles that would guide you. Role play this confrontation with one of your classmates.

6. A young couple, who has a newborn with multiple anomalies and deformities decides against any extraordinary treatment. Using a debate format with another classmate, address these issues: (1) use of differing ethical principles, (2) arguments to support the parents' decision, (3) arguments opposing the parents' decision, (4) allocation of health care resources, and (5) role of the ethics committee.

7. You suspect that one of your staff nurses is stealing patients' drugs for personal use. Her suspicious behavior has also been called to your attention by some of her coworkers. What ethical principles are being violated by the staff nurse stealing drugs? If these drugs are narcotics, what responsibility do you have Toward the patient? Toward the nurse?

▓ REFERENCES

1. Flaherty MJ, "Ethical Decision Making in an Interdisciplinary Setting," In Sward K, (editor), *Ethics in Nursing Practice and Education*, Kansas City, MO: American Nurses' Association, 1980, p. 3.
2. Fowler M, Levine-Ariff H, "Ethics at the Bedside: A Source Book for the Critical Care Nurse," St. Louis: J.B. Lippincott, 1987.
3. Barnett CW, Pierson DA, "Advance Directives: Implementing a Program That Works," *Nursing Management*, 25:10, 1994, p. 58–65.
4. Fowler M, Levine-Ariff H.
5. Erlen JA, "The Code for Nurses: Guidelines for Ethical Practice," *Orthopaedic Nursing*, 12:6 1993, p.31–33, 46.
6. Schank M, Weis D, "A Study of Values of Baccalaureate Nursing Students and Graduate Nurses from a Secular and a Nonsecular Program," *J Profess Nurs*, 5:1 1989, p. 17–22.
7. Ibid.
8. Fowler M, Levine-Ariff H.

9. Beauchamp T, Childress J, *Principles of Biomedical Ethics*, 2nd ed., New York: Oxford University Press, 1989, p. 36.

10. Ibid.

11. Ibid.

12. President's Commission for the Study of Ethical Problems in Medicine and Biomedical and Behavioral Research, *Deciding to Forgo Life Sustaining Treatment*, New York: Concern for Dying, (1983).

13. Fiesta J, "Refusal of Treatment," *Nursing Management*, 23:11, 1992, p. 14, 16, 18.

14. American Nurses Association, *Code for Nurses with Interpretive Statements*, Kansas City, MO: American Nurses Association, 1985.

15. Ibid.

16. Agich GJ, Younger SJ, "For Experts Only? Access to Hospital Ethics Committees", *Hastings Center Report*, 21:5, 1991, p. 17–25.

17. Dalgo JT, Anderson F, "Notes from the Field: Developing a Hospital Ethics Committee," *Nursing Management*, 26:9, 1995, p. 104–106.

18. Nelson RM, Shapiro RS, "The Role of an Ethics Committee in Resolving Conflict in the Neonatal Intensive Care Unit," *Journal of Law, Medicine and Ethics*, 23:1, 1995, p. 27–32.

19. Agich GJ, Younger SJ.

20. Dalgo JT, Anderson F.

21. Nelson RM, Shapiro RS.

22. McCoy C, *Management of Values: The Ethical Difference in Corporate Policy and Performance*, Boston: Pitman Publishing, 1985, p. 186–191.

23. Drake B, Drake E, "Ethical and Legal Aspects of Managing Corporate Cultures," *California Management Review*, 30:2, 1988, p. 107–123.

24. American Nurses Association, *Sexual Harassment: It's Against the Law*, Washington, DC: American Nurses Association, 1993.

25. Bandman E, "Whistle-blowers Take Risk To Halt Wrongdoing," In Murphy C, (editor), *Ethical Dilemmas Confronting Nurses*, Kansas City, MO: American Nurses Association, 1985, p. 18.

26. Regan WA, "Nurses' Complaints: 'Going Public' Is Risky," *Regan Report on Nursing Law*, 24:4, 1983, p. 1.

27. Sheehan J, "Advice of Counsel: Putting Advocacy for Patients Against Job Security," *RN*, 59:1, 1996, p. 55–56.

28. Tammelleo AD, "Refusal to "Cover Up" Death: Whistleblower Is Terminated," *Regan Report on Hospital Law*, 36:3, 1995, p. 2.

29. Regan WA.

30. Dimotto J, "Whistle-blowing: Seven Tips for Reporting Unsafe Conduct," *Nursing Quality Connection*, 4:4, 1995, p. 8, 12.

31. Rotkavitch R, "The Power of the Nurse Executive." In Henry B, Arndt C, DiViscenti M, Marriner A (editors), *Dimensions of Nursing Administration*, Boston: Blackwell Scientific, 1989, p. 21.

32. Davis A, "Ethical Decision Making: Considerations for Future Activities," In Sward K, (editor), *Ethic in Nursing Practice and Education*. Kansas City, MO: American Nurses Association, 1980, p. 21.

33. Rosenthal T, "White Uniform Theft," *Nurs Manage*, 18:4, 1987, p. 89–90.
34. Soalri-Twadall A, "Peer Assistance: One Person's Experience," *Addictions Nursing Network*, 2:3, 1990, p. 17–18.
35. New York State Nurses Association, "Obligations and Rights of Nurses Whose Practice Is Impaired by Addictive Diseases: NYSNA's Peer Assistance for Nurses (SPAN) Program," *Journal of the New York State Nurses Association*, 26:2, 1995, p. 14.
36. LaGodna GE, Hendrix MJ, "Impaired Nurses: A Cost Analysis," *Journal of Nursing Administration*, 19:9, 1989, p. 13–18.
37. Carroll MA, Humphrey RA, "The Nurses' Professional Code of Ethics: Its History and Improvements." *In Moral Problems in Nursing: Case Studies*, New York: University Press of America, 1979.
38. Quinn C, Smith M, *The Professional Commitment: Issues and Ethics in Nursing*, Philadelphia: Saunders, 1987, p. 180.
39. American Hospital Association, 840 North Shore Drive, Chicago, IL 60611.
40. American Nurses Association, 600 Maryland Avenue, S.W., Suite 100 West, Washington, D.C. 20024-2571.
41. Hastings Center, 255 Elm Road, Briarcliff Manor, New York, NY 10510.

■ SUGGESTED READINGS

American Nurses' Association Commission on Nursing Research, *Human Rights Guidelines for Nurses in Clinical and Other Research*, Kansas City, MO: American Nurses' Association, 1985.

American Nurses' Association Committee on Ethics, *Ethical Dilemmas Confronting Nurses*, Kansas City, MO: American Nurses' Association, 1985.

American Nurses' Association Committee on Ethics, *Ethics in Nursing Position Statements and Guidelines*, Kansas City, MO: American Nurses' Association, 1988.

American Nurses' Association Committee on Ethics, *Ethics in Nursing Practice and Education*, Kansas City, MO: American Nurses' Association, 1980.

Aroskar M, "Ethics Important in Allocating Health Care Resources." In Murphy C, (editor), *Ethical Dilemmas Confronting Nurses*, Kansas City, MO: American Nurses' Association, 1985.

Benjamin M, Curtis J, *Ethics in Nursing*, 3rd ed, New York: Oxford University Press, 1992.

Canon BL, Brown JS, "Nurses' Attitudes toward Impaired Colleagues, *Image*, 20:2, 1988, p. 96–101.

Cooper M, "Gilligan s Different Voice: A Perspective for Nursing," *J Profess Nurs*, 5:1, 1989, p. 10–16.

Davidhizer R, "Confronting Employees," *AORN J*. 48:2, 1988, p. 319–322.

"Ethical Decisions Via Rounds and Consults," *Hospital Ethics*, 2:5, 1986, p. 14–15.

Davino M, "Advice of Counsel: When the Nurse with an Addiction is Your Boss," *RN*, 58:8, 1995, p. 55.

Davis AJ, "Helping Your Staff Address Ethical Dilemmas: Formats for Ethics Rounds," *Journal of Nursing Administration*, vol. 12, 1982, p. 9–13.

Fowler M, "Acquired Immunodeficiency Syndrome and Refusal to Provide Care," *Heart and Lung*, 17:2, 1988, p. 213–215.

Gilligan C, *In a Different Voice*, Cambridge, MA: Harvard University Press, 1982.

Krekeler K, "Critical Care Nursing and Moral Development," *Crit Care Nurs Q.* 10:2, 1987, p. 1–10.

Mitchell L, "Resources for Ethical Decision Making," *Journal of Cardiovascular Nursing*, 9:3, 1995, p. 78–87.

Oddi LF, Cassidy VR, "Participation and Perception of Nurse Members in the Hospital Ethics Committee," *Western Journal of Nursing Research*, 12:3, 1990, p. 307–17.

Raines C, "Personal Value Systems: How They Affect Teamwork," *AORN J.* 48:2, 1988, p. 324–330.

Silva MC, "The Ethics of Whistle Blowing by Nurses," *Nursing Connections*, 5:3, 1992, p. 17–21.

Weeks L, Gleason V, Reiser S, "How Can a Hospital Ethics Committee Help?" *Am J Nurs*, 89:5, 1989, p. 651–654.

Windle PE, Wintersgill CL, "The Chemically Impaired Nurse's Reentry to Practice: The Nurse Manager's Role," *AORN Journal*, 59:6, 1994, p. 1268–1269.

UNIT 2

An Overview of Organizations and Management

6

Organization and Management Theory

Introduction

Today's health care organizations are undergoing enormous change. As managed care and integrated health systems assume increasing dominance, health care organizations are forming different structures, serving new functions, and are considered as independent cost centers. The hospital is no longer dominant in the delivery of health care. Instead, the focal point of the new system is primary care. Despite the reorganization of health care institutions, nurse leaders/managers are expected to coordinate levels of employees and facilitate services for patients. How a complicated web of people function together to meet an organization's goal can be explained by a set of complex concepts known as organization theory. The objective of this chapter is to discuss the organization and management theories that have shaped the current understanding of modern health care organizations.

KEY CONCEPTS

Organization is a social system composed of individuals playing interdependent parts to meet a common goal.

Social System represents groups of interdependent individuals in social relationships with standards and behaviors for the group to meet a common goal.

Structure is the internal differentiation and patterning of relationships; the bony skeleton of an organization.

Organizational Chart is a graphic depiction of an organizational structure.

Power is the possession of control, authority, or influence over others.

Unity of Command is whatever action or orders that come from one command superior only.

Unity of Direction refers to one head, one plan; focus in same direction.

Division of Work is the specialization of effort to produce more and integrated work output.

Span of Control refers to how many and what levels of personnel are needed to achieve objectives; the number of subordinates managers manage.

Organizing is the establishment of a formal structure of authority through which work subdivisions are arranged, defined, and coordinated for the achievement of defined objectives.

Cost Centers are locales of service to which a fixed or preset fee is allocated.

Contingency Design is the process of determining the degree of environmental uncertainty and adapting the organization and its subunits to the situation.

Organizational Learning is a view of the organization as a living and thinking open system capable of changing based on interpretation of environmental stimuli.

Chaos Theory is a way of finding order among random events by identifying trends through mathematical analysis.

■ OVERVIEW: ORGANIZATIONAL DYNAMICS

Organizations exist in everyday life as necessary social units. For example, families, churches, and governments are forms of organizations, as well as the industries that provide employment. An **organization** is defined as a social system deliberately established to carry out some definite purpose. This purpose, or goal, is carried out efficiently and effectively using both human and nonhuman resources.[1] Most management authorities view organizations in this context while emphasizing the pattern of structured relationships, which go well beyond interpersonal and extend to interdepartmental groups. People function routinely within organizational structures, and while their behavior is orchestrated, it is often counterproductive to organizational goals. Management then becomes a necessary activity to insure that organizational goals are met. The task of management is to direct the work force and available resources within the existing structure. The task of leadership is to provide insights and inspiration to accomplish the work with enthusiasm. Leadership of and by itself is a part of management; however, it is not total management. A good leader can be a weak manager because although the strong leader gets others to follow, there is no indication that the groups are being led in the proper direction. A manager is required to plan a course of action to reach a goal, wherein the leader's primary responsibility is to challenge the group to follow. Organizational dynamics are those activities that comprise this coordinated social behavior to meet formal goals. It is in this sense that organizational dynamics interact with management and leadership processes. For example, a head nurse is confronted with the task of reorganizing a department as it merges with another nursing unit. The leader understands that the staff must be led during a period of change and disorganization while managing the day-to-day operations. Knowledge from organization and management theory will help the head nurse to be as effective as possible under trying circumstances.

■ CLASSICAL THEORY

When people group together and perform different but interdependent work to meet a common objective, this is organized human behavior. The elements of this process are differentiation of labor, a hierarchical structure, and coordination of effort. Interest in the study of organizations began in the early years of the twentieth century at the time of the Industrial Revolution when these changes fueled the growth of industries. Classical organization theory, a set of traditions, beliefs, principles, and techniques, is the earliest scholarly work that studied organized behavior in industry. Classical theory is conveniently divided into three categories: *scientific management, administrative management,* and *the bureaucratic model.* All have contributed to an understanding of organizations by identifying the organization's essential elements, including a common purpose for the organization and its subdivisions; division of labor, or the use of interdependent skills and responsibilities; and a hierarchy that determines privileges, power, and authority. This discussion will limit the study of organization theory to it's relationship with the management process.

Scientific Management

The founder of the scientific management movement was Frederick W. Taylor (1856–1915), who was an engineer and management expert. Taylor proposed a set of techniques that greatly enhanced the efficiency of the manufacturing organization. He developed techniques for systematic job study, time studies, and wage incentives, as well as standardizing methods for different types of industrial work. Scientific management focused on the organization from the manager's perspective and contributed to a more efficient organization.[2]

Administrative Management

Administrative management, another aspect of classical theory, also looked at the organization from the perspective of the administration and management, or from the top down. The primary leaders were Henri Fayol, a French industrialist;[3] Luther Gullick, an academician and public administration specialist; Lyndall Urwick, a British consultant; and James D. Mooney and Alan C. Reiley, General Motors executives. Fayol's set of universal principles of organization and management are the most commonly reported in the literature; however, all contributed to administrative management's body of knowledge. Between scientific management and administrative management, a group of principles was offered. Each theorist expressed his set of principles differently, but the following represent a synthesis of the main propositions and principles of an organization. These same principles have been criticized as being intellectual inventions and not the result of empiric work; however, much of what was devised has not been replaced in the modern organization.

Organizational Principles. The following is a synthesis of organizational principles:

- Communication
- Unity of command
- Span of control
- Delegation of authority

- Similar assignments
- Unity of purpose

1. Communication

Since a manager has to communicate with so many different persons, communication is a large part of his or her responsibility. In fact, communication consumes about half of each supervisor's work day. Therefore, the need for effective communication is paramount. To ensure effective communication, follow these guidelines:

- The nature of each position, its duties, authority, responsibilities, and relationships with other positions should be clearly defined in writing and available to all concerned.
- A clear line of authority should exist from the supreme authority to every individual in the group.
- Channels of command should not be violated by staff units. A subordinate should never be criticized in the presence of executives or employees of equal or lower rank.
- The interest of those under you should be promoted when reporting to those over you.
- Adequate reports must be made, and adequate records must be kept.

2. Unity of Command

When managerial duties overlap, there exists dual command, which confuses workers. The opposite is **unity of command,** wherein workers are responsible for a single area of responsibility and for reporting to one supervisor immediately above the employee (**unity of direction**). To achieve unity of command, observe the following general rules:

- In any organization, provision is made for centralization of authority and responsibility to the chief executive.
- No person occupying a single position in an organization should be subject to definite orders from more than one source.
- You should know to whom you report and who reports to you.

3. Span of Control

There are many factors that need to be taken into consideration when determining the number of employees that one supervisor can effectively and efficiently manage. Some of these are the level of managerial experience of the manager, the skill level of the employees, the stability of the work unit or department, the volume of work within the unit or department, the level of morale among the employees, and, lastly, the type of work managed. To determine **span of control,** keep the following guidelines in mind:

- There is a limit to the number of subordinates that a supervisor can effectively inspire, animate, direct, and coordinate.
- The supervisor should be responsible for the actions of subordinates.
- Too few immediate subordinates will result in oversupervision: too many will result in undersupervision.

4. Delegation of Authority

Delegation refers to the designated work within each position. Some amount of participation is an essential part of management. Therefore, responsibility and authority should correspond in every position, as follows:

- Accomplishment of responsibilities should be limited to only a few delegations after it reaches the operating level.
- All personnel and activities must be systematically arranged so that authority and responsibility for specific, well-defined duties can be delegated.
- Orders should never be given to subordinates over the head of a responsible superior.
- No change should be made in the scope of responsibility of a position without a definite understanding of the effects on all persons concerned.
- There must be no overlapping of authority (two or more supervisors having control of the same function).

5. Similar Assignments

The responsibilities assigned to a particular unit of an organization are specifically clear-cut and understood, as follows below:

- A function should not be assigned to more than one independent unit of the organization. Overlapping responsibility will cause confusion and delay.
- Definite and clear-cut responsibilities should be assigned to each member of the organization.
- An organization should never be permitted to grow so elaborate as to hinder work assignment.
- Every necessary function of an organization must be assigned specifically to an individual.

6. Unity of Purpose

Definite plans must be formulated that are based upon the objectives, policies, standards, and work procedures previously accepted by the organization.

- Every component should work toward unity of effort.
- Authority and responsibility for action are decentralized to the units and individuals responsible for the actual performance of operations.

7. General Rules

- An adequate number of qualified personnel (staffing) is necessary to carry out the plans and to achieve the aims of the organization. Maximum results must be obtained with a minimum of time, effort, supplies, and equipment.
- Consistent methods of organizational structure should be applied at each level of the organization.

To a great extent, the modern organization continues to implement many of the aforementioned principles because they allow work to be done efficiently. We will see, however, that because people and goals are very complex, some of these rules have been modified for today's health care agencies.

Barnard, an influential thinker, contributed to administrative management through a discussion of authority and its exercise in the organization.[4] Barnard proposed authority to be the right of the superior and maintained that authority is only effective when it is accepted and communicated within the subordinant's "zone of indifference," or willingness to comply. Barnard's work paved the way for the consideration of interactional phenomena, which is the hallmark of the modern behavioral school.

The Bureaucratic Model

The last component of classical theory is known as the bureaucratic model, which describes a particular type of structure. The prominent contributor to this theory, as well as the individual who coined the name, was a German sociologist by the name of Weber, who described the characteristics of a bureaucracy that he felt was the most efficient form of structure for complex organizations.[5] This type of organizational structure is known for the use of extensive rules and procedures to govern the work of the employees. Positions of the employees are arranged in a hierarchy with a given amount of authority and responsibility for each incumbent; positions are defined through job descriptions. To be promoted to a higher level, the employee must demonstrate a level of performance prescribed by an objective criteria. According to Weber, a bureaucracy is a rational structure in which to organize people and tasks, and it demands adherence to principles.

The bureaucratic structure exerts a constant pressure upon its members to be methodologic and disciplined to attain a high degree of reliability of behavior and conformity to patterns of action. If the bureaucracy is to function appropriately, discipline is necessary. Herein lies the basic criticism toward this structure. The emphasis is on the task as opposed to the individual. Other structures for the modern organization have evolved to deal with the deficiencies of the bureaucratic structure while trying to retain its stability and unified focus on objectives.

Contribution of Classical Theory

Classical theory provided major ideas for future theorists to consider. These ideas may be summarized to include the treatment of authority, management functions, principles of management, organizational structure, and emphasis on objectives. Classical theory enhanced understanding of efficient organizations.

■ MODERN THEORY

Modern organizational theory represented a new way of viewing people in organizations. The emphasis was on the individuals rather than concentrating on the work or the organizational structure. Modern theory is so designated because of its contribution to organizational theory rather than its chronology. In fact, modern theory has as its origin the late 1920s and continues through today. It is also referred to as behavioral, or humanistic, theory. To understand the rise of this thought, a review of the sociopolitical background is necessary. From the late 1800s to 1920, there was a rapid growth of American industry. This growth, however, was accompanied by poor working conditions, low wages, cheap immigrant labor, high profits for the owners, and the Great Depression.[6] Public sentiment moved from pro-management to pro-labor, and Congress passed the Wagner Act of 1935, which allowed for the formation of labor unions.[7] Thus, the threat of unionization, the Hawthorne Studies, and a philosophy of industrial management were the forces that focused interest on the worker.

Behavioral Science

The contributors to the behavioral school were psychologists and sociologists who studied the workings of private industry. From 1927 to 1932, Mayo and his colleagues at the Hawthorne Works of the Western Electric Company in Chicago ushered in the beginning of the behavioral school. The Hawthorne Studies were the result of Mayo's work. These studies indicated that a group can exert a powerful influence on an individual's productivity. In fact, the ability of the group to influence individuals has come to be known as the Hawthorne effect. In addition, these studies investigated group pressure, social relationships, and supervisory attitudes.[8]

Other leaders in the field who are closely associated with management theory and who made worthy contributions include Douglas McGregor, Renis Likert, Frederick Herzberg, Warren Bennis, and Chris Argyris. More recently, Thomas J. Peters, Robert H. Waterman, Jr., and Stephen Covy have provided insights into personal and organizational success. Each of their specific contributions are discussed under appropriate sections of management topics. This group, with different and interesting insights for modern organizations and management theory, shared a common, optimistic view of the worker in the workplace. They believed that the individual had the potential to be self-directed and capable of enhancing productivity. This was an important and positive perspective and stimulated the next step of the modern view, which integrates the worker and the work through systems theory.

General Systems/Social Systems Theory

The social nature of organizations allows the individual to have patterned relationships and to play a specific part in the overall mission of the organization. Social systems theory is a convenient and insightful way to understand the modern organization and how people accomplish the organization's goals. The difference in systems theory and the aforementioned perspectives is that systems theory discusses the organization and worker as a whole rather than as separate entities. A system is defined as an organized combination of united parts or events forming a complex or unitary whole that is coordinated to accomplish a set of goals.[9] This general view of a system provides the necessary overview from which a narrower definition of a social system may be derived. A social system consists of the patterned activities of people that are complementary or interdependent with respect to some common output or outcome, are repeated, are relatively enduring, and are bounded in space and time. A social system is concerned with an individual's participation in society.[10]

When groups of people are thought about in terms of systems, the concept of a **social system** emerges. This participation may be viewed as groups of individuals joined together in a network of cooperative and conflicting social relationships to achieve common goals developed around a value

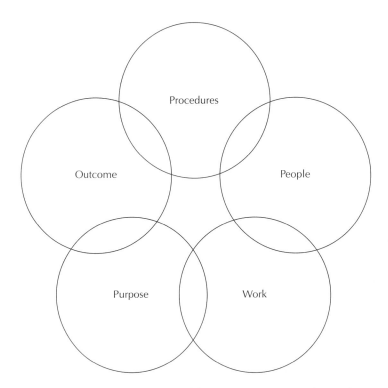

Figure 6-1. A graphic representation of the various components of a social system that are also interrelated.

system, using an organized set of practices and methods to regulate behavioral standards of the groups.[11] A group has specific patterns of associations and activity in which most persons share their abilities and talents on a day-to-day basis. This is also descriptive of modern organizational behavior. An organization is a social system that permits a structuring of events (or happenings) that have no structuring apart from their functioning. When this social system ceases to function (i.e., people stop working), there is no identifiable structure. It is a tendency to think of organizations as buildings or products; yet the essence of modern systems thinking recognizes that people are the functioning unit of an organization. Without the patterned behavior of the group, there is no social system and thus no organization (Fig. 6-1).

There are many who have contributed to our current understanding of social systems as an underlying explanatory theory to understand the modern organization. This discussion will focus on a few. Theorists such as Katz and Kahn and Tosi and Carroll break down the modern organization into subparts

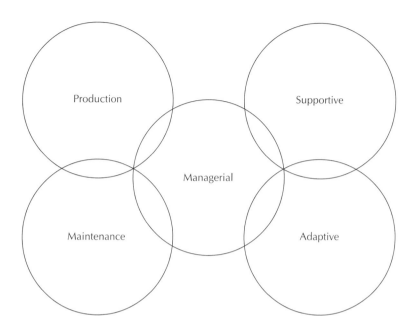

Figure 6-2. The various subsystems of an organization that are also interrelated.

that comprise a whole.[12,13] These subsystems exemplify both the real and behavioral components of the organization. This perspective combines human social behavior and the formal organization structure (Fig. 6-2).

The first conceptual subsystem is known as *Production,* or *Technologic,* and refers to those activities that are responsible for the end product of the organization, whether that be teaching in a school system, providing patient care in a hospital, or assembling an automobile in a factory. It identifies the major activity of any organization. This particular subsystem is commonly the most responsible for classifying an organization and directs the coordinated activity of the people involved to produce or to meet the goal of the organization.

The next subsystem is called *Supportive* by Katz and Kahn and *Boundary spanning* by Tosi and Carroll.[14] It involves environmental transaction, such as procuring input for production or disposing of the output. The departments that represent this subsystem are purchasing or marketing or the committee that deals with dangerous waste disposal. These activities involve interaction with the greater social system and acknowledge that the system or organization is open to the forces of change in the world outside.

Maintenance subsystems refer to the upkeep of the equipment or education of the personnel to make sure the work of the organization is properly executed. This might be continuing education or a staff development department. This subsystem keeps the organization functioning and up to date.

The next subsystem is the *Managerial*, which refers to the major activities of controlling, coordinating, and directing people, as well as the other subsystems of the organization. Every organization needs the activities of management for the completion of the work.

The last conceptual subsystem is known as the *Adaptive subsystem* and refers to those activities that ensure organizational survival in a changing environment. Nowhere is this more true right now than in health care. An example is an administration's attempt at strategic or long-range planning.

Modern Systems Theory Models

Because of the influence of the systems approach, two new variations of systems theory have evolved. The first, **organizational learning,** views the organization as a living and thinking open system.[15] Since open organizations depend on environmental input and feedback, organizations are said to learn from the interpretation of this input. Thus, organizations engage in complex processes such as anticipating, perceiving, envisioning, and problem solving. This parallels system theory from the perspective that learning is beyond an individual and includes all persons working together to process this new information for meaningful change. The other, **chaos theory,** also depends on environmental feedback.[16] Chaos theory attempts to find order among seemingly random events. The assumption is that behind every complex system is a set of rules, with its own orderliness and boundaries. The interaction and interconnectedness of the subsystems are the basis of prediction. While seemingly unrelated, all parts of the system are behaving appropriately to insure the survival of the total system. Two mathematicians, Edward Lorenz and James York have suggested that this order may be translated into mathematical principles, and the rules of probability.[17]

Social systems theory, and its variations adapted to the study of organizations, is a way to explain how organizations function through a dissection of the units of purposeful and necessary behavior. Yet to understand the practical nature of an organization, both classical and modern theory contribute to the following section of organizational concepts.

Interactional Phenomena

Organizations are so named because of the activity of organizing. **Organizing** is the establishment of a formal structure of authority through which work subdivisions are arranged, defined, and coordinated for the achievement of defined goals. This occurs through interactional phenomena, which emanate directly because of the hierarchical arrangement of interdependent people doing diverse activities. These special phenomenon include *power, authority, status*, as well as the *process of delegation*. Classical theory identified interactional phenomena but modern scholars have studied them. The following section will define the interactional concepts and consider modern contributions.

Power. **Power** is a force to meet goals and get things done. Powerful people are dominant, and as their power increases, they move upward in the group; conversely, as their power is lessened, they move downward. Power is commonly discussed through the five power bases identified by French and Raven: coercive power, reward power, legitimate power, expert power, and referent power.[18] Later, Raven and Kruglanski added a sixth power base, referred to as information power.[19] Hersey and Blanchard identified a seventh base known as connection power.[20] Since power is a transactional process to influence and requires the voluntary support of the group, it is not unlike leadership and is equally elusive. The different types of power emanate from a variety of sources and thus influence people in various ways. Definitions of the power bases follow:

Coercive power is exercised when fear is used to ensure compliance from subordinates. A nursing administrator may state that if the group does not comply with the new staffing policy, then group members will be subject to transfer to a different area of the institution.

Reward power is exercised when the leader or manager uses a position to provide something of value to the employee. A head nurse may be in a position to offer a financial reward, such as a raise, or a personal reward, such as a change in working hours, to the employees. Rewards are a very positive aspect of organizational life.

Legitimate power is comparable to authority. It is the official sanctioned right of the superior to exact rights and obligations from subordinates. This exercise of power can be used because of the position held by the leader. When power is used in this way it is because the followers are aware of the leader's position and will respond accordingly.

Expert power is the use of superior knowledge and experience to have others do as the leader suggests. The best use of expert power is demonstrated by clinical specialists who do not have line or legitimate authority in their particular institution. Rather, their clinical knowledge allows them to be influential.

Referent power is largely based on a leader's capacity to inspire others to be similar to the leader. It is a type of power that is associated with a leader's personality and the special traits the leader possesses (charisma). A head nurse who is an exceptionally skilled practitioner may be an inspiration to the staff to emulate excellence in nursing practice.

Information power is based on the leader's knowledge of or access to information. Followers want or need the information the leader holds. It has been said that knowledge is power, and in this case it is.

Connection power comes from association with a powerful figure. For example, the president's wife has power by virtue of her association with her husband. In the health care institution, an employee who is a very close friend or who is a family member to the chief operating officer may have the ability to influence a group's decision because of the leader's association.

Management experts are interested in power because it is an interactional process that can be very effective in accomplishing necessary goals. Power can be gained in a variety of ways. To help the leader or manager in the acquisition of power, suggestions have been offered in the form of a chart (Table 6-1) that summarizes this information.

Authority. The legitimate right to seek compliance is **authority,** whereas responsibility dictates the legitimate boundaries of work. There is a direct relationship between the two; thus, they should exist in equal measure. It would be a difficult situation to have responsibility for a task and not have the authority to complete it. This is the problem for temporary or acting leaders or managers. *Authority by definition is the legitimate right of the superior to exact rights and obligations from subordinates.* Authority is an integral part of the fabric of the organization and will be dispersed throughout the organizational structures by virtue of the process of delegation.

There are two ways of delegating authority within the organization, *centralized* and *decentralized.* Centralized refers to the authority of decision making remaining at the administrative level or central office. Decentralized refers to the assignment of decision making away from the central office and close to the operational level.[21] In nursing, this means close to the actual unit level or patient care division. Decentralized authority eliminates the need for levels of management because the head nurse assumes responsibility for managerial decisions that influence both the patients and staff.

Within the organization, there are two types of authority. Both forms of authority, when exercised, are able to influence members of the organization. One type is called *line authority;* the other is referred to as *staff authority.* Line authority is the formal, legitimate right of superiors to exact performance

TABLE 6-1. SKILLS AND WAYS TO ACQUIRE THESE SKILLS FOR THE PURPOSE
OF GAINING POWER IN THE ORGANIZATION[21]

Credibility	Is gained through hard work, gaining skill and becoming competitive in your work, and being very honest in your relationships with other people. Be well-informed and current through professional journals, meetings, and educational conferences. Be well-prepared for presentations using all at your disposal. Audiovisual aids, charts, and graphs provide the basis for a well-researched and documented presentation.
Interpersonal Relations	Good working relationships have to be developed with all coworkers. The suggestions offered for leadership development will help you gain good working relationships because they are built on respect and sensitivity to yourself and others.
Persuasion	To be able to convince others of the appropriateness of your point of view, your argument must be logical and show that your way of thinking is a positive solution. In addition, deal with the issues that are most appropriate for the group you wish to influence by using words that are most familiar to the group you wish to convince.
Membership	Be in a position to speak with and thus influence the group. Volunteer to be on committees and to work within the known organization's hierarchy.
Communication Network	Formally and informally talk with people on all levels of the organization. Information comes from many different sources from within the organization. Develop trusting relationships with people, be capable of discretion, and hold confidential information sacred.

from subordinates. It is represented as straight lines on the organizational chart. Staff authority is a consultative or advisory process and is represented as broken lines on the organization chart. Classical theory tended to view line authority as a commodity distributed to positions in measured amounts and did not prescribe a particularly important role to staff authority. The modern organization, however, uses line and staff authority effectively. The use and reliance on consultants demands the integration of experts to deal with modern complexities.

Responsibility. *Responsibility, also integral to organizational dynamics, is the obligation to perform according to position requirements. It is an inward obligation to perform so that the entire organization benefits.* It is the corollary of authority as well as its natural consequence.

Status. Another interesting aspect of organizational dynamics includes the awarding of status. *Status is the recognition by others that an individual possesses a superior talent or resource.* The uniqueness of the organization's hierarchy rewards individuals with varying degrees of importance. Status is a unique concept that serves as a reward, a motivator, and a goal.

Process of Delegation. *The process of delegation is the means by which responsibility and authority are entrusted and assigned to the various individuals throughout the organization.* These concepts are discussed in greater detail in Chapter 8.

The above-named, briefly presented concepts are the interactional phenomena that occur because people work together in an organized structure. They provide the basic explanation of how individuals take an active part in the operations of the organization. These same concepts also influence the establishment of the formal and informal structure the organization assumes. A **structure** provides the internal differentiation and patterning of relationships among people and especially manager and staff.

▓ ORGANIZATIONAL CONCEPTS

Organizational Chart

An **organizational chart** represents the formal organization and all its diverse relationships. It is a visual representation of the chain of authority, division of work, levels of management, and functional communication pattern from chief executive to each member of the organization. This view of the organization demonstrates the scaler chain of authority that is represented by the vertical lines clearly showing how line and staff authority has been distributed. See Figures 6-3 and 6-4 for examples of organizational charts.

Organization Structure

The organizational chart is a useful tool that shows us how the modern organization is structured. An organizational structure is the internal differentiation

ORGANIZATION OF A MODERN HOSPITAL

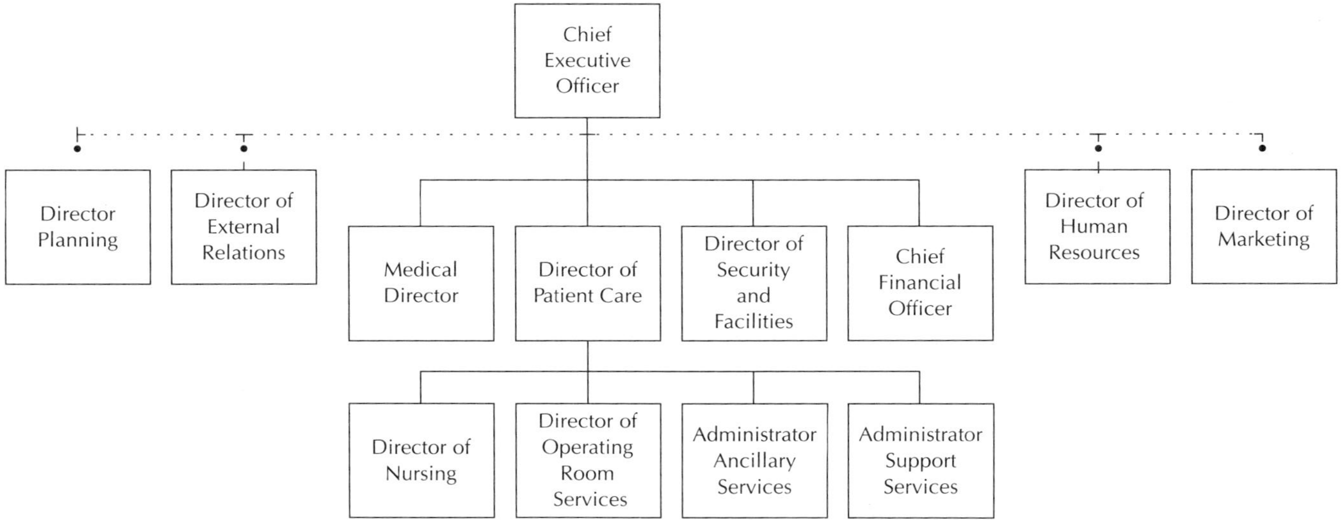

Figure 6-3. An example of the organizational chart for an entire hospital.

The chart shows the following structure:

- Chief Executive Officer
  - Director Planning
  - Director of External Relations
  - Director of Human Resources
  - Director of Marketing
  - Medical Director
  - Director of Patient Care
    - Director of Nursing
    - Director of Operating Room Services
    - Administrator Ancillary Services
  - Director of Security and Facilities
  - Chief Financial Officer
    - Administrator Support Services

NURSING ORGANIZATION AT A LARGE HOSPITAL

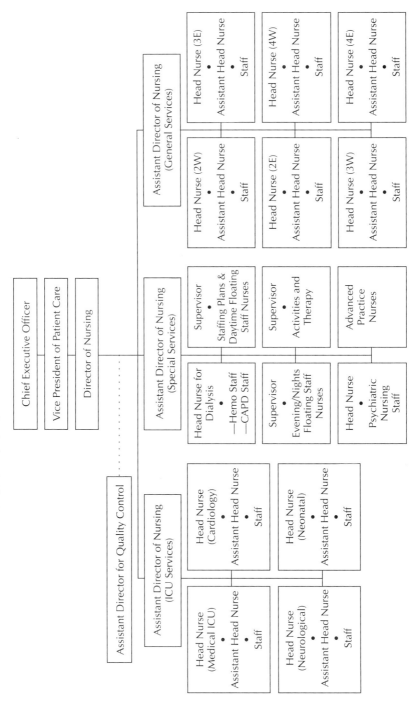

Figure 6-4. An example of a department of nursing.

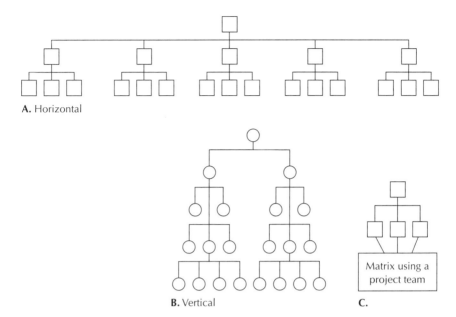

A. Horizontal

B. Vertical

C.

Matrix using a
project team

Figure 6-5. A variety of organizational structures: (A) horizontal or flat structure, (B) a vertical or tall structure, and (C) a matrix structure.

and patterning of relationships. It is the bony skeleton of the organization. The categorizing of an organizational structure is based on the characteristics of the organizing process. Structures of organizations may be categorized as tall, flat, matrix, or contingency. Organizational structures provide the means whereby the organizing process can be accomplished for the organization to meet its goals (Fig. 6-5).

Tall or *vertical* represents an organizational structure that forms when the span of control is small and may also be referred to as a pyramid, or a bureaucracy. This means that managers have fewer subordinates who report to them and likewise report to one superior. This arrangement will produce a hierarchical arrangement, regular assigned activities, written directives, and policy guidance for behavior. This particular structure was and is commonplace in health care because of the scope of responsibility and the diversity of work. In addition, this structure provides for the control of activities of employees. Communication, however, may be distorted because the message, even if written, is sent through the various layers of the organization in a long line.

A *flat* or *horizontal* structure forms when the span of control is wide. A large number of employees report to one manager. This structure is characteristically less rigid in controls, and more freedom is available to the employees.

The manager is able to communicate with less distortion through fewer levels but is not as available to the employees for consultation or supervision due to the wide span of control. Currently, health care institutions are adopting this structure in the department of nursing. This is referred to as flattening the organization by removing levels of management. This activity results in administrative staff with wide spans of control and front-line managers or head nurses with increased authority. For this structure to be useful, authority must be decentralized to the necessary personnel.

Matrix organizations are a modern organizational invention that exist within a formal bureaucracy, or tall structure, as well as within a flat structure. This structure creates groups within the organization that belong to different departments but that share common goals that affect the organization as a whole. It basically creates permanent or semipermanent departments within a structure because the needs or goals of the organization require specialized and diverse work. Organizations today are very complex, and problems faced by such institutions are not always able to be solved within traditional structures. This is because the functional relationships and communication patterns prohibit meaningful problem solving. A matrix structure provides for the creation of a group that would be instrumental in doing the highly complicated problem solving that is necessary. The formation of the new department brings together a group that ordinarily would not be in a position to relate or to communicate because they represent different factions of the organization. There is much in the literature about the advantages and disadvantages of such a structure. Simply, it is a positive way for complex organizations to deal with complex issues in a very structured and orderly way; however, it also has the potential for creating dual subordination and confusion in the institution. It is often operationalized through the establishment of project teams with a project manager. The employees are now responsible to the project manager just as they are to the manager of their division. This structure enables organizations to develop solutions to complex problems with the right group of individuals.

Contingency Structure

The contingency structure evolves in response to demands from the situation. The major factors that determine the contingent structure are forces in the environment (or market) and forces within the organization (or technologic core consisting of dominant activities). These forces are either stable or volatile (highly changeable). The resulting **contingency design** is the process of determining the degree of environmental uncertainty and adapting the organization and its subunits to the situation.[22] The types of organization structures that evolve are as follows:

- A stable environment and technologic core lead to a stable structure such as a flat or tall bureaucratic organizational design. This design, if you remember, works well where conformity to rules and regulations are expected.
- A volatile environment and stable core lead to a market-dominated structure in which much of the energy and resources of the organization are aimed at the market place. Examples of these activities would be public relations, to determine public views about the service or product.
- A stable environment and volatile technologic core lead to a technologically dominated structure in which the organization would have to continuously conform to changing technology. Major resource allocation would be aimed towards keeping the core technology current.
- Volatile environment and technologic core lead to a flexible dynamic organization in which change dominates and the structure which forms is able to adapt to information coming from either within or outside the organization. For example, at one time the market concerns would be paramount, and at another time, it would be the technologic component. The organizational structure would be one that could readily adapt to changing priorities.

■ INTEGRATED HEALTH CARE SYSTEM

The changing economic, social, and political climate (a volatile environment) has led to transformation of the health care organizations. The issues that are driving the reorganization are quality care (improving patient outcomes), reduction of health care cost, and insuring patient satisfaction (technological issues). Traditional health care organizations, such as the hospital, are now a unit within a large integrated network (resulting structure). An integrated health care system is a complex network of services to meet the consumers' health care needs. The objective is to keep people healthy and to treat them in the lowest cost setting, of which primary care will be pivotal. The restructuring of health care institutions and reengineering of the work require inventing and managing new systems to meet the needs of the future. Some of the reengineering processes include the elimination of extraneous jobs, determining work to be directed at specific outcomes of the organization, and

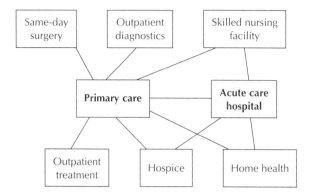

Figure 6-6. A graphic depiction of the units of an integrated health care system.

retraining individuals to have multiple skills rather than hiring highly specialized practitioners with limited skills.[23] Another technique is to reduce the number of managers and levels of management. It is desirable that decisions about work be made by the professional accountable for that decision. This is usually at the level of the operative employee. In addition, increasing the quality and utilization of data will enhance the decision-making process. Thus, decisions will be made on information rather than on circumstances.[24]

Currently, the health care system is consolidating its services in preparation for managed competition. The characteristics of this process are the formation of HMOs and PPOs, which provide cost-effective care. Primary care is emerging as the dominant delivery strategy, with health care clinics hiring primary care physicians and nurse practitioners. Patients or clients are being offered incentives to participate in formal groups where capitation is prominent and risk-based reimbursement is provided. Hospitals are joining together by linking acute care services, clinics, and ambulatory care services. To survive this massive reorganization, hospitals have had to become part of integrated health care networks, share in the financial risk of care, downsize or rightsize, and reduce personnel. See Figure 6-6.

Once consolidation efforts are complete and managed competition is the dominant health care strategy, integrated health care systems will compete for covered lives. All units of this delivery system will be **cost centers,** and the value of care will be systematically evaluated by standardized measures of quality, cost, and patient satisfaction. Organization theory explains these dynamic changes by systematically evaluating the conceptual components of an organization and relating them to the forces that are driving the changes. Organization models assist in this process.

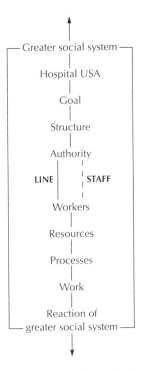

Figure 6-7. An organizational model with its components. The arrows represent the reciprocal relationship that exists between the organization and the social environment it serves.

Organizational Model

Organization models provide a representation of the conceptual areas of an organization. These components are the subsystems that together explain how and why an organization functions. Similar to a road map, organization models assist the manager to consider the effects of an action on the organization as a whole (Fig. 6-7). Throughout this text, emphasis has been placed on the importance of (1) practicing leadership and management based on a comprehensive analysis of factors found in the greater social system or the present situation and (2) forces within the participants which influence the situations. A model is offered that preserves this view by identifying those aspects of organizational dynamics that enhance or inhibit the achievement of goals. The following discussion defines the components of the model and relates them to the turbulence in the health care system.

The *greater social system* provides direction and definition to the organizational goals as well as the standards to judge the effectiveness of the work. The goal of the particular health care agency is determined by which aspect of health care is being addressed. For instance, the hospital will provide acute care to the patients. To a great extent, the current reorganization of health care has occurred because of the action and attitudes of the greater society. The need for cost containment, emphasis on health (not sickness) and growing partnerships between the health care community, providers, and consumers have revised the health care delivery in which prevention dominates and primary care is the central delivery mechanism.

The *structure* of the organization is directly related to the complexity, level, and diversity of necessary services and individuals needed to meet the particular goal or mission of the organization. The structure can take the form of a traditional bureaucratic organization, matrix, or contingency. The organizational structures within the new health care delivery system represent interdependent and integrated units of care whose aim is to provide a seamless health care delivery system. The structure provides the means whereby the mission of each aspect of the system, as well as the system itself is operationalized.

Authority represents the fundamental process that brings logic and order to the work of the organization and is integral to organizational dynamics. This authority will either be line or staff, which represents different modes of influence and different sources of power. Line authority is represented in the scaler chain. Authority, known as staff, refers to a form of influence used by specialized individuals who hold unique roles in the organization and who, while not directly responsible for employees, are involved with the outcome of the employees' work. These individuals serve as consultants or advisors to the staff and in some situations may have legitimate authority over the personnel. An example is the clinical nurse specialist who has a staff position in relationship to employees. The authority in the new health care climate is shared with the patient and decentralized to the operative employee who participates with the patient for shared decision making.

The worker or individual who performs in a particular way prescribed in part by the organization and in part by self-direction plays a unique role in organizational dynamics. The orchestration of all members or workers in the total organization in combination with available resources and the variety of processes produce the *work* of the organization. The outcome of the coordinated effort that uses the variety of people in a range of roles to complete the work of the organization is subject to further evaluation by the greater social system, representing the recipient of the service.

Organization and Management Link

This attempt to organize and to classify human behavior within the organizational context gives direction to the study of management. Organization theory in a broad and conceptual sense tells us what is involved when people come together for a similar purpose. Management theory gives us the practical knowledge and tools to meet the demands set by the goals of the organization. Specifically, management maintains the internal structure of the organization that effectively gets the job done. In addition, the manager deals with the human side of the organization: the people and their concerns. The manager also must be the leader ready to adapt to change from within and outside the organization and all for the purpose of meeting specific goals.

Properties of an Organization

Organization theory and management theory, while different, are related. There are properties of an organization that relate directly to management. These properties as summarized by Caplow follow[23]:

- **All organizations closely resemble each other so that much of what is learned by managing one can be applied to others.** These characteristics include a history, a collective identity or image, specialized activities and procedures, a set of formal rules undermined by informal rules, a special vocabulary, and division of labor which affords status.
- **Every organization except the very smallest is a cluster of sub-organizations of varying size.** Systems theory explains the interpersonal and social character of the workplace. The need for the various aspects of the organization to function interdependently produce the work output.
- **Problems of managing a large organization are similar to those of managing smaller organizations.** The role of the manager is to maintain a balance between cooperation and conflict. For a social system to thrive, conflict must be managed and meaningful communication must be encouraged, motivation opportunities offered, and evaluations provided.
- **During any given interval in an organization's history, it will be growing, stable, or declining.** Critical to the survival of any organization is regular and systematic evaluation. The cycle of an organization is to grow, stabilize, and decline. Without a concerted effort to keep an organization sensitive to its mission and constituency, it will

fail. Periodic evaluations of how effective the organization is performing is necessary to objectively consider change. Despite efforts to keep the organization flourishing, most organizations develop crises from time to time. The manner in which these episodes are managed either insures survival or hastens decline.

- **Most organizations find it easier to satisfy some of their goals more than others for reasons beyond their control.** The complexity of people and their motivation often complicates the predictability of the work outcome. However, unexpected results sometimes are extremely helpful and good for the organization.

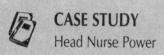

CASE STUDY
Head Nurse Power

Mrs. Jackson is the head nurse on a coronary care step-down unit. She has a habit of dictating solutions to her staff whenever a problem arises. She also publicly degrades and demeans her staff, using a rather superior attitude. Unfortunately, she also shows favoritism to some members of her staff. Those who she likes get the best hours and vacation time. The rest of the staff are intimidated by her, and those who dare to confront her to discuss their problems are assigned the worst hours or shifts, and their requests are ignored. The stress and tension on the division is great. For instance, Mary Jones, a nursing assistant, asked Pat Polk, an RN, for assistance with her patient. Pat responded, "No, that's not my patient." Conditions on the division have deteriorated, and Mrs. Jackson's response has been to be even more dictatorial.

- What type of power is being utilized in this situation?
- What are the consequences of a strong negative leader?
- Are there any advantages to an organization with this kind of manager?
- What could the staff do with a situation just described?

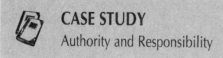

CASE STUDY
Authority and Responsibility

A small neurosurgical unit, which up until recently displayed good interpersonal relationships among the nurses and nurse aides, has suddenly developed problems. Because other hospitals in the vicinity have closed their neurosurgery units, the census of this unit has continued to increase and is usually maximally occupied. In the past, the nursing staff worked cooperatively, but recently the staff stopped working as a team. The nurse aides are expected to take eight patients, and the nurses are assigned five patients. The nurse aides have stopped completing their job responsibilities, such as bathing patients and changing beds. The nurses subsequently have had to complete the nurse aides' work. This has led to poor working relationships between the two groups. The head nurse spoke to the nurse aides at the request of the nurses a number of times. Each time, the nurse aides improved their performance for a day or two, and then fell back into the same pattern of not completing their work. The tension between the nurses and nurse aides continues to rise and the situation remains unresolved.

- Who is most responsible to correct this situation?
- What forms of power are being used in this situation?
- Would creating a work team composed of specific nurses and nurse aides be helpful?
- What situational forces led to this situation? Can they be addressed?

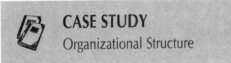

CASE STUDY
Organizational Structure

Ms. Jones, the vice president of nursing, is seriously considering reorganizing the nursing service department. Currently, the department is as follows:

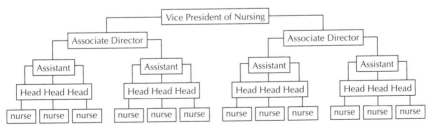

Ms. Jones wants to preserve adequate managerial control but feels that there are too many levels of management and wants to decentralize authority.

- What would the new organizational structure look like if you were consulting with Ms. Jones?

■ SUMMARY

This chapter discussed organization and management theory, looking first at classical theory's contribution and then at modern theory, with special emphasis on social systems theory. The modern organization is a source of complex relationships and functions. An organization model was presented to bring together the key concepts that define the organization and represent the source of analysis for studying organizational behavior and its consequences. To illustrate the model's usefulness, the forces that influence health care reform were used to illustrate the components of the model. Organization and management theories are presented as fundamental to the development of a manager. The relationship between organization and management theory was presented as a way to link abstract concepts to the process of management.

 STUDENT EXERCISES

1. Draw the formal organization chart at the agency you are currently working as a student nurse.

2. Examine the chain of authority in your clinical agency. Draw a representation of who influences whom. Does this match the formal chart of your agency?

3. Distinguish between the different types of power. From your clinical experience, identify individuals who use each type of power. What position does each hold and what behavior does each exhibit? Are the behaviors different?

■ REFERENCES

1. Kast F, Rosenzweig JE, *Organization and Management: A System Approach*, 4th ed, New York, St. Louis: McGraw Hill, 1985, p. 108.
2. Taylor FW, *Shop Management*, New York: Harper, 1911.
3. Fayol H, Storrs C, trans., *General and Industrial Management*. London: Pitman and Sons, 1949.
4. Barnard C, *The Functions of the Executive*, Boston: Harvard University Press, 1938.

5. Weiss RM, "Weber on Bureaucracy: Management Consultant or Political Theorist?" *Academy Manage Rev*, vol. 8, 1983, p. 242–248.
6. Kreitner R, *Management*, 6th ed, Boston, Toronto: Houghton Mifflin Co., 1995, p. 51.
7. Ibid., p. 51.
8. Stephen R, Jones RG, "Worker Interdependence and Output: The Hawthorne Studies Revisited," *American Sociologic Review*, vol. 55, April 1990, p. 176–190.
9. Von Bertalaniy L, *General Systems Theory Foundations, Development, Application*, New York: Braziller, 1968.
10. Kast F, Rosenzweig JE, p. 108.
11. Ibid., p. 109.
12. Katz D, Kahn R, *The Social Psychology of Organizations*, 2nd ed, New York: Wiley, 1978.
13. Tosi H, Carroll S, *Management: Contingencies, Structure, and Process*, Chicago: St. Claire Press, 1975, p. 156.
14. Ibid., p. 158.
15. Kreitner R, p. 52.
16. Ibid., p. 52–53.
17. Wheatley M, "Searching for Order in an Orderly World: a Poetic for Post-Machine Age Managers," *Journal of Management Inquiry*, December, 1992, p. 340.
18. French JRP, Raven B, "The Bases of Social Power." In Cartwright D, Zander A (editors), *Group Dynamics Research Theory*, New York: Harper & Row, 1968, p. 259–269.
19. Raven BH, Kruglanski W, "Conflict and Power." In Swingle PC (editor), *The Structure of Conflict*, New York: Academic Press, 1975, p. 177–219.
20. Hersey P, Blanchard K, *Management of Organizational Behavior*, 5th ed, Englewood Cliffs, NJ: Prentice Hall, 1988, p. 214.
21. Kreitner R, p. 54.
22. Porter-O'Grady T, "A Systems Approach to Managing Transformation," *Seminars for Nurse Managers*, 2:4, December, 1994, p. 191–195.
23. Ibid.
24. Ibid., p. 191.
25. Caplow T, *How to Run Any Organization*, Orlando, FL: Harcourt, Brace and World, 1976.

7

Overview of Nursing Management

Introduction

Today, nurses are practicing in new settings and organizations that require different and expanded roles. Entry-level nurses need management skills to perform their responsibilities with patients and personnel. Clinical management of patients and clients involves the maintenance of quality patient care, judicious use of scarce resources, and provision of cost-effective nursing services. Simultaneously, nurses will be required to supervise licensed and certified practitioners within their scope of authority. The time, energy, and resources spent on developing management skills are worthwhile investments in the future of health care. The dividends are great in terms of successful patient care outcomes, as well as motivated and competent employees.

Today's health care system and tomorrow's challenges provide opportunities for nursing management. Undoubtedly, the role of a nurse manager is and will be one of the most challenging of any industry. To become a manager a new process must be learned, new skills must be acquired, and new attitudes must be adopted. Much of what is known about professional management has been derived from work in other disciplines. However, the nursing profession is developing its own unique and innovative management strategies as nurse researchers and administrators study the management process. This chapter will provide an overview of the management process and what it entails.

KEY CONCEPTS

Management is a process with both interpersonal and technical aspects through which the objectives of an organization (or part of it) are accomplished by efficiently and effectively using resources.

Planning is the primary management function that decides in advance what needs to be done and charts the course for future action.

Organizing is the management function that provides the relationship between people and activities in such a way as to fulfill the organization's objectives.

Staffing is the management activity that ensures the proper ratio of workers to work.

Directing is the management activity that gets work done through others by (1) giving directions, (2) supervising, (3) leading, (4) motivating, and (5) communicating.

Coordinating is the management activity that assembles and synchronizes people and activities so that they function harmoniously in the attainment of organizational objectives.

Controlling is the management function that regulates activities with plans according to standards.

Systems of Nursing Care are the organizational and professional structures that provide delivery of nursing care. They are (1) the case method, (2) functional nursing, (3) team nursing, (4) primary nursing, (5) modular nursing, and (6) case management.

■ MANAGEMENT PROCESS

Management is defined as a process with both interpersonal and technical aspects through which the objectives of an organization (or part of it) are accomplished efficiently and effectively by using human, physical, financial, and technologic resources.[1] The management role is dedicated to facilitating the work in the organization through one's own and the efforts of others. Transition to a management role means assuming a position of authority, with its inherent complexity. The new manager is cast into a role whose tasks are conceptual. The problems that are experienced are often long term, and satisfaction also becomes delayed and abstract. Because of the new responsibilities, a status differential often results that produces a distance between the manager and staff. However, the linking nature between the manager and the group necessitates new skills. This is accomplished through the management process, which consists of:

- Establishing the organization's objectives
- Developing plans to meet the stated objectives
- Assembling the necessary resources
- Supervising the execution of the plans
- Evaluating the progress or outcome of the stated plan[2]

Management is an essential activity for organizations. Systematic study of what managers do and how the manager uses this process provides the necessary information to increase the overall efficiency of the organization.

■ LEVELS OF MANAGEMENT

Managers are expected to make decisions about how others will use their time and be responsible for the supervision of others. Professional nurses and other members of the health team (operative employees) who are not managers are expected to perform those activities that constitute the work (or part of it) for the organization. It is in this capacity that the professional nurse will either manage employees or care for patients. Since the organization is a hierarchy, the work of management is divided into levels of responsibility. Managers at all levels, top, middle, and front line, do the work of management. Top management, or the administrative level, is composed of the board of directors, the president, and the vice presidents. The vice president of nursing is among this group whose responsibilities include managing managers. Middle management includes division heads and directors of nursing (and evening and night supervisors). This group manages front-line managers. Front-line, or lower-level, managers, sometimes called unit managers, are head nurses; they manage staff employees. The various levels of managers use the management process in accord with their scope of responsibility. These levels are pictured in Figure 7-1.

Renes Likert's Four Systems of Management

System One	System Two	System Three	System Four
Exploitive Authoritative	Benevolent Authoritative	Consultative	Participative

Leadership
Motivation
Communication
Decisions
Goals
Control

Figure 7-1. Likert identified four systems of management. The differences among the systems were based on the way managers dealt with the above factors.

■ MANAGEMENT SCIENCE

Management has been studied by scholars from business, sociology, psychology, and the military. Different theorists offered frameworks to study the process of management and administration, resulting in a general body of management thought. For instance, McGregor and his Theory X and Theory Y approach to the supervision of people suggests that there are two classes of supervisors.[3] Theory X assumes that people hate work and as a result have to be coerced, controlled, and directed by their supervisors. Theory Y, on the other hand, assumes that people take to work like play and as a result are self-directed, responsible, and capable of solving problems. Other theorists elaborated on this work by placing emphasis on positive relationships between the superior and subordinate.

Herzberg provided assumptions about motivations of people, namely that most people are motivated by intrinsic factors rather than extrinsic factors.[4] Intrinsic factors are associated with self-actualization on the job and include achievement, recognition, responsibility, growth, and advancement. Extrinsic, or maintenance, factors are those that had been traditionally perceived by management to be motivators and include company policy, supervision, working conditions, salary, and job security. Both McGregor and Hertzberg are discussed in Chapter 10.

Argyris looked at the effects of organizational life and motivation to facilitate a consistency between the organization's and the individual's goals.[5] In his book *Personality and Organization*, Argyris stated his concern with the employee's psychologic growth. The concern centered around the employee's ability to self-actualize within a system that by and large was in

Top	Board of Directors
	President
Vice presidents	Vice presidents

Middle	Supervisory staff	Directors of nursing service
	Department heads	Supervisors

Front line	Head nurses
	Staff

Figure 7-2. The various levels of management: top, middle, and front line.

conflict with this need. Argyris argued that the challenge to modern organizations was to allow the maturing person to grow in an environment that was basically immature.

Likert set out four detailed systems of management that ranged from the highly autocratic to the highly participative.[6] The four systems include:

- *System 1:* Exploitative-authoritative
- *System 2:* Benevolent-authoritative
- *System 3:* Consultative
- *System 4:* Participative

The system of participative management has been suggested to be one of the most successful, and those companies that have employed it report positive results (Fig. 7-2). Nursing researchers have attempted to provide empiric data to evaluate the effectiveness of management styles, using Likert's systems, and staff reaction. Results overwhelmingly support the participative style of management as the most desirable style that produces staff satisfaction and retention.[7]

Recently, Peters and Waterman, management scientists, conducted a study of the sixty-two best-run companies in America, and concluded eight principles of excellence.[8] This has become known as the excellence approach. While not all eight attributes were present in every successful company, a preponderance of them were reported. The proposed attributes of excellence are as follows:

1. "A bias for action" refers to involved managers. Managers are visible and close to the work unit. These managers are ready and willing to become involved.

2. "Close to the customer" refers to a need to seek customer satisfaction above all else. Active input is sought on a regular basis from those who are served.
3. "Autonomy and entrepreneurship" refers to the encouragement of risk taking, and the tolerance for failure among employees.
4. "Productivity through people" concerns the emphasis of respect for individuals in the workplace. Enthusiasm, trust, and a family feeling are fostered.
5. "Hands-on value-driven" refers to a clear company philosophy that is disseminated and followed. The organization's belief system is reinforced. Leaders are positive role models, not rigid authoritative managers.
6. "Stick to the knitting" means managers manage and employees do what they do best. Emphasis is on internal growth of the company.
7. "Simple form, lean staff" refers to decentralizing authority as much as possible. Management staffs are kept to a minimum, and talented employees are at the work site.
8. "Simultaneous loose-tight properties" refers to stringent strategic and financial control counterbalanced by decentralized authority, autonomy, and opportunities for creativity.[9]

The various insights represented by the different management theorists have been both praised and critiqued in the management literature. Nevertheless, they share some common views, and may be summarized by the following assumptions:

- Managers must trust the employees to be responsible for the performance of their jobs.
- Organizational structures must be flexible enough to allow the employees to function well.
- Managers must have some input and control over the employees' work for the work to be effective.[10]

These beliefs have guided the development of managers in all fields, including nursing. Based on the assumptions of professional management, nursing has expanded the role of manager to include patient welfare.

■ MANAGEMENT IN NURSING

A philosophy of service is what differentiates nursing management from professional management in other fields. Because of nursing's social responsibility toward the health and illness of individuals, families, and communities, a unique approach is required. The quality of care to be delivered is as important a consideration as the staff and resources used. Thus, success depends on quality of service as well as ability to deliver care within a given set of resources. This dual goal of management demands thoughtful and specific professional strategies.

Evolution of Nursing's Management Role

In the new health care environment, the role of management and manager is changing. The middle management level has been dramatically downsized, and the administrative level is often responsible for a multiple of units within a network. Downsizing and flattening the organization have stimulated reconceptualization of the manager's role. In the past, nurse managers supervised one or two levels of employees, and often relied on an authoritative style. This style emanated from legitimate organizational authority and positional power. The majority of these managers learned their skills by watching their immediate supervisor. They believed there was a need for control and felt an overwhelming sense of responsibility for everything that happened. This control method was a readily accepted practice during these earlier times, and keeping people in line became the norm of a manager's work life.[11] It was an illusion of control and power over employees.

In the mid-1980s, a new concept known as shared governance introduced the idea of shared decision making. This concept suggested that decisions be reached by consensus, not by vote. Staff members were invited to share their views and give input into problem solutions. Despite some hesitation and problems, this methodology was viewed as a transition to a positive and inspiring managerial style. Contrary to past belief, the more staff knew, the better and informed were the decisions. The activities that cultivated shared decision making created a profound impact on the managerial role. Managers needed to learn methodologies that would facilitate staff participation and staff development.[12] Instead of controlling the staff behavior, managers were expected to help staff be responsible for their own behavior. Thus, managers needed education to cultivate a style that would empower the staff. In the current system the manager is expected to be a team facilitator.[13] This means managers have the responsibility to help the staff become successful in their endeavors, which is the work of the organization.

▓ OBJECTIVES OF NURSING MANAGEMENT

Nursing, a service field, is highly labor-intensive, making nursing management particularly challenging because of the wide variety of experience and educational backgrounds of the employees in the health care setting. The work, as well as the workers, challenges the nurse manager to create the kind of environment that facilitates quality nursing practice. The nurse manager has specific responsibilities to the organization and to the staff. The staff in turn have responsibilities to the organization and to the manager. The beginning nurse will contribute to the success of the unit's efficiency by being aware of the manager's role. In general, the manager has certain responsibilities. They include:

- Accomplishing the goals of the organization or nursing division
- Maintaining the quality of patient care within the financial limitations of the organization
- Encouraging the motivation of the employees and the patients in the area
- Increasing the ability of subordinates and peers to accept change
- Developing a team spirit and increase morale
- Furthering the professional development of the personnel[14]

These objectives are met in varying degrees of efficiency and effectiveness, depending upon the same framework espoused throughout this text. The successful manager is one who is keenly aware of those forces that are relevant to the managerial situation.

The manager should accurately understand the goals, the relationship between the manager and employee, the special abilities of the employee, and those relevant organizational and social factors that impact the situation. Analyzing the managerial situation and using the appropriate management tool will assist in accomplishing the organization's goals. A managerial assessment tool is offered at the end of this chapter to highlight essential factors so that positive action can be taken. The managerial role involves making good decisions based on the management process and the use of management functions.

■ MANAGEMENT FUNCTIONS

Success of management depends on an individual's talent, motivation and opportunity to manage. The first step in developing talent is to become familiar with the traditional management functions (Fig. 7-3). These functions, which are expected of managers, include **planning, organizing, staffing, directing, coordinating,** and **controlling.** Managers develop skills in the implementation of these functions as they gain experience in the role

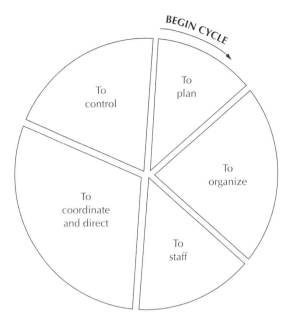

Figure 7-3. A graphic depiction of the management functions.

of manager. Nurse managers also use the same functions as they fulfill their responsibilities.

Planning

The most basic and essential activity of management is planning. Planning is the primary management function that decides in advance what needs to be done for the day, month, or years ahead. It charts the course for future action. Planning is also an activity of the practitioner. To manage care for a patient or a group of patients, planning will facilitate the use of time, activities, and resources. If there is a deviation from the overall plan of care (similar to a critical path), understanding the problem and what to do will be greatly assisted. Just as a patient's condition alters activities for the practitioner, so too will unusual events change the plan for the manager.

Planning will provide the overall structure for the accomplishment of necessary work and, properly, should include possible problems. Specifically the reasons for planning are:

- To focus attention on objectives
- To offset uncertainty and chance

- To gain economic operation
- To facilitate control

Planning requires a thoughtful reflection of what it is you want to accomplish and how to accomplish it within a given set of resources. Careful analysis of the managerial situation will provide the basis for a well-developed plan for action and will reveal problems that require solutions. Analysis is the related activity that provides the leader or manager with essential elements of the plan. The greater the analysis, the better the plan. Experience and knowledge facilitate the acquisition of this skill.

Types of Planning. Various types of planning strategies are available to the manager, namely standing, strategic, and long range. The most basic is a *standing plan,* or a stable plan, which lists daily or standard activities. The practitioner uses standing plans similar to a nursing care plan. The manager will use standing plans as a way of organizing time and activities. This may include monthly meetings, weekly staff sessions, and daily review of the patient/client services. This type of plan will provide the manager with a general framework for the purpose of allocating time.

Strategic planning is market- and future-oriented, intended to provide a plan for the life of the entire organization or network. Such planning is part and parcel of an organization's attempt to remain competitive. This kind of planning occurs at an administrative level or at top management and includes an in-depth analysis of those factors within and outside of the organization. Today, strategic planning is involved with methods to increase revenue, consolidate services, reduce loss of profit, and provide income-producing services.[15] Administration alone has the authority to initiate and to commission such comprehensive plans. However, since the mid-1980s, middle- and front-line managers are more frequently being involved in strategic planning efforts.

Long-range planning is also a form of future-oriented planning but is more general and provides a direction for organizational growth. A plan of this nature elaborates 1-, 5-, and 10-year goals. The goals are subject to change as relevant circumstances change. Administration of organizations routinely have long-range planning meetings to continually develop goals for the future. All managers (front line, middle, and top level) will use planning as an important tool, but will keep in mind that different types of planning will be determined by the responsibilities of the manager. The vice president of nursing who has a broad scope of responsibility uses planning differently than the new front-line manager or head nurse.

Organizing

Organizing is the management function that relates people and activities in such a way as to fulfill organizational objectives. An organization provides a mechanism through which this can be accomplished, known as vertical and horizontal differentiation.

Vertical differentiation refers to the establishment of a hierarchy, or number of levels, needed to do the work of the organization. Management must decide on a tall or flat structure. *Horizontal differentiation* results from the need to separate activities for more efficient and effective performance. This occurs by forming departments within an organization, enabling work to be accomplished through differentiation of labor or provision of different services. Take for instance the number of units necessary to provide care for surgical patients. The laboratory, radiology, preoperative, and postoperative nursing divisions are but a few. Then consider outpatient as opposed to in-house surgical services. Through the process of integration, both levels of differentiation succeed in meeting the needs of the surgical patients and organizational goals.

At the unit level, the manager maintains the structure that facilitates nursing care. The manager does this by using the system of nursing care adopted by the organization as a whole. Team nursing, primary nursing, modular nursing, and case management are some of the possible models for nursing care delivery. The manager is responsible for the integrity of the model that had been chosen and also for the evaluation of its general effectiveness. *Case management* as a nursing care delivery system has the capability of being a very efficient method for organizing health care services. Traditional boundaries are crossed when the hospital-based services are arranged to respond to the hierarchy of patient needs.[16] The organization and monitoring of services provided by case management ensures both the vertical and horizontal integration of the necessary departments. The above-named models are discussed under "Systems of Nursing Care Delivery."

Staffing

Staffing is the management activity that provides for appropriate and adequate personnel to fulfill the organization's objectives. The nurse manager decides how many and what type of personnel are required to provide care for the patients. Usually the overall plan for staffing is determined by nursing administration from among several models. The nurse manager is in a position to monitor how successful the staffing pattern is as well as to provide input into needed change. Staffing is a complex activity that involves ensuring that the ratio of nurse to patient provides quality care. An ideal staffing plan would provide the appropriate configuration of caregivers for patients based on data that predict the census. In addition, this same pattern would eliminate or minimize the problems of overstaffing or understaffing while providing flexibility for the individual needs of the staff members. Staffing is discussed in greater detail in Chapter 14.

Directing

Directing is a function of the manager that gets work done through others. Directing includes five specific concepts: *giving directions, supervising, leading, motivating,* and *communicating,* as described below:

1. Giving directions is the first activity and suggests that directions should be clear, concise, and consistent, and should conform to the requirements of the situation. The manager should be aware of the tone of the directive. Different types of situations require different emphasis. For example, an emergency situation calls for different inflections of voice than does a routine request. Whenever possible or appropriate, the reason for the directive should be given.

2. Supervising is concerned with the training and discipline of the work force. It also includes follow-up to ensure the prompt execution of orders. Fourteen qualities necessary for a highly successful supervisor were identified by Dr. Eugene Jennings of Michigan State University in his now classic work. A successful supervisor consistently demonstrates the following:

   a. Gives clear work orders; communicates well.
   b. Praises others when deserved.
   c. Is willing to take the time to listen.
   d. Remains cool and calm most of the time.
   e. Has confidence and self-assurance.
   f. Has appropriate technical knowledge of the work being supervised.
   g. Understands the group's problems.
   h. Gains the group's respect through personal honesty.
   i. Is fair to everyone.
   j. Demands good work from everyone.
   k. Gains the group's trust by representing their view to higher management.
   l. Goes "to bat" for the group.

   m. Is approachable, friendly, yet retains some distance.
   n. Is easy to talk to about concerns.[17]

3. Leading has been discussed in Chapters 2 and 3 as the ability to inspire and to influence others to the attainment of objectives.
4. Motivating is the set of skills the manager uses to help the employee to identify his or her needs and finds ways within the organization to help satisfy them. Motivation will be discussed in Chapter 10.
5. Communicating is the last activity and involves the what, how, who, and why of directives or effectively using the communication process. Communication was discussed in Chapter 3.

Coordinating

Coordinating is by definition the act of assembling and synchronizing people and activities so that they function harmoniously in the attainment of organizational objectives. In essence, coordination is a preventive managerial function concerned with heading off conflict and misunderstanding.

Think about the situations in your own life when you have had to coordinate the multiple activities for an important event. A school or community event involves the process of coordinating just as completely as formal managerial situations. The manager is aware of who is doing what and what the outcome should be and has the responsibility to make sure the specific and interrelated tasks are accomplished. This is not the easiest activity to accomplish, but accompanied by a thorough knowledge of the staff's responsibilities, the manager is in a good position to meet the appropriate goals.

Controlling

Controlling is the regulation of activities in accordance with plans. Controlling is a function of all managers at all levels. Its basic objective is to ensure that the task to be accomplished is appropriately executed. The three basic elements of control include *standards* that represent desired performance, *a comparison of actual results against the standard*, and, if necessary, *corrective action*.

■ STANDARDS

Sets of standards are available for the nursing profession to establish a standard for excellence. Standards for organized nursing services were developed

TABLE 7-1. THE STANDARDS FOR ORGANIZED NURSING SERVICE
AS DEVELOPED BY THE ANA

Standard I	The division of nursing has a philosophy and structure that ensure the delivery of high-quality nursing care and provide means for resolving nursing practice issues throughout the health care organization.
Standard II	The division of nursing is administered by a qualified nurse executive who is a member of corporate administration.
Standard III	Policies and practices of the division of nursing provide for equality and continuity of nursing service that recognize cultural, economic, and social differences among patients of the health care organization.
Standard IV	The division of nursing ensures that the nursing process is used to design and to provide nursing care to meet the individual needs of patients/clients in the context of their families.
Standard V	The division of nursing provides an environment that ensures the effectiveness of nursing practice.
Standard VI	The division of nursing ensures the development of educational programs to support the delivery of high-quality nursing care.
Standard VII	The division of nursing initiates, utilizes, and participates in research studies or projects for the improvement of patient care.

by the American Nurses' Association (ANA) Commission on Nursing Services to provide a framework for nurse managers and administrators.[18] These standards are exhibited in Table 7-1. These standards guide and direct nursing practice by the establishment of a professional and positive environment. In addition, the ANA developed standards for the different practice domains. For instance, the standards for cardiovascular nursing regulate, in a general way, what is expected of nurses caring for patients with cardiovascular problems. These standards serve as a general guide to focus attention on the important responsibilities entrusted to the nurse. The various sets of professional standards serve to facilitate control of nursing practice. In addition, individual organizations or institutions modify or elaborate on the expectations of a nurse's performance through institutional standards of nursing care. This is intended to make clear the expectations held for the professional nurse. This in turn facilitates the manager's function of control by knowing what is expected of the staff nurse's performance.

◼ POLICIES

Standards that deal specifically with conduct are sometimes referred to as policies. Within the organization, these policies are rules and regulations that regulate both broad and narrow aspects of an employee's position. The broad category includes the interpretation of legislation, or Labor Law, that impacts all employees, including nurses. Usually this kind of policy interpretation is handled through the legal/personnel department. Nursing as a profession is also subject to a nurse practice act that differs in wording from state to state but represents the legal boundaries for professional practice. Interpretation of this act by nursing administration committees with legal advice provides for general policies for nursing practice within institutions. Thus, the professional nurse who is employed in an organization is subject to general labor laws and to the state's professional nurse practice act.

The narrow aspects of what it is the professional nurse is expected to do is stated through the establishment of policies regarding nursing practice. These policies are derived from the profession's standards and the nurse practice act. Laws, standards, and policies are the basis for job descriptions and performance appraisal systems. Deviation from a stated, expected behavior alerts the manager to a problem. Since regulation of behavior is a part of management, control is exercised when the manager corrects the problem.

The functions of management are the skills the nurse manager uses to facilitate the mission, goals, and work of the organization. Management is a process, and as such knowledge and skills are developed over time. Throughout this text, information is provided that elaborates on these functions. However, head nurses and vice presidents of nursing make management come to life.

■ SYSTEMS OF NURSING CARE DELIVERY

Effective management makes the organization function, and the nursing manager of today has a heritage of nursing care delivery systems that demonstrate ways of organizing nursing's work. Within these systems are advantages and disadvantages for quality of care, use of resources, and staff growth. In reviewing the history of nursing, systems of nursing care delivery evolved from the existing social and professional environment of the time. Each nursing system was organized as a means of managing the delivery of care, and because these systems existed in an organizational setting with its various characteristics, management was an essential ingredient. These **systems of nursing care** are presented in chronological order, and though different, the systems share the unique perspective of nursing management that combines the concern for quality of care with the best use of available resources.

Case Method

The case method, traced back to Florence Nightingale, began in the early days of the nursing profession and was the convenient and appropriate way to manage care. Individuals were assigned to give total care to each patient, including the necessary medicines and treatments. The nurses reported to their immediate superior, who was the head nurse. The disadvantages of this system were that all personnel may not have been qualified to deliver all aspects of care, and depending on the structure, too many people were reporting to the head nurse (overextended span of control).

Functional Method

The functional method evolved as a way to deal with multiple levels of care-givers. Assignment of tasks rather than patients was the way in which care was provided. Each caregiver performed one certain task or function in keeping with the employee's education and experience. Nurse aides gave baths, fed patients, and took vital signs. Professional nurses were responsible for medications, treatments, and procedures. The head nurse was responsible for overall direction, supervision, and education of the nursing staff. The obvious problem with this system was the fragmentation of care. This complicated the process of coordination leading to reduction in the quality of care and a high level of dissatisfaction among the staff.

Team Nursing

A dramatic change occurred after World War II between 1943 and 1945. The level and number of auxiliary personnel began increasing, and the professional nurse was assuming more and more of the management functions. Because of the changing configuration of the work group and the dramatic social upheaval, a study was commissioned to devise a better way to provide nursing care. Dr. Eleanor Lambertson of Columbia University in New York and Francis Perkins of Massachusetts General Hospital were the authors of the system known as team nursing. Team nursing was developed to deal with the influx of postwar workers and the head nurse's overextended span of control. This was accomplished by arranging the workers in teams. The teams consisted of the senior professional nurse becoming the team leader; the members of the team were other registered nurses (RNs), licensed practical nurses (LPNs) or vocational nurses, and nurse aides and orderlies. Each was given a patient assignment in keeping with the employee's education and experience. The team leader made the assignments, delegated the work through the morning report, made rounds throughout the shift to make sure patients were being cared for properly, and conducted a team conference at the end of the shift to evaluate the patient care and plan and update nursing care plans. By 1950 team nursing was becoming a popular way to structure nursing care.

Team nursing was a pattern of patient care that involved changing the structural and organizational framework of the nursing unit. This method introduced the team concept for the stated aim of using all levels of personnel to their fullest capacity in giving the best possible nursing care to patients. The structural and organizational changes necessary for this method included the introduction of the nursing team with the team leader assuming responsibility for the management of patient care. The head nurse decentralized authority to the team leader to direct the activities of the team members. The head nurse was no longer the center of all communication on the division because the members communicated directly with the team leader. The team leader had the responsibility for synchronizing the abilities of her team members so that they were able to function effectively in a team relationship. Emphasis was placed on the ability of all participants of patient care to plan, administer, and evaluate patient care.

The team approach to patient care represented more than a reorganization or restructuring of nursing service. Instead it was a philosophy of nursing and a method of organizing patient care. This particular model was widely used and, as all models, was adapted for individual organizations. The difficulty with this method was the nurse's absence at the bedside; the nurse was directing the care of others and thus not using nursing's specialized knowledge as the best provider of patient care. Problems with this system became the stimulus for a new system.

Primary Nursing

Primary nursing as a system of care provided for quality comprehensive patient care and a framework for the development of professional practice among the nursing staff. Primary nursing was a logical next step in nursing's historic evolution. By definition, primary nursing is a philosophy and structure that places responsibility and accountability for the planning, giving, communicating, and evaluating of care for a group of patients in the hands of the primary nurse. Primary nursing was intended to return the nurse to the bedside, thus improving the quality of care and increasing the job satisfaction of the nursing staff.

Definitions related to primary nursing are:

- *Primary nursing*—the hospital unit organization and philosophy that places on the RN responsibility and accountability for the planning, giving, communicating, and evaluating of care for a caseload of patients.
- *Primary care*—the community contact by a patient seeking entrance to the health care system. He or she may see a physician, nurse practitioner, dentist, etc. and have his or her care given in the office or clinic or be referred into a hospital.
- *Primary nurse*—an RN, usually full time, who is assigned specific patients to whom he or she will provide primary nursing care during their stay in the unit.
- *Associate or secondary nurse*—any nurse caring for patients whose primary nurse if off duty; he or she provides total, 8-hour care.
- *Total care*—the provision of all professional nursing care needed by the patient during an 8-hour shift. This includes medications, treatments, hygienic and comfort measures, teaching, support, charting, reporting, and changing the care plan if necessary.

The basic concepts of primary nursing include fixed, visible accountability of the nurse for the care of assigned cases and inclusion of the patient in his or her own care. The primary nurse is expected to give total care, to establish therapeutic relationships, to plan for 24-hour continuity in nursing care through a written nursing care plan, to communicate directly with other members of the health team, and to plan for discharge. The patient's participation is expected in the planning, implementing, and evaluating of his or her own care. Perhaps the best aspect of primary nursing is the improved communication provided by the one-to-one relationship between nurse and patient. Associate nurses are involved with this method by caring for the patients in the absence of the primary nurse. Their responsibilities include continuing the care initiated by the primary nurse and making necessary modifications. It is conceivable that the primary nurse for a group of patients may be an associate nurse for other patients. The role played by the professional nurse is determined by the assignment of patients, which is made by the front-line manager or head nurse.

Primary nursing was adapted in organizations to fit the staffing patterns and general nursing philosophy. Because of the need for a high percentage of professional nurses, other modifications of the system were developed, such as modular nursing. See Table 7-2 for the responsibilities of the primary and associate nurses.

TABLE 7-2. RESPONSIBILITIES OF THE PRIMARY AND ASSOCIATE NURSES IN THE PRIMARY NURSING MODEL

Primary	Associate

1. Patient and family teaching
  • Carries out necessary aspects of patient care
  • Delegates and ensures continuity through care plan
  • Documents, evaluates, changes plan
2. Nursing care plan
  • Assesses patient initially and continually to write care plan
  • Updates, evaluates effects of care
  • Confers with staff if they do not follow through
  • Receptive to peer advice
3. Collaboration with physician
  • Seeks to be on physician rounds as possible
  • Knows current medical plan
  • Can intervene for patient when his or her goals conflict with medical goals
	1. Patient and family teaching
	  • Provides patient education because of patient need or through delegation by the care plan
	  • Reinforces plan of primary nurse
	  • Advises primary nurse on changes
	2. Nursing care plan
	  • Follows suggestions of primary nurse
	  • Changes plan when condition warrants
	  • When in conflict with controversial directives, discusses with primary nurse; may follow primary nurse's orders and then evaluate.
	3. Collaboration with physician
	  • Refers primary nurse's concerns to physician
	  • Answers physician's questions about daily status of patient
	  • Plans with physician when changes in patient care are necessary in the absence of primary nurse

Modular Nursing

Modular nursing is not a response to inadequacies in primary nursing but rather a practical way to combine primary and team nursing. It is a way of dealing with inadequate staffing for primary nursing. It involves the assignment of patients to nurses by geographic location, usually 8 or 12 patients, and uses the services of a variety of health care providers such as LPNs and nursing aides or assistants. This is a practical solution to deal with a scarcity of nurses.

Case Management

More recently a new method of nursing care delivery has evolved known as case management. The ANA has defined case management to be a system of health assessment, planning, service procurement and delivery, coordination, and monitoring to meet the multiple service needs of clients.[19] Case management systems address the potential mismatch between client needs, services offered, and increasingly limited health care resources.[20] This system provides care that minimizes fragmentation and maximizes individualized care, as well as an all-inclusive and comprehensive model, not restricted to the hospital setting. The model may be operationalized in a variety of ways, but the usual approach involves a case manager in a matrix organizational structure who follows a caseload of patients according to a specialized plan. When a patient deviates from the usual expected course of recovery or health, consultation ensues to quickly correct the problem. This requires a great deal of systematic knowledge about a patient's problems and putting that knowledge into a type of nursing care plan (case management plans) with time lines to demonstrate progress or deviations from the critical paths. This particular system of care has been used for many years in the public health domain and recently has been introduced into the acute care institution. What is so exciting about this concept is that it builds on the primary nursing model and improves on its efficiency. It retains the accountability and responsibility of the professional nurse but creates a more orderly way of evaluating the patient's response to therapies. It goes without saying that in this age of financial concern, this system, with its built-in radar, prevents or recognizes complications and identifies costly problems for earlier treatment.

The organizational and structural configuration of case management involves the following:

- *Case manager*—a nurse responsible for evaluating care of patients.
- *Care plan*—composed of (1) critical paths, (2) objectives of care, and (3) time lines.
- *Evaluation of variance*—if the patient varies from critical path, a report is made to reduce the impact of the complication.

The head nurse or unit leader, as the *case manager*, directs the actions of subordinates to provide managed care to a group of patients. The case manager functions are:

- Establish rapport and trust with patient/family
- Collects comprehensive assessment data including:
    Physical status
    Mental status
    Emotional status
    Family, community, and financial resources
- Communicates problem statements to appropriate sources
- Develop a plan of care in collaboration with patient, family, and other health care workers

- Establishes goals and objectives
- Considers cost containment
- Intervenes/monitors delivery of care
- Achieves case coordination
- Makes referrals/provides follow-up care
- Assesses/monitors patient outcomes

The group of patients is subject to an ongoing and comprehensive evaluation involving multiple services known as a *care plan*. The care plan is based on accumulated data and is presented as *critical paths* that determine the ideal patient reaction. In addition to the nursing and medical services that are required for patients, other services are included, such as physical therapy and respiratory therapy. These services are identified according to what most patients experience at every critical point of their hospitalization, rehabilitation, or stage of illness. Since the care plan includes the usual reaction of patients to all interventions by all essential services according to critical paths with *time lines*, the staff nurse recognizes deviations quickly. The case manager is notified, and appropriate interventions are initiated. The comprehensive plan that is used as the source of evaluation is constructed by representatives from the various services. This particular system requires cooperation and teamwork from the practitioners and is capable of ensuring quality care and cost effectiveness. Using the individual practitioner's knowledge and skill is a way of building professional autonomy.[21]

In all the named systems for the delivery of nursing care, consideration for the quality of care and resource utilization remains the underlying motivation for the nurse manager. Elements of the positive qualities in the early systems were retained, and the problematic or negative aspects of the preceding model usually was the impetus for the development of a new system.

Transition to Manager

The transition from a staff member to a manager requires the assumption of authority. There is inherent complexity in an authority role that is unique.[22] By assuming authority, the manager is the custodian of the mission, traditions, rules, and responsibility associated with the organization. Thus, the manager is able to make decisions over subordinates' time, assignments, and all other aspects of work. Since there is a potential for confusion or conflict among the subordinates, the manager facilitates the individual and group to meeting stated objectives. The manner in which the manager chooses to keep the group on track may vary from individual to individual and from situation to situation. This responsibility to maintain order differentiates the manager from the staff, and herein lies the real issue. The staff's reaction to the manager will be reflective of the staff's confidence that they will be able to control their decisions and work.

The new manager may face situations very differently than an experienced manager. The behavior of some staff members may be critical, protective, or hostile. New managers should avoid the tendency to take this as a personal assault; rather, they should understand this is defensive behavior aimed to maintain personal control of the work or work related activities.

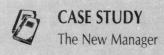

CASE STUDY
The New Manager

Mary Jones, the new clinical director of a coronary care step-down unit has noticed that some of the staff members have been behaving in negative ways. Mrs. Green has been very sarcastic in interactions with Mary. Mrs. Green had competed for the role of clinical director and was very disappointed not to receive the promotion.

Mary has also noted that some of the older employees are acting strange. They are excluding her from social conversations, and suggesting "they hope things don't change around here."

In addition, Mary has overheard people compare her to the previous director, who had been in the position for ten years and was well-liked and respected. Mary felt she was capable of fulfilling the new role, but knew she had to deal with the individual reactions of the group.

- How should Mary deal with jealousy? Competition? Resentment? Managing older employees? Comparisons to a previous manager?

Suggestions to manage these problems include:

- Review communication techniques and conflict-resolution strategies. (Remember: ignore what isn't important, and that mature, disciplined behavior and emotional control will strengthen self-confidence. In situations where new leaders are being challenged, simply because of their newness, temper any response with a non-answer and don't provoke further argument. This demonstrates emotional control and distance from the attack. Where possible, use the challenging person's experience, talent, or help, and follow up with public praise.)

TABLE 7-3. THE ESSENTIAL ELEMENTS A MANAGER SHOULD CONSIDER WHEN ANALYZING A MANAGEMENT SITUATION. THESE ELEMENTS HAVE BEEN SUMMARIZED IN THE MANAGERIAL ASSESSMENT TOOL.

- External environment: What factors impact the current situation?
  - Identify regulatory bodies such as laws, professional standards, and government regulations.
  - Identify stability or volatility in the external environment that may impact on the current situation.
  - Identify relevant characteristics of the environment:
    Geographic and cultural considerations
    Population dynamics
    Political and financial dynamics
- Internal organizational characteristics
  - Identify the boundaries of the unit of analysis.
  - Identify the existing climate of the unit of analysis.
  - Identify the nursing care system being used.
  - Identify the staffing pattern for the organization and the specific area.
- Mission and goals
  - Identify the general goal and structure of what is to be accomplished.
- Manager and employee relationship
  - Identify the participants, clients, or patients and personnel.
  - Identify formal and informal goals of the organization and the participants.
  - Identify the employees: education, experience, and level of performance.
- Resources
  - Identify the necessary resources, both human and nonhuman.
- Barriers
  - Identify possible barriers to the completion of the work: time, insufficient or inadequate resources, inadequate ratio of patient/personnel.

■ MANAGEMENT ASSESSMENT GUIDE

Nursing models provide the nurse manager with a way of organizing the work of nursing, but the manager still is faced with the complexities of the modern health care institution. Despite uncertainties in the workplace, it is still possible to be an extremely effective manager. It requires taking into account the essential elements of the managerial situation and using the appropriate management function and skill. The managerial situation consists of relevant factors in the greater social and organizational environment as well as the immediate situation. Factors in the manager and employees that enhance or inhibit the achievement of goals also must be built into the equation. For the manager to be truly effective, information must be available to use the various resources properly. The Managerial Assessment Guide presented in Table 7-3 is offered to highlight those essential variables that will focus on meeting managerial goals. In conclusion, for a manager to manage there must be an assessment of the work and adequacy of the personnel and resources to provide prepared employees in the proper ratio. Once an assessment has been made, the proper managerial decision and plan can be made. The subsequent chapters will detail what the nursing manager does and will provide some suggestions to facilitate modern-day nursing management.

■ SUMMARY

This chapter has presented an overview of the management process. The management process is a specific form of problem solving that enables the manager to make wise decisions concerning the use of resources and to supervise staff for the purpose of meeting goals. Functions of management include planning, organizing, staffing, supervising, directing, coordinating, and controlling. Systems of nursing care are organizational frameworks to structure the work of nursing and are facilitated by the role of a nursing manager. To allow a thorough assessment of the managerial situation, a Managerial Assessment Guide (Table 7-3) is offered to focus on the essential factors providing information for a proper managerial decision.

 STUDENT EXERCISES

1. Early in the chapter, nursing management was differentiated from professional management on the basis of a general philosophic position. Develop a position for nursing service. State simply, but clearly, why your nursing department exists.

2. Develop a managerial orientation including a course outline of what the nurse manager needs to know.

3. Divide the class into three groups. Have each group represent a different level of management. Give each group time to devise a plan that would reflect the type of planning expected at each level.

4. Observe a manager using the functions of management. Think about what it is the manager does while performing each of the following: (1) directing, (2) coordinating, and (3) controlling.

5. Take a real-life situation from your current clinical agency and apply the managerial assessment tool to identify relevant information. Select a management decision that you think would be best.

■ REFERENCES

1. Drucker PF, *Management, Tasks, Responses, Practices*, New York: Harper & Row, 1990.
2. Kreitner R, *Management*, 6th ed., Boston, Toronto: Houghton Mifflin Co., 1995, p. 5–7.
3. McGregor D, *The Human Side of Enterprise*, New York: McGraw-Hill, 1960.
4. Herzberg F, "One More Time: How Do You Motivate Employees?" *Harvard Bus Rev*, vol. 65, 1987, p. 109–120.
5. Argyris C, *Integrating the Individual and the Organization*. New York: Wiley, 1964.
6. Likert R, *New Patterns of Management*, New York: McGraw-Hill, 1961.
7. Volk MC, Lucas MD, "Relationship of Management Style and Anticipated Turnover," *Dimensions of Critical Care*, 10:1, January-February, 1991, p. 35–40.
8. Peters TJ, Waterman RH, *In Search of Excellence*, New York: Harper and Row, 1982.
9. Ibid., p. 13.
10. McClure M, "Managing the Professional Nurse," *J Nurs Admin*, February 1984, p. 15–19.
11. Peterson AA, "The Changing Management Role: Autocratic Doer to Team Facilitator," *Seminars for Nurse Managers*, 2:4, 1994, p. 209–212.
12. Ibid., p. 210.
13. Ibid.
14. Adapted from Tannenbaum R, Schmidt W, "How To Choose a Leadership Pattern," *Harvard Business Review*, 1965, p. 121.
15. Curtain L, "Strategic Planning, Asking the Right Questions," *Nursing Management*, 22:1, 1991, p. 7–8.
16. Schull DE, Tosch P, Wood M, "Clinical Nurse Specialists as Collaborative Care Managers," *Nursing Management*, March, 1992, p. 30–33.
17. Jennings EE, "The Anatomy of Leadership," *Management of Personnel Quarterly*, 1:1, Autumn 1961, p. 213.
18. American Nurses Association Commission on Nursing Service, *Standards for Organized Nursing Services*, Kansas City, MO: ANA, 1982.
19. American Nurses Association. *Case Management*, Kansas City, MO: ANA, 1988.
20. Strong A, "Case Management and the CNS," *Clinical Nurse Specialist*, April 1992, p. 64.
21. Sterling Y, Noto EC, Bowen MR, "Case Management Roles of Clinicians: A Research Study," *Clinical Nurse Specialist*, 8:4, 1994, p. 196–201.
22. Schmeidling NJ, "The Complexity of an Authority Role," *Nursing Management*, 23:11, 1993, p. 57–58.

8

Delegation
The Manager's Tool

Introduction

Every organization, from a multipurpose institution to a small health care clinic, exists to do work. This work is coordinated and executed through the different efforts of individuals who have the responsibility to make sure the various and diverse aspects of the work are completed. Delegation is the link that joins organizational concepts with the management process; it is that which allows a manager to manage. This chapter will deal with the specialized management activity of delegation.

KEY CONCEPTS

Delegation is the process of entrusting or assigning responsibility and authority to members of the organization.

Responsibility is the inward obligation to perform so that the entire organization benefits.

Authority is the right to give orders and power to exact obedience.

Accountability is the process of furnishing a justifying analysis or explanation for behavior/actions of self or subordinates.

Scalar Chain is the vertical line of authority within the organization from the chief executive to subordinates depicted in the organization chart.

Decentralization is the delegation of authority away from the central office to the operating units.

■ DELEGATION

Delegation is the use of personnel to accomplish a desired objective through allocation of authority and responsibility (Fig. 8-1). Delegation is the process that facilitates complex organizations to accomplish work through the coordinated and differentiated efforts of others, and it is the manager who uses the process of delegation. Delegation is pivotal to organizational dynamics because it is the direct outcome of planning and results in a system of differentiation of labor. Thus, it involves the assignment of work and the giving of orders, enabling the manager to operationalize the plan of the organization through the staff.[1]

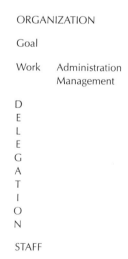

ORGANIZATION

Goal

Work   Administration
          Management

D
E
L
E
G
A
T
I
O
N

STAFF

Figure 8-1. Graphic depiction of delegation as the process that links the organization with work and with the staff.

Much of a manager's success is dependent on the efforts of the team, or how work is assigned, and delegated. New managers can learn the art of skillful delegation. Experience has shown a remarkable capacity in people at all levels of the organization to shoulder responsibility and to get results. The best way to ensure organizational effectiveness is to delegate appropriate authority to the lowest level of employee. The proper use of delegation is an important tool for staff participation that will build morale.

Assignment of Work

The organizational structure is a formal plan for arranging people in order according to their authority and responsibility to achieve defined objectives. A closer look at responsibility will shed light on understanding the conceptual basis of delegation. **Responsibility** is dependent on three coexisting concepts: **authority,** delegation, and **accountability** (Fig. 8-2). For example, if a manager is given responsibility for a task, the manager will delegate the responsibility and the necessary authority to the appropriate employee. In turn, the employee is accountable to the delegator for completing the task satisfactorily. Accountability is the process of furnishing a justifying explanation for behavior of self or for others.

The delegator or manager, however, does not give up all responsibility but retains overall responsibility and authority consistent with the manager's position. What this means is that a manager at a higher level of the organization is willing to accept and to support the decisions and actions of others lower in the organization. The manager remains accountable for those below to superiors of the manager. Delegation is not a system to reduce responsibility but for making it meaningful. The process of delegation based on the above-related concepts forms the basis for the assignment of work throughout the entire organization.

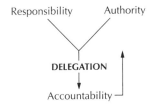

Figure 8-2. Graphic illustration of the relationship among responsibility, authority, delegation, and accountability by demonstrating the direction each takes in an organization.

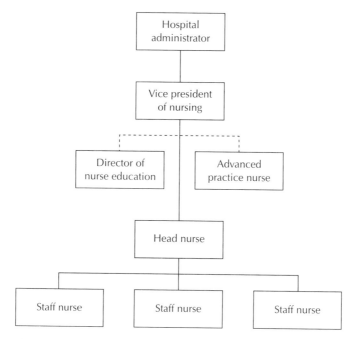

Figure 8-3. The scalar chain of authority depicted through the vertical lines on the organization chart.

The Scalar Chain

In classical management theory, the line of authority from the top on down is referred to as the **scalar chain.** It is illustrated on the organizational chart in the form of vertical lines that link the level of manager with subordinates and clearly shows the divisions of responsibility, from the broad total responsibility of the administrator to the specific responsibility of personnel in a given department. This also represents line authority, or the direct relationship of a superior to a subordinate. This is in contrast to staff relationships that are consultative or advisory. See Figure 8-3 to illustrate the scalar chain.

To exemplify, a head nurse, who is responsible for all patient care on a particular unit, cannot possibly perform all that is required for the group of patients. Thus, the head nurse delegates responsibility to the appropriate caregivers to do what is necessary for the patients as well as the necessary authority to enforce the specialized functions. The head nurse who has the legitimate right to give directives provides an opportunity for professional nurses to give care. The caregiver now has an obligation to perform. The major rule of delegation is that authority and responsibility must be delegated equally. The staff nurse, who accepts the responsibility, is accountable to the head nurse not only for what has been accomplished but also for the methods used to deliver care. In the scalar chain, authority and responsibility flow downward and accountability moves upward.

Decentralization

When delegation occurs on the face-to-face manager-to-employee level, it is referred to as general supervision. When delegation occurs on the organizational level, it involves giving more autonomy to subunits and is called **decentralization.** The movement in health care toward decentralization has occurred due to the reduction of managers and the goal to empower professionals at the operative level. Authority is delegated as a way of increasing productivity and managing cost.

Currently, decentralization is occurring downward and outward in health care organizations. Decentralization is often termed *horizontal management* because it aims to flatten the hierarchical organization structure and allows the staff nurse the opportunity to take more initiative and to become more autonomous. The practical result of this practice has been to eliminate or to reduce middle management and to give the front-line manager more authority and responsibility.

The Purpose of Delegation

The proper use of delegation serves a variety of purposes. Among them are a means for promoting internalized motivation and job enrichment by giving employees a sense of being his or her own boss through the opportunity to exercise control over his or her work. Some of the other reasons for the use of delegation include: *cost savings, time savings, professional growth for employees,* and *professional growth of the manager.*

Cost Savings. Cost-saving strategies are being used by literally every health care organization today. The easiest and most efficient way to save on cost is to use resources properly, which ensures that the right person is doing the right work. This simply means that the manager should manage and the professional nurses should provide the nursing care. Managers are expected to increase the overall efficiency of their division. This cannot be accomplished if the manager is doing the work of the staff.

Time Savings. In the same vein, *time* is another commodity that will be conserved if the manager allocates time and uses it properly for the general direction of the staff. The converse is true for the staff; time is best used when tailored to meet the individual's workload requirements.

Professional Growth for Employees. Increasing the self esteem of employees is an important reason to use the process of delegation. *Personal and professional growth* is expected as personnel experience the development of their talents and abilities by taking pride in the results of their efforts. This comes about in response to the decisions they have made. For the most part, it is difficult to expect people to take the risk of decision making without putting them in a position to make decisions. Delegation provides the opportunity to make decisions, and the employees' decisions are reflected in the outcome.

Delegation, by its very nature, allows the subordinate to make decisions that might result in mistakes. To minimize the possibility of serious error, the manager must use all aspects of the management process (in particular assessment of staff capability). Growth can occur in either case, however, and mistakes can sometimes lead to even greater professional change. Other advantages for the employees include the possibility that the subordinates' sense of responsibility and autonomy will grow, thereby enlarging the employees' sense of leadership, job satisfaction, and knowledge of organizational goals.

Professional Growth of the Manager. Effective and successful delegation centers around effective manager and staff relationships. The personal relationships that exist influence the work result. For example, the manager is accountable for certain results and gives permission to the staff members to perform part of the work and to take certain action. There are growing and shifting relationships between the manager and staff; the freedom and initiative exercised by the staff varies and cannot be spelled out in explicit detail. Thus, work habits and attitudes can be influenced by the interplay with the manager. In facilitating the staff's growth, the manager is truly fulfilling a major responsibility of the manager's role.

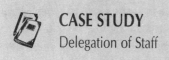

CASE STUDY
Delegation of Staff

Bob Jones is the 3 to 11 P.M. charge nurse at General Hospital's coronary care step-down unit. Due to a computer glitch, the staffing pattern for the institution became a nightmare: not enough RNs were assigned to care for the patients in the ratio Bob preferred to provide quality care.

At the beginning of the shift, Bob called his coworkers and explained the staffing problem and the reason for it. Due to the computer problem, the float pool was also unavailable, so Bob proceeded to rearrange the usual assignments. He delegated functional tasks to the LPNs and reorganized the assignments for the RNs to maximize his staff and to provide quality of care.

Following the shift, Bob met with his coworkers for feedback. They were very positive and appreciated Bob's solution.

- What would you have done?
- Did Bob have the right to change the pattern of care delivery and to reorganize the work of the unit?

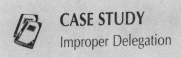

CASE STUDY
Improper Delegation

In all fields, different level employees have different tasks to do. For the nursing assistant, typical duties include giving bed baths, serving meal trays, checking vital signs, and completing a variety of other important tasks. Registered nurses, on the other hand, are expected to assess the patients, determine nursing care, delegate tasks to nonprofessional employees, and supervise their work. As in all cases, the nurse is ultimately responsible for the care received by patients.

With this in mind, consider the following situation: Jane Newnurse RN, BSN, accepted a position in a skilled nursing facility and was expected to work with nursing assistants. On her first day, Mrs. Oldtimer, an experienced nursing assistant, and Jane were to work together. Jane began giving Mrs. Oldtimer a report, when she was interrupted. Mrs. Oldtimer said that she would not complete her assignment because, Jane, as a new nurse, needed to have experience. When Mrs. Oldtimer was sure Jane was proficient with the work, then and then only could she accept an assignment. In essence, Jane was told by the nursing assistant, she had to do the work of an RN and nursing assistant.

Jane was overcome with anger and confusion. She wasn't sure what to do. She replied, "I am ultimately responsible for the nursing care of your patients and mine. I would like to share the work with you. I cannot possibly comply with your suggestion. If you have concerns about my ability to provide nursing care, please feel free to discuss them with me, after you have completed the assignment I am delegating to you. Since we are going to work together, we need to understand each other."

- What is your analysis of this situation?
- What would you have done?
- How does understanding the process of delegation assist in conflict resolution?

The Process of Delegation

The process of delegation is predominantly results-oriented. The delegator or nurse manager makes relatively few decisions alone but frames orders in broad, general terms, allowing the subordinate to work out the details of the work. The delegator or manager does the following:

- Sets goals
- Tells subordinates what is to be accomplished
- Fixes the limits within which the subordinate can work in accord with job descriptions and the job assignment
- Allows employees to decide how to achieve goals

The process of delegation allows the manager to assign responsibility, give authority, and create accountability within the subordinate. All three aspects of the process of delegation involve a degree of risk that necessitates the manager to know an employee's ability and to plan a program to increase his or her skill and knowledge levels. Successful managers systematically plan for delegation by determining what kinds of tasks can be delegated, who is ready to assume additional tasks, what assistance is needed, and what outcomes are expected. These managers view delegation as a means of helping their staff achieve their own objectives for growth and development.[2]

Guidelines for Effective Delegation

For the beginning manager, some guidelines are offered to help when delegating to employees:

- Give a clear description of what it is you want the employee to do. Describe the overall scope and background of the current task. Give the reason for the assignment, and tell the employee if other departments or people are involved to achieve the desired outcome. If there are special problems, share this information with the employee.
- Share with the employee the outcome you expect and by when.

- Discuss the degree of responsibilities and authority that the employee will have.
- Ask the employee to summarize the main points of the delegated task.
- Know what cannot be delegated. This includes confidential matters, contractual responsibilities, discipline of the workforce, and ultimate responsibility for the work output.

As an example, you are the head nurse of a busy step-down unit of cardiac surgery patients. Your division is well-staffed with registered nurses (RNs), and you feel it is time to give additional responsibility to your charge nurse. To use the appropriate guidelines, your conversation might go something like this:

> Sharon, I need help with the orientation of our new staff members, and I would like you to take on this new responsibility. The orientation process is one month long, but if you could shorten that period, it would be very helpful. The new nurses need the information in the orientation manual, but feel free to use your own ingenuity to help them gain information. Their work will be evaluated at two-, and four-week intervals. In addition, I think you would find it helpful to learn the orientation program that we are currently using. I will make arrangements for you to attend such sessions. You will have the authority to advise the employees of their positive performance and discuss with them areas of improvement. I feel confident that you will be able to do this very well, and I will be available for any questions you might have. Do you have any questions now? Would you please share with me your understanding of this new and important responsibility?

The delegator explains the task to an assistant by giving all the necessary information so that the task can be completed appropriately. In addition, the delegator delegates the necessary authority to accompany the responsibility. By delegating to the staff, the manager is helping them to develop their talents.

Barriers to Delegation

Often managers are reluctant to delegate. Some of the common reasons for failure to adequately delegate vary from manager to manager. Some of these reasons are as follows:

- *"I can do it better myself" fallacy.*
  It has been found that nursing personnel with high standards of performance naturally are tempted to perform any activity that they can do

better themselves. A nurse manager must reconcile turning over the task to someone whose performance will be "good enough." The comparison is not between the quality of work, but the *benefits* to the total operation when the manager devotes attention to planning and supervision, which only the manager may do. Only after the manager accepts the idea that the work gets done through other people will the manager be able to make full use of delegation.

• *Lack of ability to direct.*
The manager must be able to communicate to the staff, often in advance, what is to be done. This means that the manager must (1) think ahead and visualize the work situation, (2) formulate objectives and general plans of action, and (3) communicate to the assistants. In essence, the manager must identify and communicate the essential features of the work plan. All too often administrative personnel have not cultivated this ability to direct.

• *Lack of confidence in staff.*
To remedy this situation, either education through staff development or programs should be offered to help the employee to improve on the performance problem or to help the employee to find the proper role in the organization.

• *Absence of controls that warn of impending difficulties.*
Care must be taken that the control system does not undermine the very essence of delegation. The nurse manager cannot completely delegate responsibility unless the manager has confidence in the controls.

• *Aversion to taking a risk.*
The manager may be handicapped by a temperamental aversion to taking a risk. The greater the number of subordinates and the higher the degree of delegation, the more likely it is that sooner or later there will be trouble. The manager who delegates takes a calculated risk. Over a period of time the manager may expect that the gains from delegation will far offset the troubles that arise.

In addition to managers having problems with delegations, staff members may also have some difficulty accepting responsibility. Some of the more common reasons offered are as follows:

• *Easier to ask the "boss."*
The staff may find it easier to ask the manager than to decide how to deal with a problem. For some, making a wise decision may be hard

work. Making one's own decision carries with it responsibility for the outcome. Asking the boss is one way of shifting or sharing this burden. This is known as upward delegation.

- *Fear of criticism.*
The fear of criticism for mistakes keeps some people from accepting greater responsibilities. A great deal depends upon the nature of the criticism. Negative criticism may be resented, whereas a constructive review might be accepted.

- *Lack of necessary information and resources.*
A belief that employees lack the necessary information and resources makes effective delegation difficult. The frustration that accompanies inadequate information and resources creates an attitude that might convince the staff person to reject further assignments.

- *May have more work than the employee can now do.*
If the employee feels overburdened, he or she will probably shy away from new assignments that call for thinking and initiative.

- *Lack of self-confidence.*
Lack of self-confidence stands in the way of some people accepting responsibility. A staff person who is unsure of his or her ability does not like to assume more responsibility. Self-confidence must be developed by carefully providing experience in increasingly difficult problems.

- *Positive incentives may be inadequate.*
Accepting more responsibility requires more mental work and emotional pressure. Positive inducements for accepting delegated responsibilities include access to better personnel policies, opportunity for advancements, more desirable working conditions, prestigious title, recognized status in the organization, or other rewards.

Barriers to delegation can be overcome, but the first step is to understand the nature of the problem and how willing the manager or employee is to deal with the problem. The critical issue in delegation is decentralization of authority, and depending on the manager's attitude, delegation will be a productive activity or a frustrating experience. Effective management recognizes the strengths and capabilities of the staff and uses this talent appropriately. You, the new manager, in this dynamic health care system have the capability of transforming the work place into an area where employees can be autonomous and challenged through effective delegation.

■ SUMMARY

Delegation is an extremely important process that the effective manager must learn to skillfully handle. Delegation exists because the manager's personal responsibility exceeds the capacity to perform the necessary work. Ideally the manager should concentrate on what is expected of a manager and delegate those activities that the staff is qualified to perform. Despite barriers to the process of delegation, guidelines are offered to facilitate the new manager's ability to delegate successfully.

 STUDENT EXERCISES

1. Identify three tasks or projects that a vice president of nursing and a head nurse might wish to delegate to their subordinates. Are the tasks different? If so, why are they different?

2. From your clinical practice, observe and identify how the nurse managers delegate. Note the process and techniques that an effective delegator uses. Notice the same when ineffective delegation is used.

3. List three tasks that you would consider easy to delegate and three that you would consider difficult. Would you use the same technique for both?

4. How does delegation relate to the leadership process? the management process and organizational dynamics?

■ REFERENCES

1. Kreitner R, *Management*, 6th ed, Boston, Toronto: Houghton Mifflin Co, 1995, p. 316–318.
2. Frohman AL, Johnson L, *The Middle Management Challenge: Moving from Crisis to Empowerment*, New York: McGraw Hill, 1993.

■ SUGGESTED READING

Wick J, Calhoun W, Lu Stanton L. *The Learning Edge: How Smart Managers and Smart Companies Stay Ahead*, New York: McGraw Hill, 1993.

UNIT 3

Special Responsibilities of the Manager

9

Maintaining Standards

Introduction

Managers of patient care units are concerned with the delivery of comprehensive care that is beneficial to the patients. These managers are required to know the care contributions and the practice boundaries of each of the health care practitioners who come in contact with the patients. Most patient care units, especially those in long-term care and hospitals, are primarily nursing labor-intensive (persons assigned to work are nurses, patient care associates, nurses' aides, or licensed practical nurses).

The boundaries of work for different health care practitioners are established on the basis of an intricate framework composed of professional, societal, ethical, governmental, legal, and organizational inputs. At first glance, to act within such a complex set of norms, values, and regulations seems difficult; and to direct and guide others within this same framework seems even more so. Specifically, the integration of this framework exists for the maintenance of quality. The focus of this chapter is the professional and legal bases for the maintenance of standards that ensure quality nursing care. Other regulating bodies such as the federal and state governments are presented to show the forces that affect the boundaries of nursing practice.

KEY CONCEPTS

Accreditation refers to the approval of an organization by an official review board after having met specific standards.

Answerability is a matter of legal or ethical responsibility.

Certification is a process by which a nongovernmental agency or association certifies that an individual licensed to practice a profession has met certain predetermined standards specified by that profession for specialty practice. Its purpose is to assure the public that an individual has mastered a body of knowledge and acquired skills in a particular specialty.

Criteria refers to predetermined elements, qualities, or characteristics used to measure the extent to which a standard is met.

Incident Report is a written record of an event with possible or real untoward effects.

Indicator is an aspect of health care process or outcome that signals whether or not the appropriate interventions were provided.

Liability is the condition of legal risk due to the obligation of professional personnel obliged to provide reasonable care.

Malpractice refers to negligence, carelessness, or deviation from an accepted standard of practice by a professional.

Monitoring is observing and evaluating the degree to which a standard has been achieved.

Negligence is the carelessness or failure to act as a prudent person would ordinarily act under the same circumstances.

Outcomes Management is a management approach that focuses on the interrelatedness of clinical concerns of quality with cost effectiveness of care.

Performance Standards are specific written statements of nursing behaviors that further define what a nurse in a specific area of nursing should be doing; derived from standards of nursing care.

Practice Guidelines are standardized specifications developed through a process that uses the best scientific evidence and expert opinion for care of the typical patient in the typical situation.

Problems are questions or situations relating to patient care that are raised for inquiry, consideration, or resolution.

Quality is "The degree to which patient care services increase the probability of desired patient outcomes and reduce the probability of undesired outcomes given the current state of knowledge." (JCAHO)

Quality Management is a management approach that consists of systematic, ongoing monitoring and constructive actions to improve the quality of practice.

Registration is a process by which qualified individuals are listed on an official roster maintained by a governmental or nongovernmental agency. It enables such persons to use a particular title and attests to employing agencies and individuals that minimum qualifications have been met and maintained.

Risk Management is the function of planning, organizing, and directing a comprehensive program of activities to identify, evaluate, and take corrective action against risks that may lead to patient injury, employee injury, and property loss or damage with resulting financial loss.

Standards are agreed-upon levels of excellence; established norms.

Standards of Nursing Practice are written statements of the expectations of the care the nurse should give; process standards.

Standards of Patient/Client Care are written statements of expectations of the care the patient should receive (or results of care received); outcome standards.

Structure Standards are written statements addressing the organization's culture (i.e., the mission, philosophy, goals, and policies).

■ THE CLIMATE FOR NURSING PRACTICE

Each component of regulation adds a different dimension toward the maintenance of **quality** in nursing practice (Fig. 9-1). To begin, society recognizes the need for nursing's contribution, ultimately legitimizing nursing as a service profession and in turn requiring **answerability.** Professional standards guide appropriate nursing practice and to some extent are modified within specific organizations. A legal framework exists that grants nurses the right to practice through each state's nursing practice act. The government has a general responsibility for the health of its citizens and thus provides federal and state rules and regulations regarding health care delivery. For example,

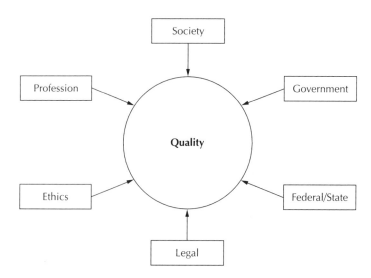

Figure 9-1. The variety of forces that create the climate for the establishment of standards of practice that ensure quality patient care.

hospitals must meet specified standards, which include the number of beds they possess.

The nursing profession is subject to these rules and regulations. Ethical standards rooted in professional, organizational, and personal values give another dimension to the boundaries of nursing practice. This chapter deals with these regulatory bodies in order for the student to formulate an approach to management. The factors cited formulate the boundaries of professional practice and thus quality assessment.

■ PROFESSIONAL BASIS FOR QUALITY ASSURANCE

Professional nurses have a responsibility and accountability, as well as answerability, for their professional actions. This necessitates the establishment of *standards of practice* to make an appropriate judgment as to what constitutes professional nursing practice. A **standard** is an agreed-upon level of excellence, or an established norm. In addition to a set of standards, **criteria** are also necessary. Criteria are predetermined elements or qualities or characteristics used to measure the extent to which a standard is met. Criteria are needed to make the standard measurable. If the standards do not lend themselves to measurement, and specific criteria cannot be written, **indicators** are used to show that in all probability the standards were met. An indicator is an aspect of health care process or outcome that signals whether or not the appropriate interventions were provided.

Standards of nursing are usually classified in one of three ways: structural standards, process standards, and outcome standards.

Structure standards address the environment, instrumentation, qualifications of personnel, job categorizations, number of staff, and committee structures. Several structural standards usually address the integrative mechanisms of an organization (i.e., those that promote communication and decision making such as committees and the divisions of work). Structural standards are influenced by regulatory bodies such as the federal government, state and licensing agencies. For example, if an agency serves persons with Medicare (the federal insurance for the elderly) as the source of payment, the agency must meet the Medicare regulation that requires the services of a registered nurse for specific times and functions.

The Joint Commission on Accreditation of Healthcare Organizations (JCAHO) has an impressive, comprehensive set of standards that must be met to receive **accreditation.** This commission is a voluntary agency rather than an official governmental agency granting accreditation. The accreditation of this body has traditionally focused its standards on quality concerns rather than fiscal or administrative concerns. The explicit mission of JCAHO is to improve the quality of care provided to the public.

Certification is another example of a structure standard. Certification reflects certain qualifications of an individual rather than an agency.

Process standards address nursing activities that nurses perform. These written statements include nursing actions of assessment, diagnosis, interventions, and evaluation. These **standards of nursing practice** emanate from patient needs and are captured in guiding documents such as the American Nurses' Association (ANA) specialized group of standards, the medical-surgical standards, or cardiovascular nursing standards.[1] Many of the specialty nursing organizations such as the Emergency Nurses have published standards of practice for their specialty.[2] In addition to the ANA standards and the specialty organizations' standards, nurses have the Agency for Health Care Policy and Research (AHCPR) **practice guidelines.**[3] These guidelines are intended to assist practitioners in the prevention, diagnosis, treatment, and management of clinical conditions.

Outcome standards address the end results of patient care. These groups of standards are patient centered and usually are identified along with the process standards. In other words, to what end are the nursing activities directed? How do nurses evaluate their work? These **standards of**

patient/client care are frequently written in terms of the behaviors of patients (for example, regular cardiac rhythm). An indicator would be the strip of the electrocardiogram that shows normal sinus rhythm.

■ PRACTICE FRAMEWORK

If standards are indeed agreed-upon levels of excellence or established norms, then it seems reasonable that the organizational structure should be based on these agreed-upon levels of excellence or established norms. To this end, the following model has been developed to demonstrate the inter-relatedness of all standards: structure, process, and outcome.

The standards framework model shows the various types of standards that are derived from the definitions of structure, process, and outcome (Fig. 9-2). At the heart of the model is the nursing care needs of patients. These needs directly influence all standards of the model. The standards of patient care and the standards of nursing practice are developed from the identified patient care needs. From these standards, which create the direct work of nursing, the additional process standards of procedures and job descriptions/ **performance standards** flow. In addition, the structure standards (i.e., policies) should flow from the patient care needs. Policies should be developed to facilitate the implementation of care and process standards.

Moving upward on the model it is noted that the objectives of the department of nursing are considered outcome standards, whereas purpose, theory of nursing, and philosophy are considered structure standards. This model and the definitions are shown to demonstrate that the many different terms used in most organizations are really variations of standards. There are different levels of abstraction used in the formulation of statements in that a philosophy statement is usually broader in scope and less definitive then a procedure. The standards framework model allows one to see the intercon-nectedness of various standards.

■ LEGAL BASIS OF NURSING

A nursing practice act is a legal statement that defines nursing, and what nurses may do. Nursing practice acts differ from state to state in text but generally represent that which the ANA has set forth. All professional nurses have a responsibility to be aware of their individual state's nursing practice act. The wording of each nursing practice act is by design general, since this allows growth within the profession without enacting new legislation for every minor change.

Standards Framework for Nursing Practice

Purpose

Theory of Nursing

Philosophy of the Department of Nursing

Objectives and Goals of the Department of Nursing

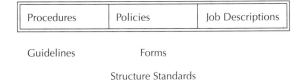

Nursing Care Needs - - - - - - ▶
of Patients

Standards of patient care

Standards of Nursing practice

Objectives of Specific Nursing Units

Procedures	Policies	Job Descriptions

Guidelines   Forms

Structure Standards

Figure 9-2. A graphic of a quality assurance model.

Typically, nursing practice acts address definitions of practice and practitioners, allowable titles, licensure requirements, and qualifications/appointments of the Board of Nursing. Licensure allows a nurse to use the title of "registered nurse." Licensure is given after successful completion of the State Board of Nursing examination. **Registration,** which is tied to licensure, means that a qualified individual's name is listed on an official roster maintained by a governmental agency. Nursing practice acts also spell out the duties of the State Board of Nursing.

The interpretation of the act occurs at a state and organizational level for the purpose of creating policies to guide professional activities. For example, the profession of nursing is generating new and useful knowledge for patient care, and this explosion of knowledge has the potential for changing the work of nursing. A process known as research utilization is attempting to develop operational models that will incorporate clinical research findings into the usual and expected care of patients. Nurses must be allowed flexibility in practice based on sound research while at the same time be assured of freedom from legal sanction.

Ethical and Societal Concerns

Ethical and societal values influence health care legislation. This legislation often deals with particular populations and accordingly can be a powerful determinant of who and how we care for individuals. The growing number of elderly in the United States and the moral conflict surrounding legalized abortion are but two complex concerns for health care. The rationing of health care is another ethical and societal concern exemplified by the State of Oregon's plan to limit services.[4] Rationing deals with distribution of resources and is currently used in health care practice. For example, triage and even some health insurances are forms of rationing. Active congressional legislation is attempting to correct some of the existing problems in insurance coverage, but enactment of law is a slow process, and those who lack insurance coverage experience a form of rationing. Literature is sparse on the rationing of nursing care. However, a manager does indeed ration when he/she makes assignments, places patients in rooms, moves patients, and delegates.

Ethical analysis can be used to examine health care rationing. Ethics provides the tools (principles, such as justice and beneficence) and the framework (theories, such as utilitarianism) to address both substantive and procedural questions. (See Chapter Five for additional information on ethical analysis.) Thus, this complex network has the power to influence the profession's work requiring the nursing practice act to be broad enough to allow for the active growth and change that is mandated by issues from society.

■ GOVERNMENTAL REGULATIONS

The public concern as well as the concern of government officials in the 1970s toward the social conditions, especially a rapid growth in inflation and the rising costs of health care, led Congress to enact two pieces of legislation.

These acts tried to enforce self-regulation in the health care industry. The first act was the passage of the Bennett Amendment in 1972, which established professional standards review organizations (PSROs). This legislation provided for review of medical care at those institutions or at those programs receiving federal monies such as Medicare reimbursement. There were two purposes in this legislative act: utilization review and quality review. The focus of utilization review was the appropriate site for care while the focus of quality review was the effectiveness of care. This legislation had little effect on either medical effectiveness or control of costs. Hospitals were reimbursed on a retrospective fee-for-service basis and the incentive to change was not present or demanded.

The second piece of legislation Congress passed was the National Health Planning and Resource Development Act of 1974 (amended in 1979). The purpose of this act was to correct the poor distribution of health care facilities and health care personnel (PL 93-641, 1975).[5] Health systems agencies were established. Both of these acts focused on the maintenance of quality health care through government and professional regulation.

The most significant impact of government regulation was the enactment of the Social Security Act Amendments of 1983 (HR 1900, SI), Prospective Payment for Medicare Inpatient Hospital Services, which changed the way hospitals were reimbursed for Medicare patients.[6] The payment changed from a fee-for-service reimbursement to a prospective payment system. The basic thrust of this legislation involved the reorganization of the Medicare Trust Fund and the introduction of diagnosis-related groups (DRGs).[7] In essence, this involved the formation of DRGs, which represent a homogeneous grouping of variables for the purpose of consistent payment and to prospectively pay institutions a preset amount for each of the DRG categories. This was an attempt to limit the increases in the costs of hospital health care.

Under the DRG system, utilization review and quality assessment have taken on new and important meanings, which are to ensure that the most effective and efficient health care is being delivered. The appropriate use of resources became a critical issue. New meanings demanded new approaches to utilization review and quality assessment.

The term *quality assurance* was used in the 1981 JCAHO hospital standards to convey attempts to formalize the issues of quality-assessment programs in hospitals.[8] Currently, the terms **quality management** and **outcomes management** are used to denote the approach to quality care. Quality management is considered a pervasive, constant **monitoring** of actions to improve the quality of care. It was popularized by the late W. Edwards Deming.[9]

Outcomes management has been popularized through the demands of third-party payers for evidence of quality. It was also called for as part of the Omnibus Budget Reconciliation Act of 1986. As a result of this act, the Institute of Medicine (IOM) carried out a comprehensive review. The report of the IOM called for an emphasis on outcomes. Following the IOM report, Congress supported a number of new health care research initiatives through the Omnibus Reconciliation Act of 1989 (Public Law 101-239). Legislation was signed in March 1990 creating the eighth agency of the Public Health Service, the Agency for Health Care Policy and Research (AHCPR). The major thrusts of AHCPR are appropriateness of care and outcomes effectiveness.[10]

■ RISK MANAGEMENT

Another aspect of managing quality is the concept of **problems** or risk. **Risk management** is the function of planning, organizing, and directing a comprehensive program of activities to identify, evaluate, and take corrective action against risks that may lead to patient injury, employee injury, and property loss or damage with resulting financial loss.[11] It is apparent from the definition that implied in a program of risk management are concerns for medical and nursing **malpractice** as well as **negligence** and the issue of professional **liability.** Malpractice is a legal term that implies improper action on the part of a professional resulting in some form of injury to the patient as a direct result from care by the professional.[12] It involves deviation from a standard of usual professional conduct or interventions and results in injury. Negligence is the carelessness or failure to act as a prudent person would ordinarily act under the same circumstances.[13] Professional personnel are obligated to provide reasonable care to patients. If this care is not provided, the professional is said to be liable or at risk for legal action.[14] For the plaintiff (the individual who claims injury) to bring about a lawsuit, certain conditions must be met. The conditions include:

- Proof that the nurse owed a duty to the patient
- Proof that failure to act properly would cause harm to the patient
- Proof that the prevailing standard was not met
- Proof that injury directly resulted from the nurse's actions

In our current social climate, lawsuits are not uncommon and risk management is necessary as a hospital department attempts to manage the problem. Management of lawsuits involving malpractice and negligence fall

TABLE 9-1. THE MAJOR ELEMENTS OF A RISK-MANAGEMENT PROGRAM

Financial management
  Self-insurance program
  Property insurance coverages
  Casualty insurance coverages
  Education: Patient education
               Employee education
               Visitor education
Risk transfer
Risk identification
Risk analysis
Risk treatment
Risk evaluation

under the purview of this department as does concern for product liability, worker's compensation, director's and officer's liability.

Model of Risk Management

One way of conceptualizing risk management is through a model that identifies the essential components of a risk management system. These components are financial management, risk transfer, risk identification, risk analysis, risk treatment, and risk evaluation (Table 9-1).

Financial Management. This is by no means a simple concept, but provision has to be made in the overall budget to deal with the problem of financial loss through a crisis, lawsuit, or settlement of an unanticipated natural event such as a tornado. Insurance through a variety of companies may be the best way of managing potential emergencies. What this is doing is transferring the risk either to a self-contained fund or to insurance carriers. The individual professional is also in a position to transfer the risk of financial loss to insurance carriers. Liability insurance is available for the practicing nurse, but adherence to hospital policy and the standards of nursing care are the best insurance.

Risk Identification. Risk identification involves the finding, through the process of auditing charts or reviewing incident reports or in conversation with staff, of those problems with financial and legal risk to the institution.

Risk Analysis. To a great extent the analysis process of determining the risk is a mathematical or statistical maneuver. Information exists to determine

TABLE 9-2. AN ANALYSIS OF A RISK EVENT THAT POSES HARM AND REQUIRES
ACTION

Risk Event	Patient Given Wrong Medication		
Peril	Unit secretary fails to remove incorrect order.	Pharmacy action correct.	Nurse fails to check order and administers the wrong medication.
Hazard	Unit secretary forgets to transcribe correct order onto requisition to pharmacy.		Nurse liable for malpractice.
Outcome	Harm to patient.		

the probability of a particular event occurring in a particular institution, and
how the risk to the agency can be calculated. For example, a medical center
may incur more risk because of the nature of the care provided, such as
experimental treatments and very ill patients. This may, according to the
laws of probability, produce opportunities for a mistake or mismanagement of
patient care. The analysis process identifies this and produces data to plan for
these events. As part of the process to produce data, the analysis usually
reviews a problem in light of several factors:

- The probability of the occurrence of the loss
- The probable severity of the loss
- The possible severity of the loss
- The effects the potential loss would have on the organization clinically
  as well as financially.

For an example, see Table 9-2.

Risk Treatment. Risk treatment involves dealing with the situation in
such a way as to reduce the risk to the organization's resources, whether they
be financial, human, or intangible. The programs available to reduce the risk
depend entirely on the problem. For example, an educational program may
be necessary to prevent patients from falling, or perhaps a human relations
program is necessary to preserve and to reward staff for their contributions.
Another tool that might be employed is to maintain an active public relations
department so that the relationship with the community served is always
positive.

Risk Evaluation. As in any problem-solving method, the evaluation of the
interventions establishes the effectiveness of the interventions and methods
used to gain information about the potential problem. Evaluation usually

centers around basis issues, such as the impact on (1) the organization's assets, (2) the future credit standing of the institution and its capital worth, and (3) the relationship with the community depending on the outcome of the problem.

Impact on Nursing Management

The impact on nursing management is significant. The nurse manager is in a position to control the activities of the staff to prevent problems and facilitate the goals of the organization. Risk management and nursing management are interdependent in meeting this end.

One tool that is available to the nurse manager is the **incident report.** This serves a very important function in identifying problems of a high-risk nature and allows for documenting the corrective action taken to deal with the problem. Incident reports are also referred to as occurrence reports, which is more descriptive of the function they serve because they alert the risk manager of potential problems that may require the intervention of members of the risk-management committee.

The success of this tool is directly related to administrators' attitudes and use of the information. A punitive use could dissuade its intended use. As a nurse manager, you will want to encourage the reporting of every occurrence that could escalate into an incident. Doing this may control unexpected problems.

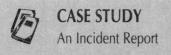

CASE STUDY
An Incident Report

Mary Reynolds, a staff nurse on a postoperative neurosurgical division, had been assigned five extremely nursing care–dependent patients. Mary was also working with one nursing assistant. She realized this was a very heavy assignment, but she decided to do her best. One of her patients, Mr. Morrow, a postoperative craniotomy who had also suffered a stroke, needed to get up in a chair. Mary and the nursing assistant got him up and restrained him in a chair because he remained listless and unresponsive. Mary checked him at 12:30, and all was fine. At 1:00, the neurosurgical resident found Mr. Morrow slumped on the floor. The resident immediately started shouting, and Mary walked in the room, and tried to explain that

Mr. Morrow was fine one half hour earlier. The resident accused Mary of negligence and continued an angry diatribe. The head nurse walked in at this point, and immediately agreed with the doctor. The arguing continued out into the nurse's station, and ended by the doctor leaving the area in mid-sentence, the head nurse slamming her office door, and Mary crying.

- What are the appropriate steps to take when an accident has occurred?
- Is an incident report required?
- What could Mary have done differently?
- What could the head nurse have done differently?

■ SUMMARY

This chapter has addressed the maintenance of quality through the process of quality management. The professional and legal bases for nursing practice are presented as the foundations for monitoring quality. Quality management as a process is a systematic, ongoing function with explicit standards and criteria. The process is highly influenced by governmental, legal, and professional bodies. To some extent, society and ethics give direction to both the government and the profession. An associated process known as risk management deals with serious problems associated with financial loss, professional and staff problems, and intangible problems such as the agency's status in the community. Quality management and outcomes management are vital activities in the current health care system. Major third-party payers are demanding data that shows quality care.

 ## STUDENT EXERCISES

1. Review your nurse practice act. Discuss in class what this act means to you as a professional.

2. Select a patient's chart, and review it to see into what classification the patient has been placed. Find out how much the hospital will be reimbursed for the care depending on the category. Make a judgment as to how you think as a manager you could shorten the patient's stay.

3. Review the written standards of your agency. Are the standards monitored? How?

4. You are a case manager, and one of the patient care associates working with you spilled a basin of hot water on herself. Complete the incident/occurrence report. What information should be included?

5. Define "nursing malpractice." What constitutes a legal transgression? What can you do to protect yourself from a malpractice suit?

■ REFERENCES

1. American Nurses Association, *Standards of Clinical Nursing Practice*, Washington, D.C.: American Nurses Publishing, 1991.
2. Emergency Nurses Association, *Emergency Nurse Core Curriculum*, Philadelphia: Saunders, 1994.
3. U.S. Department of Health and Human Services, Agency for Health Care Policy and Research, *Information Dissemination to Health Care Practitioners and Policymakers*, Rockville, MD: AHCPR, 1996.
4. Weiner JM, "Oregon's Plan for Health Care Rationing," *The Brookings Review*, 10:1, 1992, p. 26–31.
5. 93rd Congress of the United States, *Health Planning Act of 1974*, Washington, D.C.: U.S. Government Printing Office, 1974.
6. 92nd Congress of the United States. *Social Security Amendments of 1972* (PL92-603), Washington, D.C.: U.S. Government Printing Office, 1972.
7. Curtin L, Zurlage C, *DRGs: The Reorganization of Health*, Chicago: S-N Publications, 1984.
8. Joint Commission on Accreditation of Healthcare Organizations, *Accreditation Manual for Hospitals*, Chicago: JCAH, 1996.
9. Walton M, *The Deming Management Method*, New York: The Putnum Publishing Group, 1986.
10. U.S. Department of Health and Human Services, Agency for Health Care Policy and Research, *Using Clinical Practice Guidelines to Evaluate Quality of Care*, Rockville, MD: AHCPR, 1995.
11. Solomon S, *Handbook of Health Care Risk Management, Risk Management Process and Functions*, Rockville, MD: Aspen, 1985.
12. Cushing M, *Nursing Jurisprudence*, Norwalk, CN: Appleton & Lange, 1988, p. 27.
13. Ibid., p. 27.
14. Ibid., p. 26.

10

Motivation in the Work Setting

Introduction

Of the multiple, interacting forces influencing people's performance in work settings, **motivation** is among the most complex. Motivation is defined by Kreitner as a psychological process that gives behavior purpose and direction, and by Davis as caused behavior, the switch that turns the motor on.[1,2] Motivation is sparked by internal and external interacting forces that modify one's perception of and commitment to goals. Motivation is a phenomenon internal to the individual but can be influenced by a variety of circumstances, including other people (coworkers and managers) and overall conditions in a setting. Bass cites Combs and Snygg's *self-concept theory* in which they assert that the most basic human drive is to maintain, protect, and enhance the perceived self, and Purkey and Schmidt's belief that the perceived self constitutes one's self concept.[3] Along with these considerations is the assertion that self-concept is learned and modifiable. What is learned about self-concept is determined partially by time. The marked *generational* differences among practicing nurses today provides us with evidence that individuals view the same situation differently through their thinking, attitudes, and values that were formed from time-related factors. The differences have significant consequences for group efforts in the work setting and will be discussed at greater length later in this chapter under the section on organizational climate. Despite the differences that might exist between coworkers, McBurney and Filoromo remind us that in nursing, the Nightengale pledge continues to motivate and give direction to nurses today; it is not only a Victorian ideology.[4] Written in 1893, it still "serves as a professional mission statement, one that truly reflects the deep-seated vision and values of nursing. A modern analysis of this classic work creates a frame of reference to measure nursing practice." In it, one can recognize the source of many of today's nursing standards of practice statements.

The theme of motivating forces that affect individuals' performance will be carried throughout the chapter. References are made to material presented in earlier chapters, especially communication, group dynamics, decision making, conflict management, and how people function effectively in complex organizations. Descriptions of selected theories of motivation and how they apply to nursing practice follow, along with how motivational climate affects groups and individuals. Finally, common problems that interfere with productivity in the work setting are discussed.

KEY CONCEPTS

Climate is a systems concept described as the human environment in which people work.

Dissatisfiers in Herzberg's theory are factors of motivation that are extrinsic to work content. Examples are salary, pleasantness of surroundings, and policies; also known as hygiene factors and maintenance factors.

Expectancy is a term used in Vroom's theory of motivation, meaning effort-performance association.

Instrumentality is from Vroom's expectancy theory, and means perceived performance-outcome association.

Intentionally Disinviting is the level in Purkey's Intentional Model of Motivation in which the individual is dissuaded and rejected.

Intentionally Inviting is the level in Purkey's Intentional Model of Motivation in which the individual is respected and encouraged.

Macromotivation describes the expectation that personal-needs satisfaction be a part of the employment situation; also known as type B motivation.

Micromotivation describes the expectation that only work-related needs be met through employment; also known as type A motivation.

Motivation is caused behavior; a psychological process that gives behavior purpose and direction.

Satisfiers in Herzberg's theory are factors that relate to work content. Examples are responsibility, autonomy, and achievement; also known as motivation factors.

Valence from Vroom's expectancy theory means one's feeling of satisfaction/ dissatisfaction about an outcome.

X Characteristics in McGregor's theory are those characteristics that cause a person to dislike work and to be productive only through coercion.

Y Characteristics in McGregor's theory are those characteristics that cause a person to enjoy work and to seek responsibility and challenges.

■ THEORIES OF MOTIVATION

Overall, motivation theories are generalizations about the "why" and "how" of purposeful behavior. Motivation theories provide managers with a knowledge base for encouraging individuals to willingly pursue organizational objectives.[5] *Goal setting*, a part of the performance-appraisal process, is one way in which managers attempt to influence motivation. Participation in goal setting gives the individual personal ownership of them, and triggers the motivational process that improves behavior.[6] In order to be effective as motivators, goals must be (1) specific, (2) difficult, and (3) participative.[7]

Needs Theorists

In 1943, Maslow described the propositions upon which he developed his theory of human motivation, popularly known as the hierarchy of human needs theory.[8] The propositions Maslow described include the following:

1. The human organism should be treated as a whole.
2. Somatically based drives are atypical in human motivation.
3. Basic goals of an unconscious nature are more fundamental in motivation theory than conscious goals.
4. Behavior must be understood as a channel through which many basic needs are simultaneously expressed or satisfied.
5. Human needs arrange themselves in a hierarchy of prepotency.
6. Classifications are based upon goals.
7. The total situation in which behavior occurs must be taken into account.
8. Both integrated and isolated reactions explain motivation.

Motivation theory is not synonymous with behavior theory but rather motivation is only one class of determinants of behavior, including biological, cultural, and situational determinants. Maslow formulated his theory of motivation on these theoretic demands and presented it as a framework for research through which his theory would be tested and either stand or fail. Today, we are familiar with his arrangement of prepotent needs into a five-classification hierarchy from lowest to highest: (1) physiologic needs—the need for air, water, food; (2) safety needs—the need to be secure from harm; (3) belongingness—the need for friendship, affection, and love; (4) esteem—the need for feeling of self-worth and for respect from others; and (5) self-actualization—the need to make the most of one's life.[9] Lower-level needs must be partially satisfied before higher needs are activated and become the motivating force for behavior.

Over the years there have been claims that Maslow's theory has not stood the test of empiric assessment relative to distinct classifications or to an absolute, five-level, ascending hierarchy.[10] McClelland and Atkinson offer a modification of Maslow's hierarchy by stressing the influence of changing priorities in determining relative importance of needs to individuals.[11] In the 1960s, McClelland described a trichotomy of needs: (1) affiliation, (2) power, and (3) achievement.[12] According to McClelland, individuals possess high, moderate, or low levels of each as a function of personality traits. Similarly Alderfer, cited in Aldag, suggests a less rigid arrangement of needs than what is defined by Maslow by presenting them as a no-set hierarchy.[13] Alderfer arranges needs into three categories: (1) existence, (2) relatedness, and (3) growth. When frustrated in one area, an individual concentrates on another. Alderfer's theory is new (1972) and has limited empiric data. Whether there is support or criticism of Maslow's work, the important consideration is the contribution he has made to the emerging body of knowledge about motivation. An important lesson learned from Maslow's work is that *fulfilled* needs do not serve as motivators.[14]

Personality Type and Motivation

A well-known theory of motivation in the work setting is Herzberg's two-factor theory.[15] Herzberg postulates that there are two separate sets of factors that influence motivation, each having a high-through-low value on a continuum. He labeled his two sets *motivation factors* and *maintenance factors.* Maintenance factors are also known as **dissatisfiers,** or *hygiene factors.* Dissatisfiers are extrinsic influences that do not relate to job content. Instead, they relate to pay; job security; working conditions, such as lighting and pleasantness of surrounding; agency policy; and interpersonal relations with peers and supervisors. Poor quality or negative perceptions about these factors greatly dissatisfy some workers, who are called *maintenance seekers*. Improvement in the factors, even in the perception of the workers, results in a neutral state and not in improved motivation. In other words, these factors are potent dissatisfiers but not strong motivators. Motivation factors are also known as **satisfiers**. Satisfiers come from intrinsic influences, relate to work content, and, when workers have opportunities to realize them, they serve as strong motivators. These workers are called *motivation seekers*. Some examples of satisfiers are the nature of the work itself, a sense of achievement, recognition, advancement, responsibility, and autonomy.

No factor from either set is wholly one-dimensional. Individuals are affected to some degree by each. At any given point in time, each person can be identified as predominantly a maintenance seeker or a motivation seeker. A significant difference separates those who are primarily maintenance seekers (i.e., while motivation seekers desire and appreciate improved dissatisfiers, maintenance seekers tend to purposefully avoid satisfiers). This phenomenon is explained partially by the fact that innate potential limits motivation. Situational variables influence how a person acts relative to job-related factors. In times of scarce job opportunities, different motivators influence people as opposed to when such a condition does not exist. Herzberg has contributed to motivation theory by emphasizing the potential of enriched work.[16]

An example of how Herzberg's theory was demonstrated in nursing practice is the development of primary nursing as a pattern of patient care delivery. Professional and nonprofessional activities in caring for critically ill patients were scrutinized by a group of nurses, and a new system was designed to concentrate nurses' time and activities on professional responsibilities. Where primary nursing is practiced, nurses give care to the same patients over time and assume high-level responsibility for the quality of nursing care given. Nurses who helped develop primary nursing are definitely motivation seekers. Had they not been, the concern for better quality care would not have led to a new pattern of assignment of patient care. Herzberg counseled, "if you want to motivate the worker, don't put in another water fountain, provide a bigger share of the job itself."[17]

McGregor's theory X and theory Y present two contrasting sets of assumptions about human beings and work.[18] The assumptions are labeled **X characteristics** and **Y characteristics**. X-type individuals dislike work and avoid it when possible; have little ambition; need control, direction, and coercion; and respond when threatened with punishment. Their primary concern is security. Reasons for X-type behaviors vary with individuals and might be persistent or temporary.

Y-type individuals are self-directed, self-controlled, like work, seek challenges and responsibilities, and are inspired to increased commitment with success. As with individuals' preferences in Herzberg's two-factor theory, the total situation accounts for departure from one's usual characteristics. One who typically performed at peak levels might suddenly begin to behave more like an X-type person. Factors internal to nursing might be the cause of such a change. Ironically, an event intended as a reward, such as the practice of "promoting" an excellent bedside nurse to the role of first-level manager, produces the negative change in the individual's performance. If the promotion places the nurse outside her field of expertise, the move can produce widespread problems for the organization (e.g., the newly promoted nurse begins to avoid situations and responsibilities she is not prepared to meet). At one time, promoting practitioners into management positions was more commonly seen when there was no other form of reward for nurses. McGregor suggests arranging conditions and methods so that the worker can attain his or her own goals by directing efforts toward organizational goals.[19] Because of generational differences, some nurses find themselves in situations like those described above because of their different expectations about work limitations and opportunities. Mechanisms such as a practice ladder and programs to prepare nurses for new roles have made a significant difference in how nurses can be rewarded today. The concept of a ladder will be discussed in more detail in Chapter 11, Monitoring and Improving Performance.

Motivation as Rational Decision Making

Vroom's expectancy theory, cited in Aldag, views motivation as a rational decision-making process involving (1) **expectancy,** defined as effort-performance association; (2) **valence,** defined as one's feeling of satisfaction/dissatisfaction about an outcome; and (3) **instrumentality,** defined as one's perceived performance-outcome association.[20] Porter and Lawler, cited in Aldag, designed a model of Vroom's theory in which valence is the strength of one's desire for something, expectancy is the probability of getting it with a certain action, and motivation is the strength of drive toward the action.[21] The formula is as follows:

$$[\text{Expectancy} \times \text{sum of (Valence} \times \text{Instrumentality)}] = \text{Effort}$$

Motivation is high when an individual has a good chance of getting personally satisfying rewards through his/her efforts. Expectancy theory might be seen in nursing when a nurse initiates a request to be considered for more responsibility on her unit. Perhaps she sees a need for an experienced nurse, other than the head nurse, to coordinate orientation activities and functions for new graduates beginning their professional careers on her unit. Once the head nurse approves the idea, together they agree on what new competencies the nurse will need to develop to serve in the new role. They establish a time frame for readiness, and the expectancy-valence instrumentality connection is put into motion. If the unit budget permits an increase in salary for the added responsibility of the role, the nurse's valence will undoubtedly go up in the direction of satisfaction, even though salary was not the original motivating force. In this example, the nurse engaged in participative management by being instrumental in decisions, problem solving, and organizational change.

The nurse in the above example can also be viewed as (1) operating at a high-need level in Maslow's hierarchy, (2) a motivation seeker in Herzberg's theory, and (3) a McGregor's Y-type individual. The same can be said about examples given by nurses who were instrumental in designing primary nursing care and in being instrumental in development of a clinical ladder. Motivation theorists present different perceptions on the same theme (i.e., suggesting explanation of what influences performance). They are the postulates upon which theoretic demands are satisfied. While the theories presented in this chapter continue to undergo the scrutiny of empiric assessment, they provide a framework for greater understanding of the complex phenomenon of motivation. A question of motivational differences based on gender arises as the number of male nurses increases. Henderson found, however, that when correlating the need for power, risk taking, and influence, no gender differences were found.[22] Sharpening understanding of the many different internal and external forces that influence performance in the work setting remains an ongoing challenge to practitioners in striving for excellence in nursing care delivery.

■ ORGANIZATIONAL CLIMATE AND MOTIVATION

A person's interest, ability, and will to accomplish, while essential for success, are not sufficient to ensure the kind of performance needed to accomplish goals. Work-related goals are formulated and carried out in complex organizations where the worker is affected by numerous changing events over which he or she has little control. The collective events operating simultaneously create a climate described by Davis as the human environment in which people work.[23] It surrounds and affects everything that happens and in turn is affected by everything that occurs in the setting. **Climate** influences the quality of performance that can take place in a given situation. High-quality performance is more likely to take place in settings where the climate is predominantly positive relative to the organization and its goals *and* to individual workers and their needs. Climate can be the result of chance or design. Climate by design in the work setting aims to improve motivation for the purpose of improving performance. Arranging work relationships within and between departments is one way the organization can maintain some control over its internal climate. It is an important way to promote organizational goal attainment. Having an understanding of how workers and groups are alike and different from one another is critical in planning a positive work climate. The effectiveness, then, of an organization's structure is partially dependent on participation of representatives of all major work groups employed.

Qualifications of nurse representatives within the organization relative to communication, group dynamics, decision making, and conflict management were discussed in some detail in Chapters 3 and 4. The effectiveness of leaders who represent nursing in organizations greatly influence the climate in which nurses at all levels function. The climate is a strong determinant of opportunities afforded nurses in the organization, which result in high or low motivation.

Individuals working together in a work setting affect the work climate. Nurses in practice today represent two distinctly different generations, each having been groomed by different times. As a consequence, they frequently hold different values and attitudes relative to expectations in the work setting. An interesting analogy of this is presented by Toffler in his book *The Third Wave* cited in Buchholz.[24] Toffler describes three revolutionary eras in the history of humankind dating from primitive man to the present. The first two eras proceeded at a slow and placid pace, gradually introducing changes that persisted over long periods of time. The first era began when primitive, roving hunters settled into permanent communities and began to farm the land. It is the longest of the eras, lasting until the Industrial Revolution ushered in the second era. With the advent of mechanization, men flocked to cities for employment in factories where machines took over tasks previously done by hand. While short in comparison to the first era, industrialization produced changes in society that dominated the thinking, values, and attitudes of several generations, roughly for a 100-year period. Lastly, the development of cybernetics and the introduction of computers in the marketplace following World War II marked the beginning of the third era. The third era is characterized by rapidly occurring changes and shifts in individuals' expectations relative to all aspects of living, including the work setting.

Toffler refers to individuals from the second and third eras as *second wavers* and *third wavers*, respectively.[25] The terms come from the comparison of the third era to *tsunami*, the giant Pacific tidal wave set off by an underwater earthquake that caused sudden, dramatic, and permanent changes in land masses. Second- and third-wave nurses work side-by-side today with their different expectations from employers. Simon subdivides goals into personal goals and role-defined goals.[26] Second-wave nurses tend more to role-defined goals relative to their work, while third-wave nurses expect both categories to be satisfied in the work setting. The differences can be a source of conflict if not managed well.

Veteran, experienced second wavers are more likely to be in upper-level nursing management positions. They have been strongly influenced by the depression of the 1930s, with the concomitant fear of being out of work. Their experiences equip them to conform more to what is established in the work situation. The younger generation of nurses, on the other hand, are third wavers who have been strongly influenced by the attitudes of the 1960s. They tend more to question established practices, such as standard eight-hour shifts, and expect to participate actively in decisions that affect them. The outcome can be that third wavers' thinking, values, and attitudes confuse many second wavers.

Using Toffler's analogy, Buchholz suggests that it is to the advantage of second wavers to use the power of the third wave—to ride it rather than try to turn it back to sea.[27] The task, however, is a reciprocal one requiring effort from both groups. Understanding what motivates each other can bridge the gap that separates them. Focusing joint efforts on criteria that remain constant in the face of changes holds the most promise in finding a common ground that can enable the two groups to work effectively together. In nursing, the criteria are the Standards of Professional Nursing Practice. Agreement on standards is the stabilizing force that enables individuals with different approaches to the practice of nursing to work together in harmony. Each generation must respect the fact that, unavoidably, different forces produce caused behavior that is motivation. Skillful managers can predict under what conditions second wavers and third wavers will complement each other and therefore work well together and when they are serious antagonists and need to be separated. Keeping standards of nursing practice the focal issue for all nurses, requires that conflicts be managed so that they do not predominate to the point of becoming the focal issue. Maintaining positive relationships, high-quality standards, and attainment of organizational goals depends on a purposefully designed pattern of people relationships.

Relationships are established through organizational design and are depicted graphically in organizational charts.

Micromotivation and Macromotivation

When second wavers were the only practitioners in nursing, motivational efforts in the work setting were directed toward the work to be done within organizational conditions. Davis refers to this approach as *type A*, or **micromotivation.**[28] There were few problems with this system because second wavers had known or had been directly affected by unemployment. Being gainfully employed for them was highly self-fulfilling. When third wavers entered practice, work-related goals alone no longer sufficed for their felt sense of self-fulfillment. They had not been directly affected by unemployment as their predecessors had been. The experiences of third wavers permit them to think of themselves in broad terms, not only in terms of what they do for a living (e.g., a nurse or a banker). They perceive themselves more holistically and seek broader considerations in their workplace. The shift in organizations is therefore toward *type B*, or **macromotivation,** which includes outside environmental considerations that influence performance.

The shift from micromotivation to macromotivation can be seen in lengthening lists of employee benefits in organizations today. Fringe benefits have implications for motivation. They are tangible rewards, relatively easy to provide, and have the potential to produce high levels of satisfaction in workers. While fringe benefits influence climate, they are extrinsic to work and tend to add to satisfaction but do not improve performance. For example, a worker can experience heightened commitment to a disliked job because of the company's comprehensive fringe benefits. The worker does not feel a need to improve performance because the benefits are not contingent on performance.[29] This example demonstrates the real dichotomy between extrinsic and intrinsic sources of motivation. There can be serious problems in organizations where the fringe benefit package is the dominant mechanism for satisfying workers.

Aldag reminds us that one cannot generally assume that making an employee happy will in turn make him more productive.[30] Fringe benefits, such as sick leave, salary, and vacation time, are examples of extrinsic sources of motivation that are not related to the work that one does. Teachers who continue to teach primarily because summers off suit their lifestyle are extrinsically motivated. Intrinsic sources of motivation, on the other hand, are derived from the work itself because it is self-fulfilling to the individual. Teachers who enjoy teaching because their work helps develop minds remain committed to their profession despite average-to-mediocre benefits. They are intrinsically motivated in the same way that nurses who worked long hours to develop the system of primary nursing care were intrinsically motivated.

Because intrinsic sources of motivation hold more promise for improving performance, organizations must design work that will increase performance-related satisfaction. Recall what Herzberg had to say about additional water fountains versus a greater share of the work itself. In nursing, this can be done by designing a climate that will allow nurses to realize their true professional potential. Academic preparation of baccalaureate nurses equips them to move forward from an initial state of task and relationship concerns, described in the Hershey model in Chapter 2, to the mature level of independence relative to autonomous decision making in health matters that fall within the realm of nursing practice. Climates dominated by rigid bureaucratic policies and procedures that are concerned primarily with efficiency frequently frustrate the potential that professional nurses bring to their places of practice. The unfortunate consequence all too often is a willingness of many nurses to remain in the prevailing dependent role perpetuated by administrative paternalism that still characterizes some health care organizations.

■ MOTIVATIONAL PROBLEMS

It would be nice if leaders in nursing, or any other field, could develop a formula to improve motivation that would apply to all, despite their differences, or if it were possible to take what has been successful in one situation and apply it to another situation. Differences exist between individuals and groups that spring from ability, experience, preference, values, culture, ideals, time, place, and beliefs. Such wide variations make uniformity impossible. Davis points out that primary physiologic needs differ in intensity from person to person and in the same person from time to time, and that secondary psychosocial needs are vague and change with level of maturity.[31] These facts complicate efforts to improve motivation. Experience shows that the same factor exists as opposites in two different people (e.g., submission and aggressiveness). At times, several factors in combination act as a single factor to influence people, such as hunger. A behavior can be produced by several different factors (e.g., absenteeism can be due to lack of interest, conflict with coworkers, or an attempt to avoid an unpleasant or feared task).

Simon describes the responses of three bricklayers to the question, What are you doing? One said, "laying a brick"; another said, "building a wall"; and the third said, "helping to build a cathedral."[32] Obviously, each was motivated by very different perceptions of his task.

A Situational Approach

Bassett discusses the Japanese spin-off on the concept of participative management, originated in but never implemented in the United States.[33] The Japanese have used the concept successfully in industry to foster motivation that improves performance. It is frequently heard that the United States should learn from Japan how to implement participative management. Consideration must be given to the vast differences between people of these two countries. There is little in common between the two regarding societal factors or recent, major, historic events. The Japanese live in an ancient, single-culture, imperialistic society, whereas Americans live in a young, multicultural, democratic society. Recent historic events left Japan's cities war-torn and their country defeated, whereas Americans have experienced neither event. A consequence of the widespread destruction in Japan is the fact that more modern factories were built during reconstruction and newer, more modern equipment was purchased, whereas the United States continues to operate with outdated factory buildings and equipment designed early in the Industrial Age. Participative management filled a need for the Japanese to demonstrate unity and to restore some of the pride lost as a result of their loss from World War II. The differences between the two situations make it unlikely that outcomes can be duplicated. This example demonstrates that what works in one situation does not necessarily work in another.

What then is necessary to improve motivation? The answer is clear that careful analysis of all situational factors is necessary to know how to begin. Experienced, skilled managers understand that they have a first-line major responsibility to provide their staff with a climate that is conducive to the actualization of each individual's needs. In Bass is a description of Purkey's *Intentional Model* that depicts ways to influence motivation.[34] It was introduced in 1978 and has been utilized by several disciplines. Nurse managers are encouraged to make use of it as a strategy for influencing motivation within nursing. One level of functioning in the model is **intentionally inviting** and consists of four elements: (1) optimism, (2) respect, (3) trust, and (4) intentionality. In the intentionally inviting level, people are viewed as being valuable and capable of being self-directed. Their uniqueness is acknowledged through courtesy, they are trusted to choose what is best for the overall good, and actions are designed to accomplish a beneficial end. Another level, by contrast, is **intentionally disinviting** and consists of actions designed to (1) dissuade, (2) discourage, (3) defeat and, (4) destroy. People are insulted, criticized, and ignored usually through the manner in which policies are formulated and/or implemented. Naisbitt, cited in Bassett, says that "ordinary people are dying to make a commitment," and managers pave the way for them to be internally motivated to do so.[35] The most promising approach managers can adopt to influence motivation in a positive direction is to concentrate on what is central to a group's existence and develop skill in use of strategies to accomplish that end.

Issues Central to Nursing

As stated earlier in this chapter, values central to nursing are found in standards of the profession. Nurses in formal management positions must, while hand-in-hand with practitioners, design plans that can foster staff participation and shared decision making in carrying out professional standards. Some examples have been given in this chapter, such as development of primary nursing care, investigations of practice ladders, and questions surrounding work schedules.

Managers must shift from being order givers to being facilitators. Rewards to individuals from ongoing staff involvement in matters that pertain to practice are (1) improved performance, (2) increased responsibility, (3) increased independence, (4) improved knowledge of the overall organization, and (5) improved capacity to change. Benefits to the organization are (1) combined strength of several competent individuals, (2) sharpened and refined ideas, (3) incorrect ideas that are unnoticed by one are noticed by the group, (4) competition is replaced with cooperation, (5) increased morale and motivation, (6) knowledge that is gained alters opinions and attitudes, (7) clearer understanding of the nature of goals and feasibility, and (8) goals that are congruent with group-perceived values.[36]

Barriers to sharing responsibility with the staff include (1) fear of loss of control, (2) risk of not knowing what the staff will do, (3) a felt threat to authority and position, and (4) feeling that the staff is not mature enough, smart enough, or motivated enough.

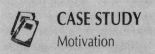

CASE STUDY
Motivation

The head nurse's seemingly diminishing interest in and knowledge about issues that directly affect patient care and staff nurse satisfaction is creating a serious morale problem. Committed and enthusiastic nurses feel extremely frustrated that their efforts to maintain high standards on the unit are being negatively affected by the lack of involvement on the part of the head nurse.

The nurses decide that the best course of action is to approach the head nurse with their perception of what is happening. They know that if nothing is done, motivation to continue to invest their energy on that particular unit will suffer and that many requests for transfer to other units in the hospital will result. As a representative of the staff, you are asked to meet with the head nurse to present a planned program for turning the situation around. The planned program has been designed by the group of staff nurses, not only by yourself.

Analyze the problem relative to the needs of the unit. Your goals are to be effectively assertive as you:

- Attempt to solve the problem at unit level.
- Offer support, rather than blame, to the head nurse by acknowledging her responsibilities as a manager that take her away from the unit.
- Maintain the high-level motivation of the staff that everyone had become accustomed to.

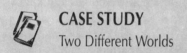

CASE STUDY
Two Different Worlds

Board members of a small community hospital are considering a major change that will bring all departments in line with more current health care organizations. With the increase in local population, the town limits are getting closer and closer to the neighboring city limits. Board members fear that without drastic changes, their hospital will become totally obsolete in the space of a few years. What they want to accomplish will require all the skill and commitment of every department in the hospital. The director of nursing service anticipates the nurses will need support to accept what the change will mean to them. The nursing staff has been virtually without turnover as far back as anyone can remember, except for retirements. They have operated in a very specific internal climate with their own definitions of professionalism, commitment, and the role of women. The director of nursing service, because of her attendance at Directors' Conferences and other meetings out of town, has a clear idea of what the new plans will mean, including hiring nurses with differences. She knows that there will be baccalaureate-prepared nurses and male nurses among those hired. Neither have been employed by the hospital in the past. She has decided that her first major task will be to influence the motivation of the staff to accept and support the change and to be able to modify their perceptions of nursing practice. She will begin with scheduling a staff development program specifically on motivation.

- Help her by recommending topics for her program.
- Prioritize them.

■ SUMMARY

In the introduction to this chapter, the reality of significant generational differences within working groups was explored as a means of focusing attention on the need for cooperative efforts to maintain standards of practice as a unifying force in nursing. Motivation was defined as caused behavior, and four theories of motivation were reviewed to provide a basis for understanding the propositions from which motivation comes. Examples were cited of how nurses have demonstrated high levels of motivation to meet their personal standards of excellence as well as those of the profession. Climate was looked at relative to its influence on group and individual motivation, and the shift from micromotivation to macromotivation in organizations was traced back to its cause. Finally, problems with motivation were explored, misconceptions of how to improve motivation in unique situations were described, and responsibilities of nurses to improve the quality of practice by taking responsibility for their own level of motivation was defined. The role of nurse management was specified for designing a climate conducive to improve motivation along with personal rewards and organizational benefits that accompany growth. Barriers to constructive climates were identified as a reminder of inadvertent behaviors that stand in the way of advancing professional practice.

 STUDENT EXERCISES

1. Think of a time during clinical practice when situational factors in your life prevented you from performing as a McGregor Y person or a Herzberg motivation seeker. To what degree did situational factors influence your professional responsibilities to your patients and the operation of the unit where you were assigned? How did you handle the situation? How did others (instructor and staff) respond to your performance? What did you learn from the experience? How will you handle a similar situation in the future?

2. You have an idea that you feel will encourage daily updating of patient care plans. You are a senior student and your instructor tells you to present your idea to the charge nurse. How will you go about this considering your level of experience compared to that of the charge nurse? What motivational factors should you stress?

3. Older nurses on a unit continually refer to younger nurses and students as being less committed to patients than their generation of nurses. This is causing a gulf between older and younger nurses, and also a morale problem. Based on Toffler's description of reasons for generational differences, propose an approach to stabilizing the conflict.

4. You overhear a group of nurses, who recently returned from a conference on improving performance, discussing their reactions to the program. Opinions vary relative to the practicality of what was presented. Reactions include:

   - "We should do what nurses in agency X did to improve performance."
   - "It is impossible to improve performance here because our benefits provide no incentives."
   - "Even though we have an outdated building and old equipment, we should be able to identify ways to improve meeting basic standards of practice."
   - "It's such a big problem, and I feel frustrated trying to balance my nursing practice responsibilities along with all the other expectations placed on me outside of work."
   - "Attending the conference was a waste of time. I went to find out how to make changes needed on our unit, and no one told us that."
   - "It was a nice day away, with pay, from the confusion of the unit."

   Respond to each reaction, giving your reasons for agreement or disagreement based on content from this chapter. Your instructor thinks it would be a good assignment for you, individually or as a group, to propose a strategy to bring some commonalty to these diffuse reactions. Using content from Chapters 1 through 10, propose a theoretic approach to the situation.

■ REFERENCES

1. Kreitner R, *Management*, 6th ed, Boston: Houghton Mifflin Co., 1995, p. 398.
2. Davis K, *Human Behavior at Work: Organizational Behavior*, New York: McGraw-Hill, 1981, p. 42.

3. Bass LS, "Motivation Strategies: A New Twist," *Nursing Management,* 22:2, 1991, p. 24.
4. McBurney BH, Filoromo T, "The Nightengale Pledge: 100 Years Later," *Nursing Management,* 25:2, February 1994, p. 72–74.
5. Kreitner R, p. 398.
6. Ibid., p. 405–406.
7. Ibid., p. 406.
8. Shafritz JM, Hyde AC, editors, *Classics of Public Administration,* 2nd ed, Chicago: Dorsey Press, 1987, p. 135.
9. Aldag RJ, Brief AP, *Task Design and Employee Motivation,* Palo Alto, CA: Scott Foresman, 1979, p. 9–10.
10. Ibid.
11. McClelland DC, Atkinson JW, *Power: The Inner Experience,* New York: Ewington Publishers, 1975, p. 585.
12. Henderson MC, "Nurse Executives: Leadership Motivation and Leadership Effectiveness," *Journal of Nursing Administration,* 25:4, April 1995, p. 45–51.
13. Aldag RJ, Brief AP, p. 11.
14. Kreitner R, p. 402.
15. Davis K, p. 56.
16. Kreitner R, p. 404.
17. Bassett LC, Metzger N, *Achieving Excellence,* Rockville, MD: Aspen Publishing, 1986, p. 86.
18. Claus KE, Bailey JT, *Power and Influence in Health Care,* St. Louis: Mosby, 1977, p. 128.
19. Bassett LC, Metzger, N, p. 86.
20. Aldag RJ, Brief AP, p. 18.
21. Ibid.
22. Henderson, ML.
23. Davis K, p. 104.
24. Buchholz S, editor, *The Positive Manager,* New York: Wiley, 1985, p. 5.
25. Ibid.
26. Simon HA, *Administrative Behavior: A Study of Decision Making Processes in Administrative Organizations,* 3rd ed, New York: The Free Press, 1976, p. 265.
27. Buchholz S, p. 9.
28. Davis K, p. 77.
29. Aldag RJ, Brief AP, p. 24.
30. Ibid., p. 23.
31. Davis K, p. 42.
32. Simon HA, p. 27.
33. Bassett LC, Metzger N, p. 86.
34. Bass LS, pp. 24–25.
35. Bassett LC, Metzger N, p. 83.
36. Ibid., p. 92.

11

Monitoring and Improving Performance

Introduction

During the formal educational experience, course objectives serve as the basis for evaluating level of academic success. Each set of course objectives contains statements of expectations and criteria for acceptable knowledge attainment and performance. The content of course evaluation forms are based on course objectives. Students are familiar with this system of evaluation and therefore have some preparation for taking an active role in judging their own performance as practitioners in work settings.

In this chapter, the focus is on monitoring performance in the work setting. Monitoring is done by self and by supervisors. The performance appraisal system is organization wide, is designed to monitor and evaluate performance, provides opportunities for improvement, and resolves identified problems.[1] Departments within organizations develop written plans to objectively and systematically oversee the effectiveness of the program. When understood and used appropriately, the system benefits patients, nurses, organizations, and the profession. Study of performance appraisal as a system is therefore important.

Performance appraisal is one element in a broader organizational system of quality assurance. It is itself a system having several interdependent parts and is designed to serve organizations and individuals. Developing an effective system is an expensive endeavor for organizations requiring time, space allocation, and qualified personnel.

The beginning nurse enters a highly complex setting and immediately becomes an active participant in the mission of the whole organization, not only that of an assigned nursing unit. Understanding the performance appraisal system and the process of implementation is important to the nurse as an individual as well as to the organization. Early involvement in functions designed to meet organizational goals can permit earlier advancement in personal career goals, since opportunities for growth and advancement are more readily perceived by those who are informed and involved. The knowledgeable individual also influences a system and makes it serve the organization better. Well-formulated and thoughtfully stated questions and comments that reflect expectations about the system can serve as a spark to turn an ineffective process toward greater effectiveness.

This chapter then serves the following purposes: (1) to stress performance appraisal as important to the profession of nursing, to organizations, and to individuals and (2) to encourage students to become familiar with all aspects of the performance appraisal process in order to advance their career goals, to contribute to organizational mission, and to advance the profession of nursing. Ultimately, all of these elements dovetail to create a system designed to protect (1) patients by insuring competent practitioners who meet professional standards, (2) nurses' rights and autonomy, and (3) the interests of the organization. There is a strong legal obligation inherent in being employed as a professional nurse. The performance appraisal system is an effective avenue for measuring the obligations of the employment agreement by employer and employee.

KEY CONCEPTS

Career Ladder is a design of a concept to select a career path beyond the basic functional level. In nursing, career paths include practitioner, educator, and manager. Masters and doctoral degrees are required as the individual progresses.

Clinical Ladder is a design of a concept to permit progression within a position category (e.g., the staff nurse level).

Disciplinary Action refers to corrective measures designed to improve performance of workers. The focus is on improvement for the future rather than punishment of the past.

Evaluation Interview is the formal evaluation meeting of a supervisor and an individual employee during which the employee's performance is reviewed relative to position responsibilities.

Grievance is a real or imagined feeling of personal injustice that an employee has about the employment relationship. The feeling of injustice is not necessarily true or correct.

Management by Objectives is the evaluation method based on attainment of predetermined goals that have been set by mutual agreement between a supervisor and an employee. A specified time frame for achieving a goal or set of goals is part of management by objectives. It is a method that fosters active participation in evaluation and self-determination in career development.

Performance Appraisal Program is the process in use in an organization by which the performance appraisal system is implemented. It is the means of redefining and improving work performance.

Performance Appraisal System is an integral function of an organization to monitor employee performance.

Reliability is a characteristic of measurement in which an instrument consistently assigns scores to an attribute.

Validity is a characteristic of measurement in which an instrument measures attributes it is intended to measure.

PURPOSE OF A PERFORMANCE APPRAISAL SYSTEM

Good performance appraisal provides a systematic, orderly source of information not available to the organization in any other way. **Performance appraisal systems,** in order to be effective, must be (1) suited to the philosophy, goals, and objectives of an organization, (2) understood by all personnel, and (3) enacted and operationalized by qualified managers and staff. Queen gives the following purposes of performance appraisal: (1) to maintain safe competent care, (2) to meet organizational goals, (3) to foster professional development, and (4) to develop ideas for clinical nursing research.[2]

In organizations today, a matrix structure is common. The **performance appraisal program** in any organization must allow for a *design* that permits each department within the matrix to produce the kind of information that identifies *its* primary contribution to the overall mission. The business office clearly contributes differently to the organization than does the nursing service department. It is important, however, that issues that emerge from a matrix structure be understood by everyone. Departments having essentially different responsibilities must work together to allow organizational survival in the volatile environment of the changing health care delivery system. Linkages between departments in organizations was discussed in Chapter 6, Organization and Management Theory.

Performance appraisal is multifaceted, dynamic, and a managerial tool designed to:

- Evaluate performance
- Identify staff development and training needs
- Identify unrecognized talent and ability
- Influence motivation
- Assign rewards
- Take disciplinary action
- Encourage career goal planning

Beck describes the development and piloting of a performance appraisal tool for use when primary nursing as a patient care delivery pattern is used.[3] The framework for developing the standards of performance are (1) 24-hour accountability, (2) case method of assignment, (3) communication among caregivers, and (4) change in the role of the head nurse. The tool, while specific to primary nursing is of value to other patterns of care (e.g., case management). Generally speaking, the hallmarks of modern performance appraisal systems are (1) performance orientation of everyone in the organization, (2) focus on goals, and (3) mutual goal setting between managers and staff.

■ CRITERIA FOR NURSING PERFORMANCE

Professional standards of nursing practice constitute the basic framework and serve as criteria for evaluating nurses' performance in the work setting in the same way that course objectives do in the classroom. Different standards serve as criteria for performance of personnel in other departments of the organization. At times, standards for other departments can appear to be in conflict with nursing standards. The concept of *tailoring* as a condition for preserving professional standards in the face of other demands may be necessary. Tailoring differs from abandoning because it preserves attitudes and values, such as caring and compassion, that are essential to the nursing profession. They are values that must not be jeopardized in the delivery of patient care due to economic constraints.

Professional standards and money do, however, frequently become competing forces in today's health care delivery. A classical example is the early discharge of patients from acute care settings as a cost-containment measure. Nurses are frequently caught in economy/quality conflicts and cost-containment/compassion conflicts. They are frequently reminded of the ethics of resource allocation in today's practice world. The economic advantage of early discharge is easily understood, whereas research on the effects it has on care outcomes for patients is lacking. While professional standards must dominate decision making relative to patient care, nurses must remember that included in professional values is the effective use of resources and prevention of waste. It is important that there be communication, collaboration, and cooperation between departments. Gropper and Skarzynski discuss interdepartmental differences in the performance appraisal system.[4] In an effort to integrate and unify the system, each departments' high-risk, high-cost, and problem-prone issues are identified. Outcomes are shared, thereby giving each department a new appreciation of the role others play in the care of the patient.

Expectations and criteria for nurses' performance, as defined by the organization, can be found in *position descriptions*. The nursing service department is charged with the responsibility to formulate position descriptions for nurses that reflect professional standards of practice. They are frequently presented in the format familiar to all nurses (i.e., the nursing process). Gregory stresses the importance of including attitudinal data into the performance appraisal tool to be a link between the quantitative requirements and qualitative environmental factors.[5] Concern for output information from the performance appraisal system is an indication of the growing appreciation for using evaluation results in maintaining standards in all departments of organizations. Knowing what is included in the position description is the first step in being prepared to participate in performance appraisal.

In the sections that follow, performance appraisal will be considered as a *comprehensive* process that demands interaction between supervisors and staff. All content of earlier chapters in the text is integral to a quality performance appraisal system. Ideally, supervisors and staff understand and continue to improve their skill in *communication, group dynamics, decision making,* understanding of *motivating* forces that influence people, valuing ethical principles, and management of conflict. Furthermore, they have an *organizational* orientation and a *professional* commitment to nursing practice. The evaluation conference is viewed comprehensively as an interactive process that takes place between a supervisor and a staff member. Planning for and participating in the conference are seen as key activities of effective evaluation.

■ ACTIVE PARTICIPATION IN PERFORMANCE APPRAISAL

Performance appraisal must be *interactive* to be effective. One-way evaluation results (1) when supervisors, staff, or both lack the knowledge or the skills needed to use the process or (2) when they ignore the process. In one instance, evaluation can be something done to staff by supervisors. This happens when the staff nurse does not actively participate in the process. In another instance, objective evaluation of performance remains an expectation of the staff nurse because the supervisor does not appropriately enact the process. Either can be the result of a variety of factors that require analysis to arrive at a cause and solution to the problem.

Two-way participation in evaluation is important from a societal and a professional perspective. Society expects professionals to maintain high standards of performance. This expectation is indeed challenging in light of today's rapidly changing knowledge and technology advances. Toffler's depiction of the *third wave* generation takes on new meaning when applied to accountability in nursing today. There is the real possibility that supervisors, who are the evaluators, are significantly influenced by *second wave* norms (see Chapter 10 for a review of generational differences), making active participation by the nurse in evaluation highly desirable.

A developing professional person assumes responsibility and accountability for personal growth in the ability to *assess, plan,* and *evaluate* values, skills, and interests relative to professional state-of-the-art changes. The performance appraisal program provides the opportunity for formal participation in evaluation. It is there that latitude is accorded professionals for self-determination by enactment of internal motivation. Conscious awareness of strengths and weaknesses in self and in the organization can be identified there. Through self-inspection, incongruencies between ideal and actual behavior become apparent.

Active participation in evaluation then lies at the core of professional effectiveness. For a staff nurse to participate well in the process, adequate knowledge about performance appraisal is needed. Essential elements of a performance appraisal program are presented next because effectiveness begins there.

▓ ESSENTIAL ELEMENTS

Queen identifies the elements of the performance appraisal system as: (1) position description, (2) evaluation tool in harmony with the position, and (3) planning.[6] Documents and activities of an effective performance appraisal system in any organization (1) reflect its philosophy, mission and objectives, (2) have a clear statement of purpose, and (3) are tools that produce desired information.

Philosophy, Mission, and Objectives

Each health care organization has a *philosophy* that states beliefs about health care, the nature of clients, and how it serves a defined population. State-sponsored agencies differ philosophically from privately supported agencies. While the organizational philosophy is a mandate for all departments, each fashions its performance appraisal on those aspects for which it has major responsibility. For example, the nursing department incorporates professional standards of nursing practice as guiding principles for performance but also considers the need for economy. The business department incorporates practices of sound money management as a predominant responsibility but also considers the service mission of the agency. The overall performance of the organization is contingent on mutuality between departments.

Mission statements further distinguish primary responsibilities of departments and individuals. The mission of a neighborhood clinic differs from that of an acute care facility. The mission of general acute care facilities differs from the mission of specialty acute care facilities. Mission is a determinant of clinical credentials of the staff and specifies proficiency expectations in performance appraisal statements.

Ways in which an organization plans to carry out its mission are found in its *objectives*. One objective is to implement a comprehensive performance appraisal system that reflects its philosophy and mission through the performance of competent and effective managers at all levels. Position descriptions specify competencies of personnel and the expected quality of performance. The format of departmental performance appraisal tools might differ, but each remains congruent with the total management system designed to support the organization.

TABLE 11-1. IN COLUMN 1 SUPERVISOR'S RESPONSIBILITIES TO THE STAFF RELATIVE TO THE ORGANIZATION'S PERFORMANCE APPRAISAL PROGRAM ARE LISTED. IN COLUMN 2 THE CORRESPONDING STAFF NURSE AREAS OF ACCOUNTABILITY ARE LISTED. THE INFORMATION IN THIS TABLE SHOULD BE REVIEWED PERIODICALLY AT STAFF MEETINGS TO ENCOURAGE SKILLFUL IMPLEMENTATION OF THE PROGRAM.

Supervisor Responsibilities	Corresponding Staff Nurse Responses
Informs and interprets for staff the organizational performance appraisal program, to include:	Being appropriately informed about the performance appraisal program, the nurse is accountable for:
• Its purpose	• Viewing evaluation as important
• What is valued by management	• Acting on defined priorities
• What results to expect	• Awareness of rewards and disciplinary action
• What methods are used	
• What resources are available for goal attainment	• Familiarity with the evaluation form
	• Using resources to influence personal success
• Whether active participation is expected	• Being appropriately active in evaluation interviews
• How much self-determination is encouraged	• Exercising appropriate autonomy and being accountable for own decisions

Well-Defined Purpose

The purpose of performance appraisal should be clearly stated and understood by all in the organization, and it is the supervisor's responsibility to clarify this information to the staff (Table 11-1). The effective supervisor has a staff that is informed about performance appraisal and holds them accountable for knowing the following:

- The importance of evaluations.
- What the priorities are.
- What the rewards are and when disciplinary action is enforced.
- What is on the evaluation form.
- How to influence success.
- What role they play in evaluation.
- How much autonomy and accountability they have.[7]

See Table 11-1 regarding supervisor responsibilities and staff nurse responses.

The desired outcomes of performance appraisal are:

- Wise allocation of resources.
- Motivated employees who improve performance.

- Fair distribution of rewards and use of discipline.
- Employee growth.
- Nondiscrimination.[8]

Nondiscrimination regulations protect against unfair employment practices. It is one of the areas in the system having serious legal implications. Regulations require employers to have:

- Written records of evaluations.
- Clearly stated position descriptions.
- Evaluations based on job-related criteria.
- Evidence of tool validity and reliability.
- Trained, qualified raters.

Nondiscrimination along with other legal issues are discussed in detail in Chapter 12.

See Figure 11-1 for an illustration depicting the ongoing, interactive nature of performance appraisal and the individuals involved.

Evaluations that Produce Desired Outcomes

Selection of an evaluation tool is based on what information is desired. The format should permit systematic collection and analysis of objective data. The tool should have **validity** and **reliability.**[9]

Validity refers to the extent to which a tool measures the attributes it is intended to measure (i.e., does it measure a target attribute). Validity is the correlation between a tool result and a criterion (a professional standard) against which performance is measured. For example, if a standard requirement is individualized care based on cultural considerations and the tool does not measure assessment for cultural differences, then it is not valid for that target standard.

Reliability refers to how consistently the tool assigns scores to an attribute. An automobile odometer that does not consistently measure actual miles traveled is not reliable. Tools that are not reliable cannot be valid. Validity and reliability are essential characteristics of measurement and are part of measurement theory used by managers. For staff nurses, the tool must make sense and evaluate what it is supposed to relative to position descriptions. Experience with evaluating tools provides practical reinforcement of information about measurement for the practitioner. Since the mid 1980s computer technology has become a part of the performance appraisal system in terms of collecting and storing data and analyzing the results. Stalker et al list the following ways in which a computerized system improves evaluation.[10]

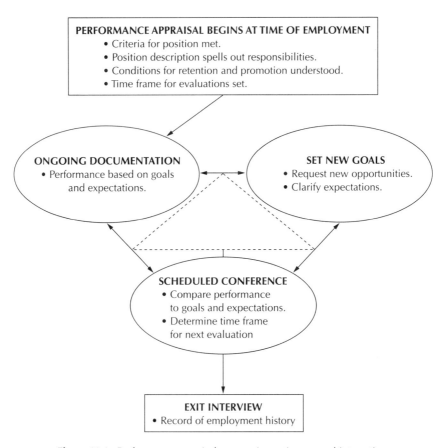

Figure 11-1. Performance appraisal process is continuous and interactive.

- Articulates and promotes professional standards.
- Integrates philosophy and practice.
- Replaces a long, redundant, confusing, and expensive system.
- Improves staff confidence in the managers as evaluators of their performance.
- Ease in weighting of categories being evaluated.
- Defines meritorious performance.
- Identifies issues for staff development.
- Identifies need for counseling.
- Predicts nurses who will be promoted in the future.

Adoption of a system that yields results similar to the above could benefit nurses who wish to remain in and be promoted within the caregiver role rather than into a management role. While technology is expensive and requires training time, it holds promise for several other positive changes in nursing in the area of personnel management.

Another factor for consideration in tool selection is whether individuals are being evaluated comparatively relative to the performance of others in their category (normative-referenced approach) or relative to accomplishment of predetermined goals (criterion-referenced approach). Both can be useful depending on what information is sought. Professionals are frequently evaluated using the criterion-referenced approach. A popular method of the approach is called **management by objectives,** a concept introduced by Drucker in 1954 and used in nursing since 1970.[11] The approach allows staff nurses the opportunity for active participation in their evaluation by increasing individuals' autonomy and accountability for their own growth. The concept forces ongoing involvement of staff in performance appraisal through goal setting, selecting methods to meet goals, and evaluating success. Therefore, performance appraisal is not an isolated, passive experience that occurs annually; instead, it is a process that becomes an integral part of everyday performance.

Normative-referenced approach is useful in situations when more than one person competes for a single position. It is competitive in nature and ranks individuals on attributes from high to low. Through normative-referenced evaluation, the best applicant can be selected for a position.

In summary, the way in which performance appraisal systems are structured is important because the system can fail if it is not a part of a total management system. It must reflect formal organizational documents—philosophy, mission, and objectives. Its purpose must be understood by all, and the tool selected must measure performance relative to each category of position descriptions. Furthermore, the system must be sensitive to legal and ethical issues as described in equal opportunity regulations.

■ PERFORMANCE APPRAISAL PROCESS

There are three main phases of the performance appraisal process: (1) planning, (2) interviewing, and (3) utilization of outcomes. Success of the process can be determined by indicators about performance in employees' files and quality care indices in unit records, such as the incidence of errors, accidents, and operational expenses.[12] Outcome indicators serve as targets for future goals, and the process is put into motion. A performance appraisal program is only as good as the process by which it is operationalized and the people who use it. A one-on-one **evaluation interview** is where the process is operationalized. The immediate supervisor and one staff nurse come together in a formal way to review past performance and to plan for the future. Each have responsibilities to make the program successful. Careful attention to each phase of the process is the key to productivity.

Planning for the Interview

Preparing for the evaluation interview is important. A period of reflective inspection of past performance by the nurse is helpful in identifying strengths and weaknesses. It is a time to revitalize ideals and commitments and to target an area for improvement. A positive approach to improving performance is better than a list of "don'ts" that are quickly forgotten. For example, a nurse might share a success through presenting an informative series of staff development sessions. In this way, leadership skills are developed while others profit from his or her experience.

Supervisors also need to prepare for evaluation interviews. A record of first-hand observations of the nurse's performance over time and a review of the previous evaluation report are necessary to focus on the individual. Judgment about performance must be related to position description expectations. Logistically, the supervisor selects a place that provides uninterrupted privacy and adequate time. The date and time are planned collaboratively with the nurse whenever possible. A reminder of the scheduled interview is sent in writing to the nurse. See Table 11-2 for a checklist for planning the evaluation interview.

Participating in the Evaluation Interview

Participating in the interview is the second phase of the process. The interview allows the supervisor to evaluate an individual staff member. It is never appropriate to discuss anyone else or allow the interview to deteriorate into a charge-countercharge situation during which the staff member becomes the evaluator. It is generally agreed that review of successes be the first topic for discussion to set a positive climate for the rest of the interview. It is important that an attitude of importance about evaluations prevail throughout the interview. Joking and idle chitchat are out of place, as are discussions of mutual social interests. Whether such events occur through nervousness or as

TABLE 11-2. COLUMN 1 IS A LIST OF RECOMMENDED SUPERVISOR BEHAVIORS PREPARATORY TO THE EVALUATION INTERVIEW. COLUMN 2 LISTS RECOMMENDED STAFF NURSE BEHAVIORS PREPARATORY TO THE EVALUATION INTERVIEW. THE BEHAVIORS ARE DESIGNED TO FACILITATE A PRODUCTIVE INTERVIEW.

Supervisor Behaviors	Staff Nurse Behaviors
• Records spaced, periodic observations of the nurse's performance relative to position and standards in a variety of situations	• Utilizes position and standard expectations daily
• Validates interpretation of important incidents in which the nurse is involved	• Documents specific patient outcomes that reflect planned nursing interventions
• Offers counsel and support as needed, citing position and standard expectations	• Asks for clarification of expectations when there is doubt, citing position responsibilities and professional standards
• As the time for a formal evaluation interview approaches, collaboratively plans a date and time with the nurse	• Summarizes accomplishments during the evaluation period
• Confirms the interview in writing	• Prepares a list of activities that could advance career to the next level, and negotiates for opportunities
• Reviews nurse's past evaluation record	• Collaborates with the supervisor relative to date, time, and expected preparation for the evaluation interview
• Completes the written evaluation form	

deliberate, time-consuming distractions to avoid addressing critical issues, they interfere with accomplishing the task at hand. Either party can and should assume the role of "gate keeper" so that the interview can proceed in orderly fashion.

The supervisor and the staff nurse have different roles and responsibilities in making the evaluation interview productive. See Table 11-2 for the roles of each. Disciplinary action is covered in more detail in Chapter 12, but some comments about it as it relates to the evaluation interview are included here. **Disciplinary action** is warranted by documented evidence of inferior performance that relates to position standards. When disciplinary action is invoked, it requires *due process* to protect the rights of the staff member. Due process (1) assumes innocence until proof of wrongdoing, (2) ensures the individual's right to be heard, and (3) assigns discipline that is reasonable relative to the wrongdoing. Disciplinary action should be instructive and corrective and aim to improve performance in the future rather than punish the past. Counseling is a positive approach to discipline based on fact finding and guidance. Counseling encourages desirable behavior instead of punishing undesirable behavior. Effective counseling preserves workers' self-image and dignity and keeps working relationships cooperative and constructive.[13]

Ways in which managers can maintain a positive climate when disciplinary action is necessary include (1) identifying resources to help the individual, (2) expressing confidence in his or her ability and willingness to improve, and (3) making a sincere offer of help and support whenever needed. Offering to schedule a follow-up interview when improvement is demonstrated lifts the staff member's stigma of being disciplined. Even with the best of efforts, however, the potential for a grievance action exists whenever disciplinary action is used. When the nurse's best efforts fail to solve a serious misunderstanding, a true grievance can exist. **Grievance** is defined as any real or imagined feeling of personal injustice that an employee has about the employment relationship.[14] The staff nurse should be aware that a grievance can be filed by anyone and does not depend on having a collective bargaining mechanism in place.

Having a grievance system is a requirement of equal employment regulations. It benefits organizations as well as individuals by bringing problems into the open so that corrective action can be attempted. Problems can be caught early and solved before they become serious. When a grievance system exists, everyone in the organization knows their actions are subject to scrutiny and they are put on guard to make decisions carefully. Disciplinary action, grievance process, and discrimination are covered in detail in Chapter 12.

The staff nurse's role during the evaluation interview is *active* participation facilitated through *planning*. The informed, constructively assertive nurse can gain more from the interview than the unprepared nurse. Interviews can boost morale or can be a source of dissatisfaction. Skillful and effective participation in the evaluation interview is important and should be a stated expectation for everyone in the organization. See Table 11-3 for a checklist of supervisor and staff nurse roles and responsibilities relative to evaluation interviews.

Using Evaluation Results

Making use of interview results is the third phase of the performance appraisal process. It is ongoing. Careful attention must be given to how the results will be used if they are to be of optimal value. Brookfield cautions that blindly rushing into action in the excitement of new insights and opportunities can lead to bad decisions.[15] Time is needed to consider alternative courses of action. All planning for and active participation in evaluations will

TABLE 11-3. COLUMN 1 IS A LIST OF SUPERVISOR RESPONSIBILITIES FOR CONDUCTING THE EVALUATION INTERVIEW. COLUMN 2 IS A LIST OF STAFF NURSE RESPONSIBILITIES FOR ACTIVE PARTICIPATION IN THE EVALUATION INTERVIEW. ALL ACTIVITIES LISTED IN BOTH COLUMNS ARE ESSENTIAL IF THE INTERVIEW IS TO BENEFIT THE NURSE AND THE ORGANIZATION.

Supervisor Responsibilities	Staff Nurse Responsibilities
• Conducts the interview • States judgments about the nurse's performance relative to position and standard expectations beginning with positive accomplishments • Provides justification for rewards or disciplinary action based on criteria • Encourages the nurse to new challenges • Specifies time period for next formal evaluation interview • Secures from the nurse specific goals to be accomplished during the next evaluation period	• Shares documented evidence of main accomplishments since the last evaluation interview relative to position and standard expectations • Clarifies circumstances of situation as necessary • States goals for the immediate future • Requests opportunities for specific activities that will promote progression • Expects guidance and direction from the supervisor • Adds comments to the evaluation form in writing, stating degree of satisfaction with the interview. Attaches any documentation needed.

have no long-range effects if results remain in the personnel office file. It is necessary, therefore, that a structured plan for using the evaluation outcomes be formulated and used.

Scheduled interim review of evaluation reports by supervisors and staff nurses permit improvements to occur in increments as each stage of improvement solidifies. The substance of an interim review could come from thinking about how much closer one is to a goal, and how much farther one has to go. Motivation is strengthened as short-range goals are accomplished on the way to reaching the long-range goal.

■ REWARDS

Rewards in nursing have become an issue in recent years and a concern of management. Recall the reorganization of patient care standards discussed in Chapter 1 and the different expectations among nurses because of their different orientations to the profession discussed in the chapter on motivation (Chapter 10). Satisfying expectations of staff nurses and meeting the needs of higher acuity-level patients as a result of DRGs forced management to reconsider the traditional single-track reward system for nurses. For decades, the only way a staff nurse could advance was vertically into an entirely different role. Staff nurses, proficient at the bedside, were "promoted" to a management or teaching position. There were few management and teaching positions available, and most nurses remained throughout their careers in staff nurse positions with the concomitant salary compression and shift change schedules.

Attempts on the part of nurse managers to satisfy different needs of individuals include experimenting with variable scheduling to replace the traditional five days a week, eight-hour shifts. Several alternatives have emerged that provide attractive incentives for some nurses to remain in nursing. Various patterns provide for:

- Four 10-hour shifts a week
- Three 12-hour shifts a week
- Two 12-hour weekend shifts every week

In some acute care settings, the latter provides a salary greater than that of a 40-hour a week schedule. The "menu" of schedules has been met with varying degrees of enthusiasm and success. The hours can be ideal for students who need to be free during the week to attend classes. Parents of young children might find the hours attractive in that they can avoid costly child care expenses. Variable scheduling has the potential to reduce dissatisfaction of nurses in patient care settings and to improve staff nurse satisfaction because it fits their lifestyles.

On the other hand, there are also problems with variable scheduling. Coordinating the schedule when nurses work different time patterns can be difficult. Confusion about patient care responsibilities during overlap hours can cause conflicts. Finally, there has been no systematic evaluation of the effect of long working hours on ability to perform quality patient care.

Another strategy for improving rewards for nurses has been the introduction of **clinical ladders** (Fig. 11-2). The concept of a clinical ladder permits horizontal advancement, keeping excellent clinicians in their chosen role. Nurses advance through a determined number of levels within a position category (e.g., staff nurse) based on predetermined criteria. At each level there are additional advantages to the nurse (e.g., fewer rotating shifts, higher salary, or fewer weekends on duty). Once the highest level in the category has been reached, advancement requires additional education, usually a masters degree in nursing.

Level One

Entry-level nurse.
—Accountable to Asst. H.N.
—Manages care for assigned patients.
—Begins unit charge role with mentor.
—Unit committee member.
—Rotates shifts.

Level Two

Minimum of one year practice in a similar setting.
—Assigned as charge nurse on occasion.
—Demonstrates consistent high-quality and innovative patient care.
—Has reduced number of rotation of shifts.
—Merit salary increase.

Level Three

Bachelor of science degree in nursing required.
—Proficient in all Level Two responsibilities.
—Serves as a mentor for new staff.
—Chairs a unit committee.
—Effective as a change agent.
—Frequent charge nurse role.
—Merit salary increase.

Level Four

Assistant head nurse responsible for all patient care matters on assigned unit.
—Accountable for quality of care delivered on the unit.
—No rotation of shifts.*
—Generous salary increases.
—Generous differential salary for evening or night shifts.

*Assistant head nurse assigned permanently to one shift, which can be days, evenings, or nights.

Figure 11-2. A diagram of levels within the staff nurse category allowing for progression without having to leave the patient care role. The levels with benefits and responsibilities depicted *are examples*. Assistant head nurse position at Level Four is considered a clinical role rather than a formal management role.

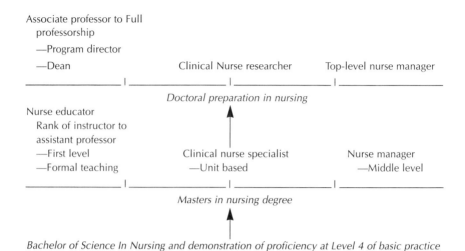

Associate professor to Full
    professorship
    —Program director
    —Dean   Clinical Nurse researcher   Top-level nurse manager

_____ | _____ | _____ | _____

Doctoral preparation in nursing

Nurse educator
Rank of instructor to
assistant professor
    —First level   Clinical nurse specialist   Nurse manager
    —Formal teaching   —Unit based   —Middle level

_____ | _____ | _____ | _____

Masters in nursing degree

Bachelor of Science In Nursing and demonstration of proficiency at Level 4 of basic practice

Figure 11-3. The path from basic clinical practice to advanced career levels in nursing. The academic preparation represents recent changes in recommended preparation for professional nurse roles.

Sometimes vertical progression is referred to as moving into a Career ladder (Fig. 11-3). Nurses move out of the basic practice levels and pursue advanced education as preparation for roles as managers, educators, or clinical specialists.

Clinical and career ladders have met with considerable success but are not totally without problems. Confusion over authority and responsibility between clinical specialists and head nurses on the same unit can cause conflicts. While the organizational chart shows what their relation is to each other, no document can clarify how to handle day-to-day events.

A menu of benefits is another way an organization can attempt to satisfy individuals with different interests and needs (Fig. 11-4). Nurses with bachelors degrees have no use for the tuition remission benefit to complete the bachelor degree. Not all agencies support graduate education, meaning a lost benefit to nurses with bachelors degrees. A married nurse whose spouse's employer provides comprehensive family health insurance coverage has little use for health insurance.

Some organizations elect to offer variable benefits that can be selected from a menu. Employees select from the menu up to a specified monetary allowance that is the same for all. In this way, the cost of the benefit package remains the same for the organization, and employees have the opportunity to meet their own individual needs. Young nurses with small children can

General Hospital
Liberty City, USA

All full-time employees are entitled to the following schedule of benefits.

Everyone receives:

- Two weeks paid vacation
- Paid holidays established by the hospital
- Participation in the retirement plan.

During the first five (5) years of employment, each employee may select thirteen (13) additional benefit points from the following list:

- 5 pts—Full family-health insurance coverage
- 3 pts—Individual health insurance coverage
- 2 pts—Individual dental insurance coverage
- 5 pts—Tuition remission for a baccalaureate degree
- 2 pts—Additional two (2) weeks paid vacation
- 3 pts—Paid life insurance equal to 3 times basic salary
- 3 pts—Increased retirement program contributions by the hospital
- 8 pts—Remission of child care costs during work hours
- 5 pts—Free meals during work hours
- 2 pts—Free parking on hospital lot during work hours

After five (5) years of full-time, consecutive employment, an additional five (5) points may be selected.

Figure 11-4. An example of what a menu of employment benefits might look like. The point system shown is a rough guesstimation of value of each benefit and has no basis in fact. A reduced benefit package can be developed for permanent, part-time employees.

choose more life insurance rather than retirement benefits. Nurses close to retirement can choose additional retirement benefits in place of life insurance or vacation time. Nurses with bachelors degrees can choose additional vacation time or additional retirement benefits in place of tuition remission. Variable benefits is an example of how organizations change to meet volatile internal and external environmental demands.

■ OBSTACLES TO PERFORMANCE IMPROVEMENT

The obvious obstacles to performance improvement are (1) a program that does not address performance requirements, (2) vagueness of purpose, (3) unqualified raters, (4) a tool that does not provide desired information, (5) poor record keeping, and (6) failure to use results. The obstacles come about for a variety of reasons, which might include any or all of the following: (1) lack of support from administration, (2) resistance on the part of raters because of the time involved, (3) rater biases and rating errors that result in unreliable and invalid information, (4) lack of clear, objective standards of performance, (5) failure to communicate purposes and results of evaluation to staff, and (6) failure to monitor the process effectively. Queen summarizes problems into three categories: (1) time, (2) paperwork, and (3) incongruent judgments.[16]

Rater biases and errors have been listed as commonly occurring distortions in performance appraisal by Stevens.[17] They first appeared in print in 1976, but readers might still find some of them familiar in their own experiences. Labels applied to the errors and distortions help explain them.

The *halo effect* is a distortion that occurs when the rater assumes that the individual who performs well in some areas must therefore perform well in other areas that have not been observed. Instead of acknowledging that there was no opportunity to observe a particular behavior, the rater assigns a high score to the behavior.

In the *recency effect*, the rater weighs recent events more heavily than other events that occurred throughout the evaluation period. Observations and record keeping can facilitate more accurate assignment of value to performance that occurred since the last evaluation interview.

Problem distortion occurs when a single, poor observed performance weighs more than good performances that went unobserved. Conferring with the staff nurse about circumstances of the problem when it happens can reduce the distortion.

The *sunflower effect* occurs when the rater grades everyone on the unit the same based on overall group performance. There is failure to focus attention on the individual. Assets go unrewarded, and weaknesses are not corrected.

Central tendency errors are the result of rating the staff nurse "average" when in fact real performance is unknown. Raters should not hesitate to record that certain behaviors were not observed during the period being evaluated. Since evaluation is interactive, the rater might ask the nurse to bring to the conference self-evaluation statements about behaviors not observed by the rater.

Rater temperament effect reflects variances in the degree of importance different raters assign to the same attribute. Prioritizing performance based on total situational factors reduces the incidence of making judgments based on predetermined expectations of a person who sees performance out of context.

The *guessing error* occurs when the rater guesses about performance rather than recording that it is unknown. All distortions and errors described are due to some flaw in the system. Rater incompetence or low priority of evaluations as an organizational attitude are some possible causes.

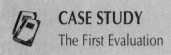

CASE STUDY
The First Evaluation

Kim Jackson, a new graduate, recently accepted her first position as a graduate nurse. When she interviewed for the position, she was given a packet of materials that described all aspects of her staff nurse position. As a part of her orientation, she was expected to become familiar with the information in the packet. A portion of the orientation period was spent in discussion and clarification of the materials.

By the time orientation was over, Kim felt confident about her preparation to function as an informed nurse in the organization. Everything seemed designed to unify the various aspects of employment to focus on delivery of high-quality nursing care throughout the nursing department. She was glad she had decided to practice in such a well-organized and high-quality organization.

After six months as a staff nurse, Kim remembered that she was due for her first evaluation as a bona fide professional. She decided to review the materials she had received at the time of her employment to be prepared for the interview with her head nurse. Two weeks went by, during which she heard nothing from the head nurse about an evaluation. She decided to ask about it. The head nurse said, "Oh yes, your evaluation form has been completed and is ready for your signature. You are doing fine. Don't forget to stop by my office soon to sign the form, or you won't get a raise."

Based on the purpose and process of performance appraisal information that was presented in this chapter, recommend a course of action for Kim.

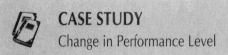

CASE STUDY
Change in Performance Level

Melanie Jamieson has a several-year history of receiving excellent evaluations. Her head nurse has appropriately used the evaluation system in describing Melanie's progression as a staff nurse, providing documentation of her behaviors as called for. Shortly after her last evaluation conference, Melanie found herself in a situation where personal responsibilities were competing for her time, attention, and energy. She knew that the quality of her nursing performance suffered as a result and was certainly not up to her personal standards or the standards of her head nurse. Consequently, she was prepared to explore with her head nurse ways in which she could resolve problems inherent in her situation. She definitely did not expect a raise because her recent performance did not warrant one. To her surprise, her head nurse was unrealistically high in her rating of Melanie's performance and recommended a raise. It is as if she were totally unaware of changes in Melanie's performance.

There are several possible reasons for the head nurse's behavior. One possibility is that she felt justified in "carrying" Melanie because of her earlier history, thinking she would "snap back." Another possibility is that the head nurse had no experience or skill in delivering a difficult message.

- What is your response to the first possibility?
- What are the problems created when the second possibility exists?
- How difficult would it be for you to deliver a difficult message?
- What would you do if you were Melanie?

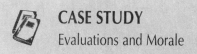

CASE STUDY
Evaluations and Morale

The morale of staff nurses on a particular unit is very low due, according to the staff, to the outcomes of their evaluation conferences. Comments by the head nurse seem "out of the blue." A single event that happened months ago became the focus of the head nurse's evaluation of the nurses. Nurses feel they enter the evaluation conference without any idea that the head nurse attached so much importance to a one-time behavior. The performances the nurses feel good about are discounted in the written report. The result is that the staff nurses feel that they are being scrutinized for errors. There is an increasing level of stress and anxiety among them. Communication is guarded, adding to the strife and poor working relationships.

- Apply principles from this chapter to analyze the problem and recommend an approach to this deteriorating situation.
- List as many causes that you can think of for the head nurse's behavior. Keep in mind that there are two sides to every story.

■ SUMMARY

In this chapter, performance appraisal is viewed as a highly valuable system designed to improve performance. While it is an expensive endeavor for the organization, it is worthy of the time and expense. The program must reflect the organization's philosophy, mission, and objectives, and a process must be developed that produces desired results. The process is interactive, consisting of three phases: (1) planning, (2) the interview, (3) using results. It should be a clearly stated expectation, understood by everyone in the organization, that all participate actively in the program. Because of complexities in organizational settings, performance appraisal must be studied to be understood by participants. Use of results is a frequently neglected phase. Failure to act on results negates the other two phases, because results are essentially the "evaluation of evaluations." Individuals and organizations benefit from effective performance appraisal programs. Individuals more readily advance in their careers, and organizations make better use of personnel strengths. Early identification of problems allows corrective action in an economic way. Problems with performance appraisal programs are described.

Throughout the chapter, the focus is on active participation in the program by informed nurses. The ultimate goal is to keep professional standards of nursing practice pivotal to evaluation of nurses' performance. Economic constraints must not significantly interfere with professional standards.

It is a firm belief of the authors that professional standards and economic efficiency are not mutually incompatible. We also believe that the new generation of nurses will meet today's challenges as successfully as past generations of nurses managed their time-related challenges. Their commitment to professional standards and values will continue to preserve the profession during times of strong outside challenges.

 STUDENT EXERCISES

1. A staff nurse is told by her supervisor to remain in the conference room after change-of-shift report so that the supervisor can give her her evaluation. It is the first time the supervisor has communicated to the nurse about the evaluation. Outline the major problems with the manner in which the supervisor is handling evaluations. Propose solutions.

2. During a floor meeting, the head nurse on a unit explains to the staff that evaluations are going to be late because she had to fill in for the

unit secretary who was on vacation for a week and then had to take a full-patient assignment due to staff vacations and nurses who called in sick. She seems to take the situation in stride even though expected salary increases and evaluation interviews will be delayed. What principles of management are being violated? As a staff nurse whose salary increase will be delayed, respond to her announcement.

3. You overhear a fellow staff nurse say that professional nursing standards of care can no longer be met because of budgetary cuts. From what you understand about professional standards of practice, respond to the nurse's comment.

■ REFERENCES

1. *Monitoring and Evaluation of Quality and Appropriateness of Care.* The Joint Commission on Accreditation of Health Care Organizations, 1988, p. 1–13.
2. Queen VA, "Performance evaluation," *Nursing Management,* 26:9, September 1995, p. 52–55.
3. Beck S, "Developing a Primary Nursing Performance Appraisal Tool," *Nursing Management,* 21:1, January 1990, p. 36–42.
4. Gropper EI, Skarzynski JJ, "Integrating Quality Assessment and Improvement," *Nursing Management,* 26:3, March 1995, p. 22–23.
5. Gregory GD, "Using a Performance Information System," *Nursing Management,* 26:7, July 1995, p. 74–77.
6. Queen VA.
7. Bassett LC, Metzger N, *Achieving Excellence,* Rockvill, MD: Aspen Publishers, 1986, p. 31.
8. Davis K, *Human Behavior at Work—Organizational Behavior,* New York: McGraw-Hill, 1981, p. 457.
9. Stamps P, *Nurses and Work Satisfaction: An Index for Measurement,* Ann Arbor, MI: Health Administration Press, 1986, p. 66.
10. Stalker MZ, Kornblith AB, Lewis PM, Parker R, "Measurement Technology Applications in Performance Appraisal," *Journal of Nursing Administration,* April 1986, p. 12–17.
11. Spitzer R, *Nursing Productivity—The Hospital's Key to Survival and Profit,* Chicago: S-N Publication, 1986, p. 101.
12. Ibid.
13. Davis K, p. 321.
14. Ibid., p. 361.
15. Brookfield SD, *Developing Critical Thinkers,* San Francisco: Jossey-Bass, 1987, p. 79.
16. Queen VA.
17. Stevens BJ, "Performance Appraisal: What the Nurse Executive Expects from It," *Journal of Nursing Administration,* 6:10, October 1976, p. 26–31.

12

Legal Issues in the Workplace

Introduction

Nurse administrators and managers need to be familiar with laws and legislation related to nursing practice, administration, labor-management, and employment. Both federal and state laws influence how health care is given and reimbursed and, therefore, they have an impact on nursing practice. Nurse administrators and managers also need to be cognizant of not only their own rights and responsibilities, but also those of their employees, particularly professional nurses, since it is the practice and welfare of this group of workers to whom and for whom they are most often accountable.

Awareness and understanding of legal issues is imperative for a number of reasons. One, these are times of considerable change and increasing complexity in the health care environment. Runaway health care costs have resulted in integrated health systems or networks. Two, work redesign has been a consequence of such restructuring. The related reductions in the work force via layoffs, decreased work hours, and/or a change in job descriptions have led to anxious and, in some cases, dissatisfied workers. Yet, in times of change, organizations depend on committed workers for their success.[1] Three, health care institutions and agencies employ racially and ethnically diverse workers, as well as large numbers of women workers. Several laws/legislation have been instituted to protect women and minority workers from discrimination. Four, litigious tendencies of the American public are widespread and have been particularly acute in the health field with multi-million dollar awards not only to patients and families for malpractice or negligence by employees but also to employees as a result of employers' insensitivity to, ignorance of, or flagrant violation of legal rules and regulations.

Consequently, it is imperative that nurse managers know the kinds of situations that can lead to **litigation** and take steps to avoid being sued. A first step is gaining knowledge about legal regulations that apply to workers and the work environment. It is not the intent of this chapter to discuss criminal problems in the workplace (for example, nursing without a license or substance abuse) or statutory law (for example, Nurse Practice Acts). Rather, it is the intent to discuss laws governing employment practices and labor laws regulating relationships between unions and employers. Nurse administrators could be held liable for violations of these laws. There are many legal issues and **legal constraints** involved in hiring and employment. Few aspects of the employer-employee relationship are free from regulation by either state or federal law.[2] Many of these relate to specific aspects of personnel management and will be the focus of this chapter.

 ## KEY CONCEPTS

Affirmative Action refers to the active legislative attempt to insure that minorities (or others so deemed discriminated against) are provided set-aside positions in the workplace. These laws were enacted to right historical wrongs.

Discrimination is an illegal act that prohibits an individual from working on the basis of gender, age, ethnic, racial, or disability status.

Collective Bargaining is an attempt by a formal group to negotiate terms of a contract.

Equal Employment Opportunity (EEO) laws refer to those legislative acts to insure fair hiring and conduct in the workplace.

Equal Employment Opportunity Commission (EEOC) refers to the enforcing agency for EEO laws.

Sexual Harassment is a special case of EEO law that prohibits unwanted sexual advances from those who directly influence the work. May be of two types: (1) *Quid pro quo*—sexual requests for privileges in the workplace; and (2) Hostile environment (blatantly offensive) refers to the creation of a workplace setting that interferes with or intimidates an individual's ability to work.

Litigation refers to the acts of bringing a lawsuit.

Legal Constraints refers to the structural limitations imposed by existing law.

Strike is an organized action and work stoppage by a formal group who uses this methodology to negotiate terms of a contract. This is usually a last resort when negotiating fails.

■ EQUAL EMPLOYMENT OPPORTUNITY (EEO) LAWS

Equal Employment Opportunity laws were the first legislation in the area of employment hiring practices and they resulted from years of **discrimination** toward persons of color. The federal government has enacted several laws to expand equal employment opportunities by prohibiting discrimination not only on the basis of race but also on the basis of sex, age, religion, physical impairment, pregnancy, or national origin. There are also state laws addressing equal employment opportunities. The nurse manager should be familiar with and abide by the following equal employment opportunity laws when hiring and assigning nursing personnel.

The Civil Rights Act of 1964

Title VII of the 1964 Civil Rights Act protects people from discrimination for reasons of race, color, national origin, sex and religion. It *prohibits* discrimination based on factors unrelated to job qualifications and *promotes* employment based on ability and merit. Executive orders by President Lyndon Johnson in 1965 and 1967 strengthened the Civil Rights Act. Because some groups had a long history of being discriminated against, the government sought to assist those groups in catching up with the rest of the work force. Therefore, the executive order created an **affirmative action** component. In most states, affirmative action plans are voluntary unless government contracts are involved. Affirmative action isn't the same as equal opportunity. EEO laws are aimed at preventing discrimination, whereas affirmative action plans are aimed at activity seeking to fill job vacancies with groups who are underemployed and have had a history of being discriminated against.

The **Equal Employment Opportunity Commission (EEOC)** is responsible for enforcing Title VII.[3]

Age Discrimination Act

In 1967, Congress enacted the Age Discrimination in Employment Act to prohibit job discrimination solely because of age (discrimination against people aged 40 to 70). This act applies to employers of 20 or more persons. An amendment in 1978 prohibited mandatory retirement for persons under 70 years of age. A second amendment in 1987 removed even this restriction except in certain job categories.[4]

Pregnancy Discrimination Act

The Pregnancy Discrimination Act of 1978 prohibits sex discrimination against women who are or might become pregnant. Under protection of this act, neither potential legal liability nor protecting the women's fetus is sufficient reason to practice sex discrimination.[5]

Americans with Disabilities Act (ADA)

Passed in 1990, the ADA mandates that people with physical or mental abilities be integrated into the mainstream of the work force. It states:

> No qualified individual with a disability shall, by reason of such disability, be excluded from participation in or be denied the benefits of the services, programs, or activities of a public entity, or be subjected to discrimination by any such entity. One who is disabled is defined as anyone who has a record of or is perceived as having a mental or physical impairment that substantially limits at least one major life activity.[6]

The act went into effect in 1992 and not only prohibits discrimination but also delineates enforceable standards.

Sexual Harassment: A Special Case of Discrimination

Although **sexual harassment** has become a newsworthy topic since such highly publicized events as the Anita Hill-Clarence Thomas Supreme Court hearing and the Navy Tailhook scandal, the sexual exploitation of women at work is not a new problem. Bularzik and Segraves cite records dating as far back as colonial times.[7,8] Further, sexual harassment was not named or made a household word until the mid-1970s.[9,10] However, approximately 40–50% of working women experience sexual harassment.[11,12]

In her influential book, MacKinnon , a feminist legal scholar, argued that sexual harassment was primarily a women's problem and should be considered a form of sex discrimination under Title VII of the Civil Rights Act .[13,14] Consistent with her position, the EEOC established its now well-known guidelines in 1980. Although the guidelines per se do not have the force of law, the courts generally rely on them. According to the EEOC, sexual harassment is defined as follows:

> Unwelcome sexual advances, requests for sexual favors, and other verbal or physical conduct of a sexual nature constitute sexual harassment when: (a) submission to such conduct is made either explicitly or implicitly a term or condition of employment, (b) submission to or rejection of such conduct is used as the basis for employment decisions affecting the individual, or (c) such conduct has the purpose of reasonably interfering with an individual's work performance or creating an intimidating, hostile, or offensive work environment.[15]

Most of the early cases were *quid pro quo* in nature ("this for that") in which there was an overt demand for sex in exchange for job privileges or promotions (*a* and *b* in the above definition). However, these cases soon gave way to *hostile environment harassment* (*c* in the definition above), which is more widespread and more difficult to prove.[16] In 1986, the landmark case *Meritor Savings Bank v Vinson* set the precedent for deferring guidelines to the EEOC when the U.S. Supreme Court concurred with the D.C. Court of Appeals' decision that sexual harassment that creates a hostile environment is just as discriminatory as *quid pro quo* harassment.[17-19] Therefore, actionable sexual harassment can include unsolicited nonreciprocal verbal and physical sexual advances, other sexual contact such as leering, gestures, touching and pinching, as well as pejorative behaviors and remarks directed at women (e.g., sexist jokes or pin-up calenders).[20] According to the EEOC, the greatest number of legal complaints about sexual harassment have occurred in the service industry, which includes health care.[21]

Employers can be held liable for acts by coworkers, supervisors, and managerial staff if the employer knew of the conduct and didn't address it. Although cases are still being decided that will give more guidance in determining the type of evidence necessary for holding the employer accountable, it is clear that employers have a responsibility for fostering a "no tolerance" environment.[22-24] Employer liability for acts against workers may be minimized by taking immediate and appropriate corrective action in instances of sexual harassment.

The emergent change in the social context of gender issues in the workplace is challenging nurse administrators as organizational leaders. This, plus the fact that nursing is predominantly a female profession, means that they need to provide a clear understanding of the complex issues surrounding sexual harassment, voice opposition to sexual harassment, and initiate appropriate actions within their organizations.[25]

Costs of sexual harassment are high, not only for the harassed individual, but also for the organization, and include not only litigation costs but also other direct and indirect costs.[26] The financial impact of sexual harassment was assessed by the federal government in a large-scale survey of federal workers: sexual harassment cost the federal government an estimated $267 million over a two-year period.[26] In another survey of Fortune 500 companies, harassment cost a typical company approximately $6.7 million per year.[27] Costs included replacing employees who left their jobs, paying employees sick leave, reduced individual and group productivity, and costs of internal complaint handling. In addition, these studies found that there were indirect costs, which included, for example, lower confidence in management in general, reduced job satisfaction, diminished commitment to the organization, and a less positive view of the organization's communication practice.

Prevention programs are the best way to avoid or reduce costs. To treat employees fairly and to avoid such costs, the administrator needs to develop a clear policy statement opposing sexual harassment, establish grievance procedures and processes for reporting harassment, take prompt and appropriate action in response to reported incidents, develop training programs for managers to increase awareness and sensitivity, and develop educational programs or workshops for all employees regarding reactions and behaviors on the part of victims that are likely to resolve or reduce harassment, reporting procedures, and disciplinary action for perpetrators.[28] Nurse administrators need to lead the way in educating nursing personnel.

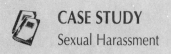

CASE STUDY
Sexual Harassment

A female staff nurse was assigned to care for a middle-aged male patient with a pulmonary diagnosis of a chronic nature. The patient has a history of frequent admissions and is often admitted to the same nursing unit. Throughout his admission, he consistently tells the nurse dirty jokes, makes intimate comments about her physical appearance and sex life, and the wall in his room sports a nude poster. The climate created by this patient makes the nurse want to avoid going into the patient's room.[29]

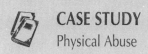

CASE STUDY
Physical Abuse

A nurse executive recounts an incident reported to her by the manager in the operating room. A physician who stated he was "just having fun" attached a vaginal clamp to the abdominal area of a staff nurse's scrub attire. The clamp pinched and broke the staff nurse's skin.[30]

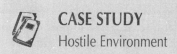

CASE STUDY
Hostile Environment

A staff nurse found a "sexual harassment consent form" posted in the women's bathroom, shortly after a legitimate notice about sexual harassment had been posted in the hospital. She called the personnel director to report it. He not only verified it but stated it originated at a department head meeting as a joke. The nurse told him she didn't think it was funny at all.[31]

- If these cases had been reported to you as the nurse manager, how would you handle each of them?

■ LABOR-MANAGEMENT LAWS

Some observers feel that employment and labor-management laws are too prescriptive and, therefore, prevent creativity. They view them with resentment and hostility. More recently, progressive managers have taken a proactive stance, adopting an attitude of acceptance and tolerance and starting to forge newer models of work structures and relationships between labor and management.

Unions and Collective Bargaining

Labor organizations have become a significant factor in hospital-employee relations. Nurse administrators must understand the impact of unionization on the health care industry and the legislation regarding employment practice. Since they may be dealing with employees represented by unions and working under collective bargaining agreements, they need to be familiar with the provisions and protections offered by law and the basic tenets of these labor relations laws.

The *National Labor Relations Act (Wagner Act)* of 1935 governs collective bargaining between employee groups (unions) and their managers or employers.[32] **Collective bargaining** includes the activities occurring between labor and management that concern employee relations, such as negotiation of formal labor agreements and day-to-day interactions. The NLRA is administered by the National Labor Relations Board (NLRB), which determines an employee's union representation status and resolves labor-management disputes.

Since its initial passage, several amendments have changed the provisions of the act. In 1947, the *Taft-Hartley Amendment* excluded not-for-profit hospitals from the definition of "employer" in the National Labor Relations Act. Consequently, unionization of workers in health care institutions was illegal until 1962 when President Kennedy amended the act by executive order to allow public employees to join unions. As a result, the first collective bargaining by nurses employed by city, county, and state hospitals and agencies began. Congress amended the act further in 1974 to allow employees of not-for-profit hospitals and organizations to form or join unions.[33]

The initial NLRA recognized only three bargaining units: all professionals, all non-professionals, and guards. However, in 1991, in a major case involving the American Hospital Association, the U.S. Supreme Court upheld the rule of the NLRB that allowed recognition of up to eight categories, including a separate one for registered nurses (RNs). This issue had an enormous impact for the American Nurses Association (ANA) and its state affiliates which act as collective bargaining units or agents for RNs. Although both the ANA and other unions began targeting hospitals and RNs for organizing since the new NLRB rules were instituted, most of the activity has amounted to "nothing more than a flurry of activity."[34]

Although union activity has increased slightly since the mid-1970s, 90% of the six million health care workers remain nonunionized.[35] Further, only approximately 280,000 RNs in the United States are represented by a collective bargaining agent: about 150,000 by the ANA and about 130,000 by other unions.[36] RNs have been ambivalent about joining unions. A recurring theme surrounding unionization is the issue of professionalism. Some argue that collective bargaining and strike clauses are contrary to professionalism, while others see it as an opportunity to improve relations with management, raise the status of the profession, resolve staffing and patient safety issues, and improve health care delivery.[37]

According to Moylan, the nurse manager must be thoroughly versed in four parts of the NLRA: Section 7, Section 8A, the definition of supervisor, and the definition of employer.[38] Section 7 guarantees employees the right to organize while protecting the rights of those who refrain. Section 8A identifies five categories of unfair labor practices that restrict employee rights. These are (1) interference with the right to organize, (2) domination (for example, the nurse administrator supports one collective bargaining agent over another), (3) encouraging or discouraging membership in a union by preferential treatment of union or nonunion employees, (4) discharging an employee for giving testimony or filing a charge with the NLRB, and (5) refusal to bargain collectively (for example, negotiate salaries or working conditions).

According to the terms of the NLRA, supervisors are excluded from coverage (that is, they have no right to organize or engage in collective bargaining). The NLRA defines "supervisor" as

> Any individual having authority, in the interest of the employer, to hire, transfer, suspend, lay off, recall, promote, discharge, *assign*, reward, or discipline other employees, or *responsibly* to *direct them*, or to adjust their grievances, or effectively to recommend such action, if in connection with the foregoing the exercise of authority is not merely a routine or clerical nature, but requires the use of independent judgment (29 U.S.C.142,11).

It also states that anyone acting in a supervisory capacity, regardless of job title, is acting as the "employer." It is this issue of the definition of supervisor that has most recently been redefined and has implications for all RNs.

For several years, the NLRB maintained that staff nurses who direct the work of less-skilled employees in the exercise of professional judgment do so with a focus on the "well-being of the patient" and are not exercising their authority "in the interest of the employer." Therefore, they were not considered supervisors by the NLRB.[39] However, this argument was rejected in 1994 when the U.S. Supreme Court upheld a decision by an appellate court in the case of *National Labor Relations Board v Health Care Retirement Corporation of America*, which ruled that nurses who exercise supervisory authority are excluded from the coverage of the NLRA.[40] In this case, the appellate court held that licensed practical nurses (LPNs) at an Ohio nursing home, who directed the work of nurses aides, acted as supervisors and, therefore, were not protected from firing when they took action to improve working conditions.[41] The confusion for nursing management is which definition is binding: the Supreme Court's definition of supervisor, which includes some staff nurse responsibilities (thus eliminating the right of staff nurses to unionize), or the NLRB's more restrictive definition of nonstatutory supervisor (thus staff nurses can unionize).

Some observers feel that the former interpretation may open the door for employers seeking to exclude RNs from bargaining units since they could argue that RNs have supervisory status when directing the work of less-skilled employees, especially since one facet of the current work redesign and restructuring in hospitals is to downgrade the number of professional nurses and increase the number of unlicensed assistive personnel.[42]

In fact, a Montana hospital has attempted to eject the collective bargaining unit that represents its RNs based on the Supreme Court's ruling on nurses' supervisory status. The hospital's Board of Trustees voted not to recognize the union after expiration of the contract ("Hospital uses top court issues," 1994). In similar situations in hospitals in Michigan and New York, the state nurses' associations have filed unfair labor practice charges.[43] Besides hindering union activities, the Supreme Court's ruling could dampen nurses' willingness to speak out when they have concerns about safety in the workplace.[44] Labor union leaders hope, however, that the NLRB will reinterpret certain provisions of the NLRA's definition of supervisor. The ANA and other labor unions have united in lobbying for an amendment to the NLRA that would guarantee nurses' protection.[45]

While this seems to be an era of uncertainty for labor leaders and formation of new collective bargaining units, several observers note that the uncertainty is part of an era of transition and change in health care that necessitates new models for labor-management relations. They advocate a model for professional collaboration for labor relations, working together to establish mutual agreements of language interpretation, and forging win-win approaches to the grievance process. The need to decrease costs is forcing employers to change the way they do business. More progressive employers are adopting more cooperative and collaborative approaches to labor management relations, such as flattening hierarchical organizations, creating self-directed work teams, and forging new partnerships with workers, which increase their ownership and participation in outcomes.

Strikes

Nurses have used **strikes** in last-resort efforts to improve care and working conditions. The law requires that there must be a ten-day notice given before a strike takes place in order to give the hospital a chance to prepare for the strike.[46] However, strikes are not a common tactic used by nurses. The ability of nurses just to threaten to strike is often powerful enough in itself to bring about change.[47] In the few instances where they have gone on strike, client safety and well-being have not been jeopardized. However, nurses who have participated in strikes have suffered retaliation, including losing gains made by seniority, being denied opportunities afforded others, being given difficult assignments and heavy patient loads, losing full-time jobs, or being permanently replaced.[48]

The U.S. Supreme Court gave employers the right to permanently replace striking workers. However, this practice did not become common until 1981 when President Reagan fired striking air traffic controllers and hired replacements. Legislation that prohibits employers from permanently replacing strikers has been rejected by the Senate twice, most recently in 1993. The ANA has supported the legislation since it was first introduced several years ago and has joined a coalition of labor unions, advocacy groups, and religious organizations. This coalition is called the Citizen's Committee for Employment Rights and is working for labor law reform.[49]

In essence, strikes are often detrimental to both labor and management. Some collective bargaining units have developed alternatives to strikes for achieving their goals. Nurses have many concerns about collective bargaining and strikes. If employers collaborate with nurses to initiate a means for them to practice professionally on a long-term basis, nurses will probably be even less likely to form collective bargaining units. It is only when they are dissatisfied with several issues and feel like pawns in the work environment that joining or organizing a union is considered.

Just as the interpretation and tenets of the NLRA keep changing and evolving, the union-management relationship must evolve and change. The old polarized approach to resolution of differences will need to give way to outcomes that benefit both. Both have a chance to be proactive as health care workplaces are being restructured. The need to control costs and depend for success on empowered workers who feel connected and invested in the workplace means labor and management have to reconsider the character of their relationship and join together in constructing new models of collective relationship.

■ FAMILY AND MEDICAL LEAVE ACT (FMLA) OF 1993

The Family and Medical Leave Act, which became effective in August 1993, was the first major initiative of the Clinton administration.[50] However, it does not preempt state or local laws with more generous provisions.[51] The original concept was directed at pregnancy and maternal leave but eventually became very broad and extended to cover the entire family.[52] The act requires employers with 50 or more workers to provide up to 12 weeks per year of unpaid, job-protected leave. Eligible employees must have been employed for at least 12 months and completed 1250 hours of service during the 12-month period immediately preceding the leave.[53]

An eligible employee is entitled to a leave under the following four circumstances: (1) upon birth of the employee's child, (2) upon adoption or foster placement of a child with the employee, (3) to care for a child, spouse, or parent with a serious health condition, and (4) when the employee is unable to perform functions of the job position because of a serious health condition.

Both the employee and the employer have rights and responsibilities. The nurse administrator needs to be aware of both parties' obligations. The employee has the right to (1) return from leave to the same or an equivalent position with equivalent benefits, compensation, and conditions of employment, and (2) take leave on an intermittent or reduced time strategy if medically necessary for a serious health condition of the employee or child, spouse, or parent. However, the employee also has an obligation to provide the employer with a 30-day advance notice if the need for the leave is foreseeable.

Employers have both the right to require the employee to provide medical certification for a claim for leave associated with a personal serious medical condition or to care for a seriously ill child, spouse, or parent and the right to require certification that the employee is eligible to return to work if leave was taken due to a personal illness. The employer can also require that the employee's accrued paid vacation time or sick leave be used in lieu of part of the 12 weeks of unpaid leave. However, the employer must maintain the employee's health benefits coverage for the duration of the leave. Records must be made, kept, and preserved. In addition, the employees' medical information must be kept confidential and in separate files from their usual personnel file.

▚ SUMMARY

The legal system is just one part of the whole health care system. Some laws relative to health care organizations are made to protect workers and promote peaceful and productive interactions between employers and employees, as well as between coworkers. Both the health care environment and legislation are constantly changing and, therefore, constantly challenging the nurse administrator to stay abreast of these changes. Effective nurse administrators must develop an understanding of the basic principles and processes of current legislation and its implications for both themselves and the nursing staff for whom they are responsible and to whom they are accountable. Developing a working knowledge of laws and legal rules and regulations related to health care organizations and their relationship to their workers has the potential to increase the quality of the work environment and, therefore, the quality of care the nurse delivers.

 ## STUDENT EXERCISES

1. List questions that can not be included in a hiring interview?

2. If you were asked any of the questions just named, how would you answer?

3. If you were in a situation in which you felt you were being sexually harassed, what would your responsibility be? (Remember assertive communication, sharing your discomfort with the individual, and suggesting "call me by name," etc, repeating if necessary.)

4. If you were physically attacked (supposedly as a joke), what would your response be? (Review dealing with difficult, verbally hostile people: stand up for yourself, don't engage in further argument, physically hostile: secure your safety, stand up for yourself, report to personnel director.)

5. What advantages do you see to joining a union? Professional organization?

■ REFERENCES

1. Porter-O'Grady T, "Of Rabbits and Turtles: A Time of Change for Unions," *Nursing Economics*, vol. 10, 1992, p. 177–182.
2. Haimann T, *Supervisory Management*, 5th ed., Dubuque, IA: W. C. Brown, 1994.
3. Equal Employment Opportunity Commission, "Guidelines on Discrimination Because of Sex," *Federal Register*, vol. 45, 1980, p. 51266–51269.
4. *Age Discrimination Act*, 1976. 29 U.S.C. 621.

5. *Pregnancy Discrimination Act*, 1978, 49 U.S.C. 2000e(d).

6. *Americans with Disabilities Act*, 1990, 42 U.S.C. 12101.

7. Bularzik M, *Sexual Harassment at the Workplace: Historical Notes*, Somerville, MA: New England Free Press, 1978.

8. Segrave K, *The Sexual Harassment of Women in the Workplace, 1600 to 1993*, Jefferson, NC: McFarland & Company, Inc. 1994.

9. Safran C, "What Men Do to Women on the Job: A Shocking Look at Sexual Harassment," *Redbook*, November 1976, p. 149, 217–223.

10. Farley L, *Sexual Shakedown: The Sexual Harassment of Women on the Job*, New York: McGraw-Hill, 1978.

11. U.S. Merit Systems Protection Board. *Sexual Harassment in the Federal Workplace: Is It a Problem?*, Washington, D.C.: Government Printing Office, 1981.

12. Gutek BA, *Sex and the Workplace*, San Francisco: Jossey-Bass, 1985.

13. MacKinnon C, *Sexual Harassment of Working Women: A Case of Sex Discrimination*, New Haven, CT: Yale University Press, 1979.

14. *Title VII of the Civil Rights Act*, 1964, 42 U.S.C. 2000e.

15. Fitzgerald LF, "Sexual Harassment: The Definition and Measurement of a Construct." In Paludi MA, (editor), *Ivory Power: Sexual Harassment on Campus*, Albany, NY: State University of New York Press, 1990, p. 21–44.

16. Frazier PA, Cochran CC, Olson AM, "Social Science Research on Lay Definitions of Sexual Harassment," *Journal of Social Issues*, vol. 51, 1995, p. 21–37.

17. *Meritor Savings Bank v Vinson*, (1986), 477 U.S. 57, 40 FEP Cases 18222.18.

18. Chan AA, *Women and Sexual Harassment: A Practical Guide to the Legal Protections of Title VII and the Hostile Environment Claim*, New York: Harrington Park Press, 1994.

19. Dowell M, "Sexual Harassment in Academia: Legal and Administrative Challenges," *Journal of Nursing Education*, vol. 31, 1992, p. 5–9.

20. Fitzgerald LF.

21. Center for Women in Government, "Cost of Sexual Harassment to Employers Up Sharply," *Women in Public Service*, Spring 1994, p. 1–4, 45.

22. Creighton H, "Sexual Harassment: Legal Implications—Part I," *Nursing Management*, vol. 18, 1987, p. 18–22.

23. Creighton H, "Sexual Harassment: Legal Implications—Part I," *Nursing Management*, vol. 18, 1987, p. 18–22.

24. Hall JK, *Nursing Ethics and Law*, Philadelphia: W.B. Saunders Co, 1996.

25. Gutek BA, Koss MP, "Changed Women and Changed Organizations: Consequences of and Coping with Sexual Harassment," *Journal of Social Issues*, vol. 38, 1993, p. 97–115.

26. U.S. Merit Systems Protection Board (U.S.MSPB), *Sexual Harassment in the Federal Workplace: An Update*, Washington, D.C.: Government Printing Office, 1987.

27. Klein F, Rowe M, *Estimating the Cost of Sexual Harassment to the FORTUNE 500 Service and Manufacturing Firms*, Cambridge, MA: Klein Associates, Inc., 1988.

28. Beauvais K, "Workshops to Combat Sexual Harassment: A Case Study of Changing Attitudes," *Signs*, vol. 12, 1986, p. 130–145.

29. King CS, "Ending the Silent Conspiracy: Sexual Harassment in Nursing," *Nursing Administration Quarterly*, 19:53, 1995, p. 48–55.

30. Ibid.

31. "Confronting Sexual Harassment," *Nursing*, 24:49, 1994.

32. Rhode DL, *Justice and Gender: Sex Discrimination and the Law*, Cambridge, MA: Harvard University Press, 1989, p. 230-237.

33. Flarey DL, Yoder SK, Barabas MC, "Collaboration in Labor Relations: A Model for Success,"*Journal of Nursing Administration*, 22:9, 1992, p. 15–22.

34. Porter-O'Grady T, p. 179.

35. Wilson CN, Hamilton CL, Murphy E, "Union Dynamics in Nursing," *Journal of Nursing Administration*, 20:2, 1990, p. 35–39.

36. Foley ME, "The Politics of Collective Bargaining," In Mason DJ, Talbot SW, Leavitt JK (editors), *Policy and Politics for Nursing*, 2nd ed., Philadelphia: W.B. Saunders, 1993.

37. Wilson CN, Hamilton CL, Murphy E.

38. Moylan LB, "Implications of the National Labor Relations Act," *Nursing Management*, 19:6, 1988, p. 80.

39. Cohen DM,Wick EF, "Healthcare in Transition: Labor Law Impact on Nurse-Supervisor Roles,"*Journal of Nursing Administration*, 25:6, 1995, p. 15–18.

40. *NLRB v Health Care & Retirement Corporation of America*, 1989, 114 Sct 1778 [1994].

41. Mahoney ME, "Supreme Court Rejects Longstanding Labor Rule for Nurses," *Health Care Supervisor*, 13:4, 1995, p. 13–17.

42. Ketter J, "Restructuring Spurs Debate on Staffing Ratios, Skill Mix," *American Nurse*, vol. 26, 1994, p. 26.

43. Ketter J, "NLRB Rules on RN Supervisory Status at Alaska Hospital," *American Nurse*, vol. 26, 1994, p. 8.

44. Wolfe S, "What Is the Supreme Court Doing to Nursing?" *RN*, vol. 57, 1994, p. 59–60, 63.

45. Ibid.

46. Califano JT, *Contemporary Professional Nursing*, Philadelphia: FA Davis, 1996.

47. Giovinco G, "When Nurses Strike: Ethical Issues," *Nursing Management*, vol. 24, 1993, p. 86–90.

48. Ketter J, "Striker Replacement Loses in Senate Again," *American Nurse*, vol. 26, 1994.

49. Ibid.

50. *Family and Medical Leave Act*, 1993, 29 U.S.C. 2601.ct.seq.

51. Ealey T, "What You Should Know about the Family and Medical Leave Act of 1993," *The Journal of Long-Term Care Administration*, vol. 21, 1993, p. 35–39.

52. Ibid.

53. "The Family Medical Leave Act," *American Association of Occupational Health Nurses Journal*, 43:10, 1995, insert 2p.

13

Managing Change

Introduction

Brookfield describes change as a societal constant evident in relationships, in work settings, and in the political process.[1] Lutjens describes change as inherent, natural, and continuous.[2] The rate and intensity of significant changes that have occurred in the past three decades remove the 1990s from the mid-twentieth century as much as other entire centuries are removed from those that preceded them. As we approach the twenty-first century, we are immersed in a kind of change turbulence that seems almost perpetual. Godfrey reports that between 1980 and 1992, 828 U.S. hospitals closed.[3] Downsizing continues as a practice throughout the country. In nursing, patient care units with very high occupancy rates have been closed because of overall organization considerations. Nursing departments are faced with unprecedented challenges to place nurses in other available positions and to help the displaced nurses work through their understandable anger and sense of betrayal.[4] Advances in computer technology seem to have endless potential for continuing to generate change. There is a sense of powerlessness relative to political and international issues that influence our way of life. All of these changes will have long-lasting effects on nursing departments as well as overall health care agencies. Consequently, knowing how to manage the pace and process of change takes on new meaning and importance.

Throughout this chapter, the active role of nurses as initiators or participants in change is focal. Their role as participants is viewed as a critical means to preserve nursing standards and values in the face of strong influences from other power bases in large organizations where nursing is practiced. Where nurses fail to influence and control the direction and extent of changes in nursing practice, changes can be imposed by nonnurse groups.

The following topics about change are covered in this chapter: a theoretical perspective, the basis of change in nursing, the change process, stages of change, characteristics of change agents, response to change, and evaluating change. Each is important and must be understood by nurses if they are to respond appropriately to proposed changes in nursing practice.

KEY CONCEPTS

Change is a dynamic process by which an alteration is brought about that makes a distinct difference.

Change Agent is someone who initiates an idea for a goal-directed change or directs stages of the change process or both.

Empirical-rational Strategy of change is based upon the assumption that people are rational and will follow their own self-interests.

Moving is a term given to the second stage of the change process during which the planned change is put into action.

Nonintervention is one way in which change comes about. Essentially nothing is done. Not doing can be planned and deliberate to accomplish some end or is a form of neglect.

Normative-reeducative Strategy of change is based on the assumption that people are motivated to commit to societal norms.

Planned Change is a deliberate course of action that results in a change.

Power-coercive Strategy of change is based on the belief that power lies with the person of influence.

Radical Change is one way in which change comes about. Action taken is quick and revolutionary. It can be legitimate out of necessity or through misuse of power and a show of force.

Refreezing is the third stage of the change process during which the new goal becomes established as the expected condition.

Risk Taking is willingness to expose oneself to the chance of some loss as a result of making a change.

Unfreezing is the first stage of the change process during which reasons for making a change are given in a way to make the change desirable.

◼ A THEORETICAL PERSPECTIVE

Change is either planned and managed, or it occurs haphazardly. The challenge to nurse executives to manage change is greater than ever before as influencing forces go beyond the confines of a local health care delivery system. The scope of influences extend to international and even global considerations. To the extent that nursing meets the challenge, professional standards, values, and interests will be preserved.

What is the contribution of beginning practitioners in the effort? The answer is by applying knowledge and understanding of the stages of change from a theoretical perspective to the evaluation of change, in order to be supportive to upper-level nurse managers who bear the ultimate responsibility for changes within the profession. Tiffany points out that all who plan change must adopt a theory to use, and in another work pointed out that research on change theory and its use in nursing is limited at this time.[5,6] In a series of articles on evaluating change theories in use in nursing, the Bennis, Benne, and Chin theory was found to be highest in significance, agreeing with nursing's perspective, clarity, economy, and practicality.[7] The views put forth in the theory synchronize well with interactionist approach. Three strategies of the Bennis, Benne, and Chin planned change theory are presented: (1) empirical-rational, (2) power-coercion, and (3) normative-reeducative. As will be shown, not all three lend themselves well to nursing.

Empirical-rational strategy is based on the philosophy that rational human beings will follow their own self-interests. If a person perceives some personal benefit or gain from an innovation he or she will support the change effort, and conversely will resist the change if the innovation causes a personal inconvenience or loss.[8] When using this strategy, some nurses welcome a change in staffing patterns, while others resist it for personal reasons.

Power-coercive strategy is an option that is adopted when there is a belief that power lies with the most influential individual. There is an assumption that the group will comply with the plans, directions, and leadership of power figures.[9] Loyalty is given to a person who occupies a position, and it shifts when a new person assumes the position. In any setting, therefore, cooperation is dependent on the groups' perception of whoever is in the position of most authority.

Rational-empirical and power-coercive strategies are not appropriate for nursing. Neither fosters the professional purpose or perspective.

Normative-reeducative strategy is based on the philosophy that humans are driven by commitment to norms and values.[10] Nurses' primary concern for professional standards and values motivates them to either support or resist change based on the kind of consequence they believe the change will have on standards and values. Reeducation insures opportunities to gain knowledge about the substance of the change and to formulate new values and attitudes. Normative-reeducative strategy is the most appropriate for nursing because it is most likely to advance the profession. Future research into change theory as it relates to nursing might produce insights not currently held. It is a rich field for ongoing investigation.

■ BASIS OF CHANGE IN NURSING

Forces internal and external to nursing form the basis for change that influences nursing practice. Need for changes are dictated internally as patient acuity levels, treatment modalities, and use of technologies increase. Externally, social and economic factors exert ongoing influence on how nursing is practiced. From systems theory it is understood the ongoing interaction between internal and external forces that influence all segments of the open system and thus the practice of nursing in organizations.

External Forces

Continuing spiraling health care costs and shrinking resources prompt vigorous efforts to conserve in all departments of organizations. Nursing represents the largest group of health care providers and therefore a sizable percentage of health care costs. The introduction of technicians for patient care activities as a cost-cutting effort has been met with resistance by professional nurses. History shows that cost considerations without quality concerns frequently produce negative results. Nursing experienced an era following World War II when technically prepared caregivers (that is, nurse aides), performed many tasks but were unprepared to interpret patient responses to the care they received. Because of concern for quality at the bedside, nurse aides were retrained for nondirect care activities, such as looking after supplies and ordering equipment and materials requested by the nurse. Consider that technicians were removed from direct patient care activities at a time when acuity level was not as high as today and treatment modalities had fewer and less severe side effects. Through the efforts of professional nurse leaders, baccalaureate preparation was recommended as an entry level into nursing, and this practice is becoming a reality in many parts of the country. This standard is worthy of guarding and preserving. Where professional practice values are threatened, the essential task of nursing is an ongoing clarification and interpretation of professional care as cost-effective. Research has demonstrated the cost-effectiveness of professional care, and nurses who make use of research findings will more effectively convey the message to others.

Internal Forces

History has shown that changes in nursing practice that are initiated and implemented by nonnurse groups fail to represent professional norms and values. Nurses are socialized in a unique way during their education and experience in practice and are therefore prepared as no other group to monitor nursing practice. A major source of strength within nursing can be found in collaborative efforts of nurses in the four functional roles—practitioners, educators, researchers, and managers. Together they can exert significant influence in maintaining professional practice. The four roles make up the acronym PERM. Figure 13-1 illustrates the interactional as well as the independent nature of the work that each contributes to nursing. Table 13-1

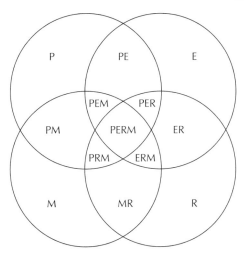

The four overlapping rings create 13 chambers:
—4 chambers with a single letter signify independent responsibilities.
—4 chambers with 2 letters each signify shared responsibilities between 2 individuals.
—4 chambers are created by the overlap of 3 rings and signify shared responsibilities among 3 individuals.
—1 chamber is created in the center and is formed by all 4 rings. It signifies responsibilities shared among all.

Figure 13-1. The PERM complex depicts the interaction among nurses in the four major functional roles.

TABLE 13-1. THE PERM COMPLEX—INDEPENDENT (I) AND SHARED (S) RESPONSIBILITIES

Practitioner

I	Accurately defines changing conditions of practice.
S	Collaborates with nurse researchers in conducting studies that relate to change.
	Collaborates with nurse educators in providing a practice setting that supports change.
	Works closely with managers in identifying ideas and supports change efforts.

Educator

I	Prepares students for the realities of changing nursing care needs.
S	Strengthens change-agent skills in students by requiring increasingly complex use of nursing research in practice.
	Communicates frequently with the nursing staff about student "change" assignments.
	Obtains management approval for student activities that relate to change.

Researcher

I	Conducts research studies or serves as a resource person to educators, managers, and practitioners who carry out research that relates to change.
S	Uses input from practitioners relative to changing conditions in practice and incorporates practitioners as participants in studies.
	Assists in the design and delivery of the research component of the curriculum.
	Designs research activities to conform to organizational policies and resources.

Manager

I	Remains abreast of issues surrounding nursing care that indicate need for change.
	Articulates clear expectations that nonoptional changes must be supported by all personnel in the nursing department.
S	Authorizes and supports research that relates to change.
	Responds in a timely way to practitioners' concerns about nursing care conditions.
	Supports the work of joint committees of service and education representatives to explore issues of common concern relative to changing nursing care needs.

describes the independent and the shared responsibilities of nurses in each of the roles.

Collectively, nurses have rich resources to bring to bear on time-related care problems and issues. Patterns of patient care delivery are constantly undergoing alterations by creative nurses to meet situational needs in a setting. Problems associated with "float pools" in critical care units and emergency rooms were handled in one hospital through a system of "self-staffing." Unit nurses assumed the responsibility for adequate coverage without having to depend on nurses with limited-to-no familiarity with the patient population. The nurses were committed to change and excellence in nursing. The outcome of their efforts, in addition to quality patient care, included (1) improved satisfaction, (2) increased morale, (3) autonomy, and (4) flexibility.[11]

Regardless of the demands for change dictated from within or without, professional standards provide the stabilizing force for preserving quality and values in a volatile environment. When standards are used, *what* nursing is does not change, only *how* it is operationalized changes when confronted with situational factors.

■ THE CHANGE PROCESS

Change occurs as a process and can be analyzed, studied, understood, and, to some extent, controlled. Lutjens says that planned change provides a way to induce structural innovations designed to make operational adjustments to meet situational demands.[12] Planned change, designed to keep the nursing department a vital influence in the organization, is presented as the ideal form of change in this chapter. Planned change (1) is based on empiric evidence of a need, (2) aims at improving a system of operation, (3) involves others in decisions, and (4) provides time for reeducation of those affected by the change. The effects of change are on a continuum of minor to major, predictable to unpredictable, and positive to negative. Daloz, cited in Brookfield, refers to change as a fusion of the old and the new rather than a total abandonment.[13] Kegan, cited in Brookfield, describes change as a process of resolving old dichotomies by integrating the new with the old.[14] In fact, success of a change effort is partially dependent on maintaining connections with what is valued. There is usually some degree of conflict associated with significant change. Risk and opportunity are presented simultaneously. There is a loss of the familiar and a venture into uncertainty. Risk taking and vision are two characteristics that are highly desirable qualities of participants in the change process.

What gets changed and *how* the change is accomplished are two major points to consider when discussing the change process. Ideally, what needs changing is based on careful analysis and diagnosis of existing practices with a view to future needs. If time permits, a thorough analysis to find the fundamental problem pays off in the form of finding a solution rather than treating symptoms of the problem. Symptoms are more obvious, taking the form of absenteeism, high turnover, and poor morale, while the fundamental problem might be felt as incompetency because of unfamiliar expectations. The solution for the problem above is appropriate inservice programs, but efforts might be in the direction of improving salaries to keep the staff happy and on the job. Such a move is counterproductive.

Problem Identification

The impetus for change has its root in some perceived conflict. The conflict can take a variety of forms, such as not enough of something, too much of something, a practice that should be and is not, or a practice that is and should not be. It is important that whatever the perceived need, the thought process must be accompanied by a strong *feeling* that a change must occur. A well thought-out problem is not sufficient for action. What is not felt, and what is not seen as improvement, will certainly produce resistance.

Individuals view situations differently. What constitutes a conflict for some is not for others. These different responses can cause conflicts regarding the change itself and thereby create resistance to change efforts. It is predictable that there will be both support and resistance from individuals relative to the same event. An important part of problem identification is to *envision alternatives* (i.e., consider a variety of alternatives to the current practice or state of affairs.) Be prepared to clarify and interpret how each alternative could improve the situation. Be realistic in acknowledging how each might produce some negative consequences, and be certain that they are only minor. Be convinced that at least one alternative is feasible and within available resources.

Gaining Support for Change

Gaining support for change cannot be left to chance. The leadership behavior of selling is an important strategy to use when resistance threatens progress in making a needed change. Selling is done by sharing with the group all known information surrounding the changing situation so that the decision to proceed becomes a shared decision. Gaining allies early on is important if time and resources are to be used to the best advantage. Some allies might come forth from the beginning, while others have to be won. One category of potential allies is individuals who initially oppose your efforts, but who are open and honest about it. Such individuals are trustworthy, will listen to clarifications, and are likely to modify their positions. Other potential allies are those who are "on the fence" and who also can be characterized as honest and trustworthy when it comes to what benefits the group. Knowing the difference between true adversaries, whose agendas lie outside the overall good of the group, and potential allies is time saving. Time is wasted on trying to win support from individuals whose self-interest outweighs group interests. Beckhard and Harris recommend a technique whereby the whole group participates in problem diagnosis.[15] What is *desired* is stated explicitly, followed by creation of a picture of the *wished-for* condition. Individuals independently make "wish lists" that, if granted, would improve their work satisfaction. A group effort is more likely to result in cooperative change efforts. An example of a situation that affects staff nurses might be something like the following: A proposal has been made by nursing administration to expand the medicine room on their unit by taking space from the nurses' conference room. Sharing documented evidence that more space is needed for safe preparation of medications, addresses a standard and is a convincing argument acknowledged by the nurses. The number of medication errors occurring during times of congestion in the medicine room cannot be ignored. However, space reallocation is only one possible solution to the problem.

How Changes Are Made

Administrators can use the information from the above example about medicine errors to mandate space reallocation without giving consideration to any other possible solution. Perhaps they see their responsibility as being swift intervention. Another intervention could be to request input from the staff for other viable alternative actions, thus providing an opportunity for their active participation in arriving at the best solution. Perhaps enlarging the medicine room is not the only way to relieve congestion during medication preparation. The nurses' conference room is used for change-of-shift reports, patient care conferences, staff development programs, and periodically for social events. Reducing the size of the conference room will definitely affect the quality of the activities that take place there.

Planned Change

An alternative plan devised by staff nurses on the unit describes how better use of space in the medicine room and spreading times for medication administration could possibly reduce congestion and thus the incidence of medication errors. All stock supplies of materials used in the medicine room could be moved to a general storage area. A nurse assistant could be assigned to restock supplies according to a schedule so that the movement of the stock does not become an inconvenience or a waste of nursing hours. Schedules for standing medications could be spread out as follows:

- TID at 8 A.M., 4 P.M., and 12 midnight
- BID at 10 A.M. and 10 P.M.
- Daily at 12 noon

A downside of a spread-out medication schedule is that patients receiving TID, BID, and daily medications would be disturbed more frequently. The plus side of the plan is in retaining use of the conference room for practices valued by the staff, and avoiding the expense of tearing down and reconstructing a wall. By inviting staff input, administration has two plans to consider before making a final decision.

Using the staff to generate ideas for alternative plans and then weighing all viable options that address quality standards makes the outcome a group decision. Such a move gives recognition to everyone who is likely to be affected by the change and addresses the need for competent professionals to be given a greater share of responsibility for the work to be done on the unit.

The example illustrates a change in which time is given to consideration of alternative actions and one in which input from the group is likely to produce support for the change. It is an example of **planned change**.

Radical Intervention

Sometimes the need for change is sudden and calls for some **radical change**. Radical intervention is an autocratic method of making changes. Sudden, drastic changes are made, usually by an individual or a select few without any input from others. Such change can have both positive and negative consequences. When used routinely as a show of force through misuse of power, thinking, competent, professional people simply move on to other employment, while passive people who relish a dependent role support the behavior. Eventually the loss of creative group members leads to diminished-quality decision making and performance and a rigid adherence to the status quo.

Legitimate radical intervention, on the other hand, is a way to ward off or to manage a crisis. A situation can call for split-second decision making where delay would only compound or create a problem. Time required for planned change is not available during crisis situations. When it is necessary to employ radical intervention, the leadership behavior of selling is again the key to gaining support from the group. This should be done as soon as possible after the decision has been made. When rationale for the sudden action is explained to a competent group, their thinking is changed and the decision retrospectively becomes theirs also. Sharing all relevant information surrounding the situation is usually adequate to gain support. Legitimate use of radical action considers others and strives to make them participants in decisions.

When radical action is used as a show of force, telling is the leadership behavior used. There is no opportunity for group members to gain the broad perspective of the situation that is needed for them to show support. Telling usually causes the loss of trust and confidence in the decision maker in future situations.

Change through Nonintervention

Nonintervention is another way in which change can come about. It can be deliberate, or it can be a form of neglect. Deliberate nonintervention is a form of planned change, whereas neglecting to intervene when intervention is warranted makes people passive recipients and sometimes victims of change.

Nonintervention as a deliberate strategy is employed to eliminate some out-of-date practice or category of worker. The unnecessary role or practice is allowed to die a natural death through attrition or depletion of materials. In some settings, not filling vacancies in the nurse aide category was the way of eliminating them as direct caregivers.

Nonintervention as a form of neglect opens the door for nonnurse groups to intervene in nursing practice issues. Although nursing was not negligent in predicting the need for baccalaureate preparation for entry into practice, forces internal to nursing caused delay in implementing the associated plan to redefine the status of workers in nursing. The move toward registered care technicians trained by nonnurse groups resulted from the long delay.

■ STAGES OF CHANGE

Once a decision has been reached to implement a change, time must be allowed for the sequence of stages designed to reduce resistance and maintain support from others. Three familiar stages in implementing change are (1) **unfreezing**, (2) **moving**, and (3) **refreezing**.

Unfreezing

During unfreezing, letting go of established and familiar practices takes place. Adequate time is needed for gradual introduction of new ideas, along with information that can serve as positive motivation for those who are going to be affected by the change. Information should include reasons why a change is needed and how the organization and individuals will benefit from it. Projecting a realistic time frame for the change to take place, giving explanations of how workers will be affected throughout the process, and being honest about temporary inconveniences can give them some sense of control. Greater control can be provided by encouraging group input through a formal feedback mechanism. Objectivity of feedback review and action taken can be ensured through representation from the group on a review committee. It also serves as testimony of flexibility in the change plan.

Commending valuable ideas submitted by the staff early on encourages wider constructive participation in feedback. Acknowledging discomfort that comes from uncertainty about a new system preserves everyone's dignity. Assurance of adequate reeducation opportunities can enable individuals to deal with their emotions over the proposed change.

Unfreezing is essentially a preparation for instituting activities to facilitate the change. During this stage, change agents have the greatest opportunity to gain allies from the staff.

Bassett says the most important element in the change process is belief in and commitment to its success.[16] Even with the best efforts to do everything right, defensive responses to being told that a system is inefficient, unnecessary, too costly, or ineffective are likely to occur. Change agents must be prepared to deal with defensiveness. All interactive processes of leadership—communication, group dynamics, decision making, and conflict management—assist change agents in overcoming obstacles to organizational change. Equally important is using systems theory and the effect of interactive parts, effective management techniques, delegation, motivation, and performance standards. At an appropriate time, a target date to begin activities of the second stage should be set to prevent nonconstructive delays. It is understood, however, that unfreezing strategies will continue to be in effect if new information surfaces that indicates a need to continue with the first stage.

Moving

The second stage of the change process is moving. Cognitive redefinition of how group goals can be met based on new understanding characterizes the second stage. The primary activity during moving is reeducation. Determining specific programs needed and for whom gives definition to what might otherwise seem like a time vacuum when the old is gone and the new is not in place. Knowing exactly what is expected during this transitional stage and how it contributes to the new system reduces insecurity that accompanies uncertainty. Beckhard and Harris caution that the transitional stage of change requires its own structure and strategies.[17] Ideally, the second stage does not begin until a roadmap checklist is complete.[18] The checklist implies that there is supporting evidence that the proposed change:

- is purposeful
- is task specific
- is integrated
- is time sequenced
- is adaptable
- has approval
- is cost-effective

The transition stage is a pilot of the larger plan and has its own temporary management structure so that there is not interference with established day-to-day operations.

Participants in the pilot project must be adequately informed as to its purpose and reeducated to be able to function proficiently. They should share the perception that the change will potentially be an improvement over current practices. A report of the pilot project should provide information on ways to avoid problems during implementation of the larger plan.

Refreezing

The third stage of the change process is refreezing. It occurs when there is consistent evidence that the new practice is stabilized, integrated, and internalized by the staff. Ongoing monitoring for continued quality must follow refreezing, since it provides valuable information about ongoing effectiveness of the change. The process is only as good as its users, and follow-up findings allow for analysis to replicate success and correct errors for the future. Keeping a written record of follow-up findings on file is helpful in remembering details. More about follow-up is discussed in the section on evaluation of change.

Knowing the ideal about the change process enables all staff to participate constructively in change efforts, either by making known their dissatisfaction through statements of their expectations or by giving their support and allegiance to change agents. Changes will continue to occur more rapidly and with higher intensity with time. Therefore, understanding change is important if nurses are to remain in control of nursing.

■ CHANGE AGENTS

Characteristics of Change Agents

Characteristics and qualities of **change agents** include (1) experience, (2) success, (3) being respected, (4) leadership skills, and (5) management competencies. Pritchett and Pound advise that individuals who have a positive attitude about work and seize opportunities to get involved in new directions are themselves change agents.[19] They are willing to spend their time in correcting problems and they deliberately choose to be positive, optimistic, and enthusiastic. Attitude is something that is under control of the individual, and developing a positive attitude can be fostered by anyone. Supporting more experienced change agents benefits the individual maybe even more than the organization.

Responsibilities of Change Agents

The change agent's first responsibility is to develop a plan for action. The plan includes (1) a description of and rationale for the change, (2) objectives expressed in measurable terms, and (3) a projected timetable for each stage of implementation, leaving sufficient flexibility to accommodate new information. Having a set deadline is a safeguard against procrastination, which can seriously compromise change efforts.

The change agent needs a keen sense of the ethical and legal elements associated with significant changes. Many people become vulnerable during change, and their rights and dignity can be unnecessarily compromised when there is insensitivity to ethical and legal factors. For example, a temporary decline in effective performance is predictable during vulnerable periods. It is therefore important that adequate time be given for personnel to assimilate all that a change incurs. Change agents must be aware of the decline in effectiveness in the early stages of change to avoid the possibility of mismanagement. He or she must know when, where, and how to intervene throughout the process.

Strategies for Change Agents

Beckhard and Harris list action strategies for change agents.[20] They are (1) defining how much *choice* there is about whether to change; (2) delivering a clear message that change action is an essential, not optional, part of work; (3) developing a system of control and information flow, (4) establishing a mechanism to monitor progress, and (5) planning for long-range evaluation. Relative to item number 3, the temporary management structure described on page 279 under MOVING should be established for the change plan. The regular structure in use for stable practices blurs differences between the new and the old. Separating management of stable and changing practices permits a clearer definition of change effects. Finally, the change agent is responsible for determining readiness for beginning the pilot project, implementing the larger plan, and determining stage progression.

Responsibilities of change agents are many and important. Selecting the best person available is an important decision. Success of a change plan is enhanced by effective change agents and informed group members who are open to new ideas and who are willing to take risks.

■ RESPONSE TO CHANGE

In field theory, described by Lewin, there are two opposing forces: driving forces and restraining forces.[21] Driving forces generate planned change, and restraining forces generate resistance to change. Planning change can be more successful when the effects of restraining forces are explored and managed. Force-field analysis is a technique used to determine the two opposing forces.

In this section resistance to change and a drive toward change are explored. With an understanding of the dynamics that create both, resistance can be reduced and drive can be increased. Individuals are dynamic, growing, social beings. At any given moment, risk involved in change can serve as a driving force, an opposing force, or even as both simultaneously. Thoughts and feelings about change and risk become modified over time with maturity

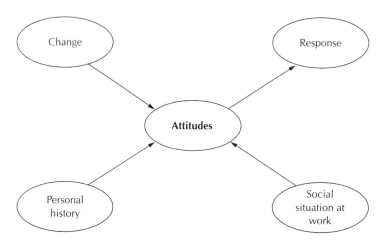

Figure 13-2. Formulation of attitudes toward change in work settings. Response is determined by attitude.

and experience. Bassett says that resistance to change lies in human attitudes.[22] Lewin, the founder of the group dynamics movement in the 1930s, created the X chart to show the relationship of attitudes and response to change (Fig. 13-2).[23] Attitudes toward change are formed by a combination of (1) the change itself, (2) the personal history of individuals who will be affected by the change, and (3) the social situation at work.

Resistance to Change

Being shown a better way to do things implies that current performance is not acceptable, resulting in embarrassment and insecurity. It is definitely not a good idea for a young nurse manager in nursing for 8 years, to tell a 20 year veteran nurse how to provide quality care. Experience is a very important qualification of change agents. Another scenario to consider is, if a proposed change is a time-saving practice, what will the staff do during the saved time? Will they be given added responsibilities without additional salary? Attention must be given to curbing rumors and speculation. When concerns such as the ones above are apparent, the staff can be asked to list important things they would like to do but do not have the time for under the current way of doing things. Maybe there are (1) activities they would enjoy but do not have time for, (2) developmental activities that would improve their personal potential, (3) quality problems that could be solved, (4) questions about how money released due to a better way of doing things could be used, and (5) questions about what stress would be reduced due to less pressure. This exercise could convince the staff that the change is designed to improve mission attainment and not to add to their work or reduce the staff size. The exercise is designed to reduce resistance.

When attempting to reduce resistance to change, nurses can be asked to reflect on *where* they learned the things they do and *why* they are done in just that way. Do they ever question them or consider a different routine? There is danger in allowing actions to become too routine, since they are then done out of habit rather than done thoughtfully. Frequently, a few simple questions about current practices can stir enthusiasm within the group to work toward making their practices flexible enough to fit the unique demands of a situation. Bassett presents a *credo* to encourage participation in change.[24]

- If you think you can't, you won't.
- If you think you can, there is a good chance you will.
- Making the effort is exhilarating.
- Reputations are made by searching for things that can't be done, and doing them.
- Aim low → boring. Aim high → soaring.

The most important element in reducing resistance is in establishing trust by (1) giving explanations, (2) requesting input, (3) acknowledging concerns, (4) making changes in small doses, (5) offering to assist, (6) explaining benefits, and (7) acknowledging success. Conversely, ingredients for resistance are listed as (1) mystery, (2) secrecy, (3) change as punishment, (4) pressure to speed up work, (5) poor planning, and (6) ignoring human nature.[25]

Davis defines three types of resistance: logical-rational, psychologic-emotional, and sociologic.[26] Logical-rational objections include (1) the time it takes to adjust, (2) the extra effort it takes, (3) the possibility of less desirable outcomes, (4) cost, and (5) questionable feasibility. All of these points have merit, and it is wise to exercise patience with logical objectors. Showing them how delay in making *truly needed* changes would be destructive to the organization and workers can help. Psychologic-emotional objections include (1) fear of the unknown, (2) low tolerance for change, (3) dislike of the change agent, (4) lack of trust, and (5) high need for security. Non–risk takers hold tenaciously to their objections. Diluting resistors among more adventurous peers might help them grow and overcome some of their fears.

Sociologic objections include (1) parochial, narrow views; (2) vested interest; (3) a wish to retain existing relationships; (4) opposing group values; and (5) political coalitions. Individuals who hold too strongly to self-interests at the expense of group goals need reminders of their employment responsibilities.

Some resistance will linger regardless of correct approaches and the best efforts of competent change agents. Human behavior and interaction is far too complex to be able to gain total support for a change. Continuing to work hard toward increasing group support is productive in reducing resistance, since in the long run the strength of group influence is the most promising force in modifying resistors' behavior.

■ EVALUATING CHANGE

How is it known that change efforts are worthwhile, whether a change works, how much outcome is due to chance, or whether a new practice will be maintained? How is change monitored? These are commonly asked questions. Answers can only be found during the evaluation stage of the change process. When evaluation is given low priority, the answers will be vague and subjective or lacking all together. When expectations are clear that evaluation is critical for effective operation, efforts are not relaxed once the change has been put into effect.

The way to arrive at answers is through design of planned, systematic data gathering and analysis that yields the necessary information. The plan for evaluation is continuous with the overall change design, with outcomes being measured against criteria found in statements of purpose and objectives for change. Implementation of the evaluation plan is carried out by everyone involved in the change process.

Responsibilities of each group member must be spelled out clearly, and individuals should be held accountable for their performance in this area as for any other expected behavior. Information must be explicit as to who is to receive data, on what dates, and by what collection method. It must be reinforced that completing reports is part of real work, not something added on to work. In other words, submitting reports is not optional. Timing of reports is important, especially when longitudinal evaluation is done. Longitudinal design requires serial collection of data at specified times to determine the effects that time, as a variable, has on outcomes. Growth grids are an example of longitudinal design. If measurement is missed at any point, a void exists in information about the individual's progress relative to the variable time.

Method of data analysis determines whether or not the analysis will indicate how many change outcomes are due to chance. The wrong method of analysis will not provide the information, while correct methods will. Courses in statistics and research methods are requirements in nursing curricula today and orient beginning practitioners to the need for precision in determining cause-and-effect relationships. They are essential for professional monitoring of practice, in the case of change, to know whether efforts are worthwhile and cost-effective.

Stability of change is the ultimate goal. Only through systematic evaluation is the degree of stability known. Accurate information from evaluation reports permits correction of neglect and inconsistencies. Problems are pinpointed early, and corrective action can be applied with precision. Change is costly, and justification of the cost can be found in well-documented evaluation reports. Change is incomplete without evaluation.

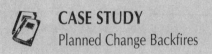

CASE STUDY
Planned Change Backfires

As patient acuity levels rose, nurses in a pediatric hospital looked for ways to reduce nonnurse activities. One area that was earmarked was the playroom. A play department was formed and staffed by trained workers, and a director was hired to oversee the functions and performance of the new group of workers. Meeting the play needs of hospitalized children was defined as their responsibility. Unfortunately, no distinction was made between "social play" and "therapeutic play." The latter is designed to assist children in coping with painful and, what is to them, frightening experiences that occur during the course of their treatment. The description of workers' job in the play department included having responsibility for the playroom, play materials, and play activities. As time went on, efforts by nurses to incorporate therapeutic play into the care of their patients' care was viewed as interference in the domain of the play department. On one occasion, a staff nurse who was caring for a long-term 3-year-old boy, requested to use some materials from the playroom for the patient's care. The response from the director of the playroom was that all play needs would be taken care of by workers in her department. The nurse explained that the patient had experienced several painful and frightening experiences and was finally showing signs of readiness to work through his feelings. The time was right for the nurse to help him gain mastery over what had happened to him by actively engaging in reenacting what had happened to him as a passive recipient. The nurse was told by the director of the playroom that using "hospital equipment for play" was scheduled for the next day at 1:00 P.M. None of the nurses efforts were met with any success. She decided to improvise with what she had on hand and proceeded with her plan of care for her patient. A major conflict ensued when the director of the playroom discovered what the nurse had done.

- In this situation, what is at stake for patient care?
- What is at stake for play department workers?
- What was missed in the change plan?

CASE STUDY
Transition from Student to Graduate Nurse

Gretchen Hoff began her first position in nursing shortly after graduating from X University School of Nursing. She did well in school, is enthusiastic, and is hoping that she fits in on the unit she has been assigned to. The topic "Transition from Student to Graduate Nurse" is on the orientation schedule for new graduates. She had never given any thought to possible differences from the ideal world presented in school and the real world of practice. There did not seem to be any need to because she had never encountered any problems relative to patient care during her clinical experiences. She overheard a discussion about quality of care issues and that how care is delivered in practice does not quite measure up to standards she learned in school. The information is unsettling to her and she becomes anxious about how she will be able to handle quality issues if she encounters them. For the first time, she will not have an instructor or assigned preceptor to guide her and to share responsibility for outcomes of a conflict situation. She decides she is being overly anxious about a bridge that probably does not exist.

Gretchen is about to embark on her first experience with change.

- What will be her best course of action when she does face a quality issue?
- How can she prevent being alienated from the group and still make her point about professional standards?

CASE STUDY
Parking Lot

Kathleen O'Toole, a nurse in her first year of practice, was surprised one day when she arrived, as usual, at the hospital parking lot. There was a sign at the entrance indicating that the lot would be reserved for administrators and physicians only beginning on the first of the next month, three weeks away. A parking attendant handed her a form describing more detailed information about the change, including the lot that would be designated for staff nurses. After reviewing this information, she realized that the parking lot the nurses would have to use is located several long blocks from the hospital. Plans included a shuttle service that would transport nurses from the lot to the hospital and back again when the work period ended. Parking had been free and now there would be a small fee charged to cover the cost of the outside shuttle company service.

Kathleen and the other nurses are understandably upset over the change. They feel that they should have some input into a solution about the parking problems the hospital is experiencing. A major concern of theirs is the safety issue of young women waiting alone in their cars for the shuttle bus to arrive. One point that stands out in their minds is that the nursing group is the largest in the hospital, and that they are essentially the "heartbeat" of the organization.

A decision is made to organize a coalition of nurses to oppose the change and to negotiate an alternative plan to solving the ongoing parking shortage. Their focus is an approach that will be fair to nurses.

• Using the content of this chapter, prepare a written statement about the nurses' concerns that is effectively assertive.

Note that the statement will be sent to top administration.

■ SUMMARY

In this chapter, change is described as an ongoing, societal phenomenon that can be controlled to varying degrees. Internal and external forces in the form of conflict bring about changes in nursing. Unmet professional standards generate internal nursing changes, while external forces tend to generate changes designed to solve economic problems. Planned change designed by nurses is presented as the most promising for maintaining vitality within nursing departments. Examples are given of changes that foster improved quality nursing care and those that threaten quality nursing care. Determining *what* should be changed is dependent on analysis of situations and predictions of decision outcomes. Only needed changes are worth the time and expense entailed in the long process. Change agents must have certain characteristics to be effective. The change plan must reduce resistance and foster support. Finally, the importance of evaluating change is stressed. The study of change is important for entry into professional practice. The reader is reminded that managing change is one aspect of a broader management system and not a discrete, isolated activity. Determining need and designing, implementing, and evaluating changes in nursing requires a collaborative effort of nurses in all categories of the PERM complex.

 STUDENT EXERCISES

In 1988, the American Medical Association (AMA) proposed a new category of care workers, registered care technicians (RTCs), to alleviate the problems associated with the nurse shortage. Two years later, on June 25, 1990, the AMA House of Delegates abandoned its plan to implement pilot sites for the training of RTCs. Opposition to the RTC came from the American Nurses Association (ANA) because the duties proposed for the RTC overlapped with roles that should be performed by RNs. With the demise of the RTC proposal, the ANA resolved to work collaboratively with the AMA and other health care groups to address patient care concerns associated with nurse shortages in acute care settings.

Two issues emanate from the described situation: (1) the AMA proposal was due to the failure of nursing to devise a workable solution to the nursing shortage, and (2) the ANA reaction demonstrates the strength of nurses' influence in monitoring standards of professional practice. Answer the following questions about the above situation:

1. Do you agree or disagree with the two issue statements? Explain your response.

2. What could have reversed the situation?

3. What are the implications for practitioners, educators, researchers, and managers in nursing (the PERM complex)?

4. In your opinion, where in the PERM complex does action for effective change begin?

5. In your opinion, how effective is collaboration among nurses in the PERM complex?

▓ REFERENCES

1. Brookfield S, *Developing Critical Thinkers*, San Francisco: Jossey-Bass, 1987, p. 51.

2. Lutjens LR, Tiffany CR, "Evaluating Planned Change Theories," *Nursing Management*, 25:3, March 1994, p. 54–57.

3. Godfrey C, "Downsizing: Coping with Personal Pain," *Nursing Management*, 25:10, October 1994, p. 90–93.

4. Ibid.

5. Tiffany CR, "Analysis of Planned Change," *Nursing Management*, 25:2, February 1994, p. 60–62.

6. Tiffany CR, Cheatham AB, Doornbos D, Loudermelt L, Momadi GG, "Planned Change Theory: Survey of Nursing Periodical Literature," *Nursing Management*, 25:7, July 1994, p. 54–59.

7. Hagerman ZT, Tiffany CR, "Evaluation of Two Planned Change Theories," *Nursing Management*, 25:4, April 1994, p. 57–62.

8. Ibid.

9. Ibid.

10. Ibid.

11. Hausfeld J, Gibbons K, Holtmeier A, Knight M, Schulte C, Stadtmiller T, Yeary K, "Self-staffing: Improving Care and Staff Satisfaction," *Nursing Management*, 25:10, October 1994, p. 74–80.

12. Lutjens LR, Tiffany CR, p. 54.

13. Brookfield S, p. 225.

14. Ibid, p. 226.

15. Beckhard R, Harris R, *Organizational Transitions: Managing Complex Change*, Reading, MA: Addison-Wesley, 1977 p. 26.

16. Bassett L, Metzger N. *Achieving Excellence: A Prescription for Health Care Managers*, Rockville, MD: Aspen Publishers, 1986 p. 94.

17. Beckhard R, Harris R, p. 27.

18. Beckhard R, Harris R, p. 57.

19. Pritchett P, Pound R, *The Employee Handbook for Organizational Change*, Dallas: Pritchett & Associates, Inc, 1990, p. 30.

20. Beckhard R, Harris R, p. 36.

21. England D, *Collaboration in Nursing*, Rockville, MD: Aspen Publishers, 1986 p. 213.

22. Bassett L, Metzger N, p. 104.
23. Davis K, *Organizational Behavior at Work: Organizational Behavior,* St. Louis: McGraw-Hill, 1981, p. 200.
24. Bassett L, Metzger N, p. 115.
25. Bassett L, Metzger N, p. 95.
26. Davis K, p. 207.

UNIT 4

MANAGING RESOURCES

14

Managing Resources
The Staff

Introduction

The issue of an adequate staff has never been more seriously considered than in this era of health care reform. New structures with new missions coupled with the increased utilization of nonprofessional personnel has put pressure on nursing service. Nursing continues to hold quality patient care as a value, and inadequate staffing poses a threat to this concept. Today's nurse manager has a major responsibility to know what personnel are doing and where they spend their time. This allows the manager to justify the appropriate case mix and insure that nursing and support staff are being used to the greatest advantage. As decentralization of authority and responsibility continue, managers are mandated to allocate available resources. **Resources** are limited commodities that allow the work of the organization to be completed, and no resource is as important as the staff. This chapter will discuss the management of resources with specific attention to the staffing process.

KEY CONCEPTS

Resources are commodities in limited quantities that allow the work of the organization to be performed.

Staffing is a complex process that determines the appropriate number and the nursing resources necessary to meet the work-load demand for nursing care at the unit or department level.

Staff Plan is the actual pattern of staff distribution based on an underlying methodology.

Descriptive Methodology is a staffing pattern that results from variables selected by the manager.

Industrial Engineering is a staffing plan that results from techniques used by industry (i.e., time-and-motion studies).

Management Engineering is the staffing plan that results in a staffing index based on usual managerial data.

Expert Panel Method is the staffing plan that utilizes a variety of experts to examine service- and unit-specific needs related to structure, process, and outcomes, and subsequently suggests an appropriate staffing plan.

Work Load of nursing is determined through an assessment of the patients' severity, and an estimate of the indirect and unit-based work requirements.

Case Mix refers to the type, number, and ratio of staff necessary to perform the established work; this includes the optimum ratio of professional nurses to licensed or certified support personnel for a particular unit of patient service.

Scheduling Pattern represents the actual assignment of personnel by unit or department and time.

▧ STAFFING

Process and Staffing Plan

Staffing decisions require judgments to allocate and juggle personnel between the projects and processes of the organization. This is done by the process of **staffing,** or the determination of the appropriate number and the mix of nursing resources necessary to meet work-load demand for nursing care at the unit or department level (Fig. 14-1).[1] **Work load** is a function of two elements: the number of patients and a measure of work. Typically, the work load of nursing is determined through the use of a patient classification system, which documents the patient severity and accompanying requirements of care (also called the direct work of nursing), as well as instruments that estimate the indirect and unit-based work requirements.[2] The purpose of using such a system is to be able to predict the correct staffing plan.

The **staffing plan** is the recommended case mix of individuals needed to provide safe and appropriate nursing care.[3] **Case mix** refers to the type, number, and ratio of staff necessary to perform the established work; this includes the optimum ratio of professional nurses to licensed or certified support personnel for a particular unit of patient service.[4] A case mix ratio may vary from department to department. However, the factors that generally predict a case mix are as follows:

- Average daily occupancy trends and fluctuations.
- Patient classification data.
- Average length of stay.
- Staff distribution patterns for the type of health care institution.
- Type of health care being delivered.[5]

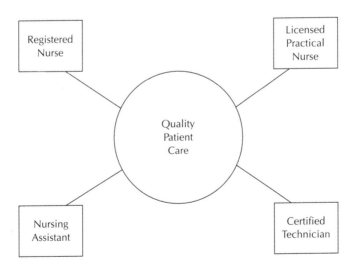

Figure 14-1. An ideal ratio of professional staff to licensed practical nurses to patients will lead to quality patient care. This ratio varies according to situational, nurse, and patient requirements.

Since the mid-1980s and through the 1990s, staffing plans within health care institutions have been and will continue to be influenced by current issues. They include reimbursement arrangements, new health care structures, early discharge for patients, and a new professional work force with changing work values and expectations. Staffing plans today require nontraditional and new staffing patterns, or the actual way staff is distributed throughout the organization. The American Nurses' Association (ANA) suggests four questions that direct the staffing plan. These questions include:

1. How many patients can one professional nurse properly plan for, supervise, and evaluate in terms of nursing care provided?
2. How many associate nurses can one professional nurse direct, supervise, and evaluate?
3. How many patients will require the direct care of a professional nurse, and how much nursing time is involved in this care?
4. How can the autonomy of nursing practice and acceptance of accountability for results be fostered?[6]

These questions provide the structure for the database upon which the actual plan will be based. The responsibility of nursing administration as stated by the ANA is to develop and execute a rational program. The objective of the staffing plan is to ensure that nursing care is safe, responsive to patient needs, and scientifically and technologically sound.

▨ STAFFING METHODOLOGIES

The development of a staffing plan is based on an underlying logic or methodology. Staffing methodologies fall into the following categories: descriptive or consensus methodology, industrial and management engineering, and expert panel method.[7,8] They vary according to a rationale that distinguishes the resulting pattern.

Descriptive methodology refers to a staffing pattern that is based on subjective data. This means that the appropriate staffing pattern is recommended on the basis of the manager's experience and intuition. For example, using the average acuity level of patients on a unit, the manager determines that a particular ratio of staff to patient maintains quality of care, based on institutional audits. The information that is gathered to determine the staffing plan is organized around the variables selected by the manager. These variables may vary from department to department within the same institution (Fig. 14-2).

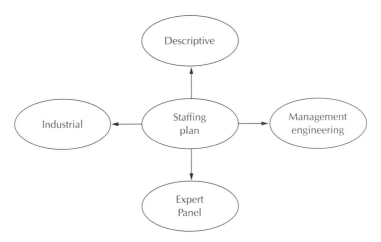

Figure 14-2. The most common staffing methodologies that lead to a staffing plan.

The **industrial engineering** methodology is a technique or group of techniques developed by industry to improve productivity. Typically, these techniques include task analysis, review of work distribution, and measurement of the staff work through work sampling and time-and-motion studies. *Work sampling* offers the possibility of an ideal staffing pattern and, even more importantly, provides empiric evidence for the establishment of a theoretic basis for staffing procedures.[9] Work sampling combines many of the aforementioned techniques, especially time- and-motion studies. Results of these methods provide information about the time it takes to do specific work.[10]

Nursing departments have used these techniques to develop appropriate staffing plans. The work of the unit is defined in terms of tasks to be accomplished, and the level of the employee who is needed to perform the work. The problem with this precise methodology is that the complex nature of professional nursing is not entirely amenable to this type of measurement. Nursing is more than a list of tasks to be performed; rather, it involves use of the nursing process, which is analytic, instrumental, and evaluative. While aspects of this methodology are useful, relying on this exclusively would be too limiting to all that is required of the professional staff.

The **management engineering** methodology optimizes the nursing work load by developing a staffing index model. Using similar techniques of industrial engineering and a variety of other information (quality nursing care; a general description of the type and volume of patients serviced;

information about institutional characteristics, such as census, bed capacity, daily visits or admission; and operating budget), a systematic analysis yields a projection for an appropriate and cost-effective staffing pattern. This methodology is as successful as the information that is provided.

The newest approach, referred to as **expert panel nurse staffing method** can be used to allocate resources and staff.[11] Using this model, a manager is able to examine service- and unit-specific needs related to structure, process, and outcomes. An expert panel, composed of nurse leaders within and related to the organization, is appointed by the chief executive nurse, and they examine the separate divisions of the organization. Data (also called minimum unit-based data set) examined by the panel differ by the mission of the organization and unit of care but usually include the patient classification system, tasks, direct and indirect costs to the delivery of care, prospective payment, availability and type of nursing and support staff, and quality-assessment findings. Following analysis of the data, staffing needs are predicted to provide coverage of the unit with calculation of a replacement factor (an estimate of the need for additional staff due to vacation, sickness, or turnover). In addition, staffing requirements are considered, which allow existing staff to participate in professional and educational meetings. The outcomes of care are predicted based on increasing or decreasing the staff, and non–unit-based staff (central staff consisting of administrators, advanced practice nurses, and staff development and support employees) are projected, which insure all necessary nursing care is provided throughout the organization. The expert panel in essence recommends an ideal, professional and support staff for the entire organization.

Nursing administration, with input from the lower-level managers, ultimately has the responsibility to determine which staffing methodology will be used by the department of nursing. Variables such as occupancy rate, salary scales, availability of nurses, organization of the department of nursing (structure of authority, centralized or decentralized), and type of institution influence the subsequent decision about the staffing pattern.

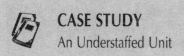

CASE STUDY
An Understaffed Unit

Michael Clay, a registered nurse on the 10th floor ICU, had just completed his fifth night of work and was looking forward to the next two days off. The unit had been completely filled to capacity and extremely busy. As Michael was leaving, the charge nurse approached him and asked him if he would work one more night because they were really short-staffed. He paused and looking exhausted said, "OK, but this is it." At the same time, Stephanie, another RN, walked into the report room, and was greeted with "What are you doing here today? I thought you were off." Stephanie said, "I was called at 5 A.M. this morning to come in and help." Another nurse, Jane, joined the group and said, "I feel like quitting, I couldn't even take a break last night."

The charge nurse who overheard the conversation said, " You are aware of the fact that we lost three permanent staff members, and their positions have not been filled, and frankly, I am not sure if those positions will be filled by RNs or technicians." She went on, "Several proposals are being considered, including flexible hours, innovative staffing patterns, and self-scheduling. The aim is to provide autonomy and flexibility to the current and potential staff."

- What kind of staffing patterns should be offered?
- How much flexibility should be suggested?
- How would you handle financial compensation for part- and full-time staff?

Scheduling Patterns

Following the establishment of the number and type of personnel composing the case mix, a pattern of scheduling is proposed. **Scheduling patterns** comprise the actual assignment of personnel to units or departments. The goal of the pattern is to provide the correct configuration of personnel for the work to be done, eliminating understaffing (not enough staff) or overstaffing (too much staff), while accommodating the individual needs of the staff.

■ WORK SCHEDULES

Work schedules provide a plan by which personnel are assigned in time periods for which the organization provides service. Take, for example, an acute care institution that provides 24-hour, 7-day-a-week service to patients. Nurses in particular are responsible for this type of coverage. This responsibility has presented some problems. In the past, nurses assumed responsibility for other departments that did not provide continuous service despite patients' requirements. For example, a nurse would provide respiratory therapy treatments for patients because respiratory therapy did not cover patients on the night shift. For the most part, this is changing because the system does not use personnel properly. In essence, it is not cost-effective or time-effective. Nurses practice nursing, and other disciplines are responsible for their specific service.

The second type of problem arising from this situation involves the issue of 24-hour coverage. Inflexible work schedules made it difficult for many professional nurses to adhere to rigid, organizational staffing requirements. As a result, new and innovative scheduling patterns have been proposed to induce nurses to be able to practice.[12]

Examples of work schedules include:

- *The traditional 40-hour-a-week, 8-hour shift.* An effective scheduling plan, this has been used for a long time and provides coverage for the work to be accomplished. Most flexible plans are in some way a deviation from this particular model. Often the manager assigns the full-time staff to the 7-day-a-week and 24-hour-a-day coverage implied by this model. In fact, this pattern of scheduling work has been the impetus for the creative and exciting changes that are occurring in staffing opportunities.

- *Ten-hour shift.* In this plan, a full-time employee is able to work a 4-day 10-hour-a-shift week. This has advantages for personnel in providing a shortened work week. It also gives the added benefit of allowing enough time to ensure that the necessary work is completed for patients. The drawback to this model, besides the longer work day, has been the added expense to the personnel budget. A reduction in personnel has not been realized, and a problem of overlap exists. Fatigue has been cited as a problem for staff that needs further study. This is, however, a plan that is very attractive to many professional staff.

- *Twelve-hour shift.* Some options within a 2-week pay period are (1) seven 12-hour shifts, (2) seven shifts on and seven shifts off, (3) three shifts per week in a 72-hour pay period.[13] This plan presents many of the advantages of the 10-hour-a-week plan. It provides an intense work period and more free time while securing benefits for a full-time position. The disadvantages are also the same, particularly fatigue.

- *The Baylor plan.* A very interesting alternative staffing plan is the Baylor plan. In essence, it is a weekend alternative plan. The idea, originated at Baylor University Medical Center, consists of a staff for a traditional 40-hour-a-week, 8-hour-a-shift plan during the week and a second staff for weekends who work two twelve-hour shifts and are paid for a 40-hour week. Its advantages include ensuring adequate weekend coverage and working fewer hours for greater pay. A problem with this method is that there is a high turnover rate due to the undesirable hours.

- *Job sharing.* This implies two people sharing a position, which has obvious advantages for people who desire a part-time position. This works very well at many levels of the organization and has been reported to be quite successful in the position of clinical specialist. It does require that the two individuals sharing the position be cooperative and compatible.
- *Part-time work.* Part-time work falls into any category. Professional staff are able to select working hours that are compatible with their personal needs. The hours of work may be consistent with any of the preceding models or may be fewer working hours per day. This allows professionals with multiple responsibilities to still be part of the professional work force. This has advantages for both the person and the organization.
- *Combination plan.* This plan combines part-time or full-time work with a variety of staffing schedules.

Flexibility and versatility have to be characteristics of today's staffing schedules. Providing options for professional nurses is an excellent way to prevent attrition and to enhance work satisfaction. Giving autonomy and decision making about working conditions to the staff is good management.

■ MANAGEMENT'S ROLE: PLANNING FOR STAFF

The role of management in dealing with the staffing issue depends on the level of management. Top-level management provides general guidelines for the selection of a staffing plan. Front-line managers implement the staffing plan and give input as to its effectiveness. The challenge of the task is great due to the uncertainty of environmental and professional concerns. No longer can managers rely solely on last year's data about patients' admission, treatments, and discharges.

Any strategy that management adopts takes into account a variety of real issues that affect the organization and professional nursing. The first of these issues focuses on those environmental forces that directly affect the specific organization. These forces are, for the most part, *economic* and *regulatory*.

Economics dictates to what extent staff may be procured. Budgetary restrictions exist that allocate percentages of the operating budget to deal with personnel salary and benefits. In the current environment, budgets have been drastically revised to adjust to a different system of reimbursement. Every professional and nonprofessional position has to be justified as to its ability to meet the mission of the organization. Hiring of key personnel has never been more carefully scrutinized.

Economic policies from government to the variety of insurance plans direct, in part, the limits of how much and what kind of staff is economically possible. Regulations about safety, infection control, and quality-control measures also play a part in quantifying staffing plans. A certain level of environmental quality must exist for any agency to be accredited. Some of these regulations have more to do with staff issues than with real environmental problems. Thus, to some extent, regulatory bodies add a dimension to "safe" staff distributions.

The second set of issues involves the *organization's database*, which predicts a staffing model for the desired level of quality nursing care. Some of these measures have been mentioned. Allotted money and available human resources are foundational to the development of a staffing model. The philosophy of nursing care held by the department is extremely important to the case mix. This philosophy is the foundation for standards of nursing care upon which quality will be evaluated. Remember that quality also involves input from the community served, professional organizations, and federal and state governmental sources.

Information regarding the patients and services offered are also instrumental in developing an appropriate staffing model. Type of patients, acuity levels, and prospective prediction of anticipated patients and services offered provide baseline data for predicting staff requirements.[14]

The third set of issues involves *professional concerns* that address working conditions. These conditions include the ability to self-assign for both shift and day. Flexible staffing is more a requirement today than a perk (special bonus). Salary demands and a salary wage scale that reflect rewards for experience are important aspects of recruiting and retaining staff. Opportunities for advancement within the organization and ongoing educational programs are important considerations for a motivated staff.[15]

Recruiting, providing, maintaining, and retaining staff involve a mutual agreement between management and personnel. Involving staff in decisions concerning their working hours can create a positive work climate. Allowing autonomy in decision making facilitates staff growth and enhances morale. The most expensive personnel costs to an organization, besides providing benefits, comes from staff turnover and absenteeism. These activities require that additional personnel be hired for temporary or permanent positions.[16]

▓ SUMMARY

This chapter has dealt with the most important resource to any organization: the staff. Staffing is a highly complex process that, because of the volatility in health care today, requires management know-how. Staffing is the process that provides adequate personnel to do the work of the organization. This is based on a staffing plan that uses a particular methodology. These methodologies include descriptive or consensus, industrial engineering, management engineering, and the expert panel method.

Following the development of a staffing plan, which includes an acceptable case mix, a scheduling plan is provided that allocates personnel to a time frame. The role of management includes the choice of a staffing plan and the evaluation of its effectiveness. Issues to keep in mind for the choice of a proper professional staff model are environmental, organizational, and professional working conditions. Staffing is the means by which the work of the organization is operationalized.

 STUDENT EXERCISES

1. Plan a staffing pattern for a 30-bed, step-down, coronary care unit for 24 hours per day for 7 days. Which staffing methodology did you use? Why?

2. What would you do to recruit and retain staff?

3. What working conditions are the most important to you?

4. What do you consider to be the major problems with staffing? What can be done about them?

▓ REFERENCES

1. Strickland B, Neely S, "Using a Standard Staffing Index to Allocate Staff," *Journal of Nursing Administration*, 25:3, March 1995, p. 15–21.
2. Dunne MA, Norby R, Cournoyer P, et al, "Expert Panel Method for Nurse Staffing and Resource Management," *Journal of Nursing Administration*, 25:10, 1995, p. 63–67.

3. Pederson A, Hoover C, Kisiel T, "Redesigning a Skill Mix in the ICU," *Nursing Management*, 26:7, 1995, p. 32J–32P.

4. Shinn JA, "Impact of Staffing Levels on Job Stress, Injuries, and Quality of Care," *Progress in Cardio-Vascular Nursing*, 26:7, 1995, p. 47.

5. Dunne MA, p. 66.

6. American Hospital Association, *Managing under Medical Prospective Pricing*, Chicago: AHA, 1983.

7. Strickland B, Neely S, p. 31.

8. Dunne MA, p. 67.

9. Quist B, "Work Sampling Nursing Units," *Nursing Management*, 23:9, September 1992, p. 50–51.

10. Mayer GG, "Work Sampling in Ambulatory Care Nursing," *Nursing Management*, 23:9, September 1992, p. 52–57.

11. Dunne MA, p. 64.

12. Loevinsobn HT, "A New Perspective on Scheduling: Freedom and Cost Control," *Nursing Management*, July 1992, p. 56–61.

13. Hung R, "A Cyclic Schedule of 10-Hour, Four Day Work Week, " *Nursing Management*, 22:9, September 1991, p. 30–33.

14. Cardello D, "Monitoring Staffing Variances and Length of Stay," *Nursing Management*, 26:4, April 1995, p. 38–41.

15. Williams C, "Why Nurses Leave the Profession: Part One," *Nursing Standard*, vol. 3, June 26, 1991, p. 33–35.

16. Taunton R, Hope K, Woods C, Bott M, "Predictors of Absenteeism among Hospital Staff Nurses," *Nursing Economics*, 13:4, 1995, p. 217–279.

Managing Resources
Time

Introduction

Effective managers use time efficiently. In essence, taking control over time gives them control over the work. Time refers to the number of seconds, minutes, hours, or days available to the manager to accomplish a given task. Using time profitably has implications for both the manager as well as the professional staff. The objective of this next discussion is the process of time management.

KEY CONCEPTS

Time is the number of seconds, minutes, hours, or days available to the manager to accomplish a given task.

Time Management is based on principles and is a variety of techniques that facilitate the best use of time.

Time Styles are predispositions (action, idea, logic, or people) of behavioral patterns that influence how a person uses time.

Stress is the sum of all the nonspecific biologic phenomena elicited by adverse, external influences. Stress may be either physical or psychologic or both.

Self-Management is an individualized approach to use time best according to one's particular needs.

Crisis Control refers to the communication and delegation of a new plan reorganized around priorities to manage an unexpected and untoward event.

Efficiency refers to the resource utilization of doing the right task.

Effectiveness refers to the quality of doing the right task correctly.

■ TIME MANAGEMENT

Time management is composed of a variety of principles and techniques to facilitate the best use of an individual's available time. It is intended to foster good work habits that use time productively. The activities for organizing time should take into account a variety of principles, including:

- *communication*
- *planning*
- *delegating*
- *prioritizing goals*[1]

■ PRINCIPLES OF TIME MANAGEMENT

Communication

Effective communication facilitates time management. Use of the communication process is an important tool to provide complete and appropriate information. Managers need explicit and correct information to plan and order work. Managers deal with information and make decisions based on changing and shifting information. Errors can lead to wasted time and useless expenditure of energy. Proper information guides correct action. Communication should include clear messages and feedback in order for correct perceptions. Decisions about the work to be completed should only be made after the necessary information is known. Poor decisions and indecision are time wasters. Good communication is fundamental to effective use of resources. Time is a resource that when managed well will enable the process of management.

Planning

Planning is the essential ingredient for effective use of time. Managers spend a major part of their time in the planning process, which may actually exceed the time required to implement the activity. The ability to plan effectively is essential to the effective use of time. Planning charts the course of action in order of importance. Every minute spent in planning saves time in the execution of activities. The fundamental issue in "time-saving" planning is that optimal results occur with the least amount of effort and consumption of resources. Planning also involves the creation of objectives and goals in accord with a time frame. If the plan includes realistic deadlines (not underestimating or overestimating the time needed), there will be less stress associated with the implementation of the work. Stress refers to the sum total of all the nonspecific, biologic phenomena elicited by adverse, external influences. Stress may be either physical or psychologic, or both. In every plan of action the possibility of unanticipated consequences should be considered. By constructing alternatives and adopting an attitude of flexibility, the manager will be able to cope with forces beyond control.

The manager who uses planning properly is in a position to not only manage his or her time well but also that of others. This manager does not procrastinate because it will prevent others from doing their work. Building in alternatives facilitates the work of others in the face of barriers. A manager who routinely reviews plans on a daily, weekly, and monthly basis is using planning properly. Planning is a key ingredient to successful time management.

Delegation

Delegation is used by the manager as a way to ensure that the work of the organization is completed on schedule. The most efficient and effective use of time is when the manager manages, and the professional staff does the operative work. Efficiency refers to doing the right task with the least amount of resources, and effectively refers to doing the right task correctly and securing good outcomes. The manager who is results-oriented executes the plan of the organization through the appropriate use of delegation. Delegating the work of the department to others is not only a part of management but also a strategy for time management.

Prioritizing Goals

By establishing a hierarchy of goals and developing a plan of time to meet them, the manager is in a position to selectively allocate varying amounts of time and energy to goal accomplishment. Prioritizing involves ordering goals, tasks, and responsibilities from the most important to least important. This process involves knowledge about the managerial role and the nature of the work to be completed. Spending time thinking through how best to meet the goals is time well spent. It is far more efficient to spend time planning for problems than to spend time to correct them.

Matching the managerial goal with monitoring criteria to ensure appropriate progress is a useful way to map the best use of time. Take the following example: the manager has a goal of having all performance appraisals completed within a three-month period so that pay raises will be on schedule. This is an important responsibility with implications for the nursing staff. The manager plans how best to proceed by completing all performance evaluations and conducting scheduled interviews in accord with mutually established dates. The manager also knows that other activities impinge on the manager's time, and must allocate time each day to complete the evaluation forms and schedule ample time for the performance appraisal interviews.

■ TIME MANAGEMENT STRATEGIES

Time management strategies are practical techniques to preserve, conserve, structure, and use time well to meet goals. These strategies are, in large measure, ways to individualize the best use of time according to one's particular needs (**self-management**). How an individual best manages time can vary and is referred to as a time style.

Since managing time is a personal experience, one must know what his/her time style is, and how time is spent. **Time styles** are based on personality characteristics and habit. These styles have been categorized on dominant behavioral preferences and are named the following:

- *action*
- *idea*
- *logic*
- *people time styles*[2]

Action-oriented people tend to view time in the present and organize activities one at a time to be completed immediately. This individual is not comfortable with unexpected tasks, and tends not to prioritize, as each task is seen as important. Idea-oriented persons are creative and don't usually pay attention to time. They have a hard time meeting deadlines and estimating proper time use. Logic-oriented persons are orderly, rational, sequential planners who are comfortable with and able to use time well. Lastly,

Goals
1. Plan patient care
2. Attend inservice
3. Evaluate nursing care

		Time/activity
Start time		*Activity*
7:15	Receive Report	
30	Give Report	
45		
0		
15		
30		
45		
0		
1:15	Attend service	
30		
45		
0		
4:00	*Day ends* Discuss patient care	
	Evaluation	

Time savers—Planning activities
Time wasters—Unnecessary trips to Central Service

Figure 15-1. An example of a time-analysis worksheet.

people-oriented people are most effective at team building and may not see time as a priority. Often these individuals are over-committed and over-extended. They tend to underestimate the amount of time required to complete tasks. Most individuals tend to have a dominant time style.

Strategies have been devised to help managers and professional staff use their time wisely and productively, no matter their personal preference. Suggested strategies are discussed below.[3]

Time Analysis

To discover your own style, a time analysis may be used. This is a personal diary in which all activities are recorded in 15-minute blocks for approximately 1 week. This log will become the basis of analysis. It will be apparent where time is spent, wasted, and properly used. For those who wish to enhance their use of time, this method will allow them to examine their individual time style and where they might be able to use time more effectively. It has been advised that this procedure be repeated yearly to discover if bad habits remain. A typical time analysis sheet is pictured in Figure 15-1.

	Morning	*Afternoon*	*Late afternoon*

Goals
1. Begin performance appraisal evaluations
2. Prepare budget for next quarter
3. Review quality assurance records

Activities
1. Review anecdotal performance records
2. Review budget report
3. Prepare a report to staff on quality scores

Figure 15-2. An example of a time-management daily planner.

Daily Planning

Planning is effective when time frames correspond with the manager's responsibility. This means daily, weekly, and monthly plans. Ultimately all long- and short-range goals and activities become subject to daily planning. Prior to the implementation of a project, time lines may be applied so that activities can be broken down into daily segments. It is recommended that the daily plans be formulated or reviewed the preceding evening by the manager. In this way, the manager is prepared to make sure certain activities are completed. This may be through the process of delegation or the manager's own effort. An example of a daily plan is pictured in Figure 15-2.

Crisis Control

No amount of planning can prevent periodic crises. In any social system, crises do occur from time to time. It is during a crisis that time-management skills are the most important. Keep in mind the principles of time management: communication, planning, delegation, and prioritizing. **Crisis control** is accomplished when communication and delegation of a new plan is reorganized around priorities to manage an unexpected and untoward event. In a crisis, certain people will be involved in its resolution. These people should be informed at once with the necessary details of the problem. Ordinarily, this group will be composed of superiors and selected subordinates.

The plan that has been established may have to be rearranged to deal with priorities. Other work may have to be delayed until a later date. Sound planning will guide the necessary day-to-day activities while effort is directed at resolution of the crisis. The manager may have to delegate tasks to the professional staff while dealing with the impending problem. The manager is in a position to communicate, reorganize, and delegate. In a crisis situation, the manager's flexibility and ability to activate alternative solutions is good management of time.

Problem Analysis

Problem analysis is essential to be an effective manager as well as to use time properly. Managers must be able to distinguish a *crisis* from an *urgent* or an *important event*. Each type requires a different type of response. The crisis requires major reorganization of priorities. The urgent situation requires immediate action. The important event requires analysis and planning.

Another aspect of problem analysis that has implications for the manager's time is that not every problem requires an immediate solution. Some problems go away with little or no intervention. Managers, in making decisions about what to do or not to do, are also making decisions about effective or ineffective use of time.

Task Analysis

One of the most efficient ways to save time is to evaluate the tasks that are performed. By reviewing tasks, the manager may discover which tasks are of low value and therefore could be eliminated, consolidated, or delegated. Similar or related activities may be able to be grouped in such a way as to allow a more efficient performance from manager or from personnel. This is very much like functional assignments on a nursing division. One individual takes vital signs for all patients on a postoperative step-down unit. Tasks can be more efficiently handled if all the necessary "tools" are available before beginning the activity. Assembling essential equipment prior to implementing a nursing skill saves time, energy, and frustration.

Time Control

Periodically, the manager should simply be unavailable by planning office time to think or to clear up pressing business. In this way the manager controls interruptions except for important messages. Planned office time should be built into the manager's plans and communicated to staff.

Time Evaluation

Periodic evaluation of how time is spent is a helpful technique to assess use of time. The ability to organize and use time effectively is the hallmark of good management. Thus time-analysis techniques can be helpful guides to improve both **effectiveness** and **efficiency**.

■ BARRIERS TO EFFECTIVE TIME MANAGEMENT

In the development of new skills, barriers may exist. Being aware of problems alerts the manager to possible pitfalls. In addition, considering problems will be helpful in the evaluation process. Some barriers to the effective management of time are discussed below.

Habit

People are creatures of habit. Habits are comfortable ways of behaving because they do not require conscious thought. It is also very difficult to change habits. Because of this, certain behaviors, while comfortable, do not use time effectively. Time analysis will show exactly where habitual behaviors take precedent over time-efficient behaviors. The manager should be mindful of negative habits, particularly procrastination, and make time more productive.

Work Expansion

Work sometimes takes on a life of its own. If 3 hours are allotted for a specific task and one hour is sufficient, the work may take 3 hours. Time frames attached to work will provide realistic guidelines.

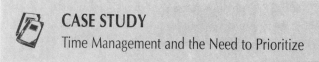

CASE STUDY
Time Management and the Need to Prioritize

Joanne Burns is a new graduate and has begun her career in the cardiac thoracic intensive care unit (ICU). Joanne has finished her orientation and is working with experienced professional nurses.

Joanne feels relatively secure with the responsibilities of the position. She knows she has a great deal to learn and is open to suggestions. She hopes her transition period from new member of the team to experienced registered nurse (RN) will be smooth. She is pleased that her first assignment includes two fairly stable patients.

The first day of her new position, Joanne is assigned to two postoperative patients. Everything proceeds smoothly until one of the patient's blood pressure drops and bleeding is suspected. Joanne is a wreck. She becomes disorganized and anxious. The other patient is neglected while she cares for the patient in crisis, who eventually returns to the operating room.

Following the episode, Joanne, who had not gone to lunch or had a break, overhears the assistant head nurse say, "I am just not sure about Joanne. She didn't have anyone take over for the other patient, and she was really shaken and disorganized." Joanne feels that the assessment of her performance was unfair, but she does not say anything.

- What would help Joanne to be more organized in the future?

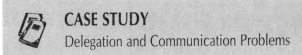

CASE STUDY
Delegation and Communication Problems

Cindy Smith, a new RN, and Kim Jones, RN, were finishing work on the day shift of a postoperative surgical floor when a new patient arrived from the emergency room. Cindy stopped what she was doing, calculating Intake/Output ratios, and proceeded to admit the new patient. When Cindy got to her room, the transporter allowed the new patient, a woman, to get up off the cart and walk to her bed which she did easily. Cindy helped her get settled, noting no acute distress, and told her she would return in ten minutes. The patient said, "Fine, I don't need anything." Cindy went back to finish the end-of-shift duties.

Just as Cindy was about to finish her last room, Kim walked in and asked her, "Where's the admission sheet you started on the new admit?" Cindy stated she hadn't started one yet, she wanted to finish these tasks before report, and planned on admitting the patient next. Kim walked abruptly away from Cindy and began the process of admitting the new patient. Cindy walked into the room and tried to help, when Kim said, "You should always take vital signs immediately when a new patient is admitted."

Outside the patient's room, Cindy tried to explain herself, when Kim screamed at her. "You don't do anything right. I hate to work with you. You are lazy, and you put a patient at risk." Cindy didn't know what to say. She completed the admission, gave report, and left the division.

- What is your analysis of what happened in this situation?
- Are new patient admissions a priority?
- What could Cindy have done differently? What could Kim have done differently?

Oversupervision

The manager must be mindful of what the employee is to accomplish and how much supervision is necessary. To give too much supervision to a competent professional presents interpersonal as well as time problems. Allowing the staff to complete their work is the best use of everyone's time.

Underdelegation

The manager who does not delegate appropriately ends up with more work than is necessary. A manager has enough responsibility without assuming that of subordinates.

Losing Sight of Objectives

A manager who loses sight of the work that has to be accomplished will surely waste time. An important element of the managerial role is maintaining a course of action. Periodically reviewing what and how objectives are to be met is a productive use of time. Suggestions to help the new manager develop time-management skills are summarized below:

1. Analyze your time for an average week. Use the time analysis tool.
2. Plan your work day the evening before.
3. Know your peak energy time. Do the most difficult work then.
4. Begin with the most important job.
5. Start the day by reviewing what you will be doing.
6. Don't *waste* time at work by too much socializing.
7. Give yourself time each day to think, plan, and create.
8. Organize the necessary "tools" to complete a task.
9. Consolidate similar tasks or work.
10. Eliminate unnecessary work.

■ SUMMARY

This discussion has provided an overview of time management. Using time properly involves prioritizing goals and applying time-management principles and strategies. The principles of time management include effective communication, planning, and delegation. Strategies are methods aimed at facilitating self-management of time. Barriers exist that are problematic to the effective use of time. The manager who uses time efficiently and effectively is managing a personal and group resource in an appropriate manner.

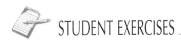

STUDENT EXERCISES

1. Keep your own record of time for an average week. Identify where you could save time.

2. Observe someone whom you believe uses time well. What is the most significant activity this individual uses?

3. In your clinical experience, try to utilize (1) time analysis, (2) daily planning, and (3) task analysis for one week. Is there a difference in your efficiency?

4. Consider this situation: Ms. Smith, the head nurse on a busy surgical division, notices that for the next two days, staffing will be slightly inadequate for the acuity of the patients on the division. This also happens to be during summer vacation. What might be done to deal with understaffing for a very short period of time and yet ensure quality of service. Since the example is general, provide a solution that deals with principles.

■ REFERENCES

1. Blanchard K, Johnson S, *The One Minute Manager*, New York: Berkley Books, 1986.
2. Tager MJ, *Time Styles, Time Management, Personal Action*, New York: Great Performances, Inc, 1992.
3. Day Timers, Inc., May 1996, Allentown PA.

■ SUGGESTED READINGS

Barkas JL, *Creative Time Management*, Englewood Cliffs, NJ: Prentice Hall, 1994.
Haynes ME, *Practical Time Management*, Los Altos, CA: Crisp Publications, 1991.
Matejka JK, Dunsing RJ, "Time Management: Changing Some Traditions," *Management World*, 17:2, 1988, p. 6–7.
Simpson RJ, "Case-Managed Care in Tomorrow's Information Network," *Nursing Management*, 24:7, 1993, p. 14–16.

16

Managing Resources
The Budget

Introduction

Financial concerns are a major force in today's health care industry. It is not surprising that health care personnel on all levels are aware of and participate in cost-saving strategies. The new nurse manager must also be aware of economic issues. The role of all managers demands that attention be directed toward the organization's financial status. This chapter will discuss financial management with special attention to the budget. Even though all nurse managers may not be responsible for the formation of a budget, it is helpful to understand the underlying dynamics to provide meaningful input when called upon.

KEY CONCEPTS

Financial Management is a major department and an activity that handles financial resources in an organized manner.

Financial Structure represents the components that are essential to managing finances and includes centralized policies, decentralized operations, and the interrelated responsibilities of those who play a part in financial management.

Financial Management System is the result of the actual plan to use and maximize the economics of the organization.

Budget is a planning document used by a department or organization that forecasts both receipts and expenditures.

Budget Process refers to those activities and steps needed to be taken for the manager to formulate a budget. The most common types of budgets are zero-based or flexible-based budgets.

Accounting is the activity that records and reports all financial transactions.

Standard Accounting refers to those procedures that prepare reports on a monthly, quarterly, or yearly basis to show financial performance.

Cost Accounting is that activity that reports to the organization or department how much it is costing to provide specific services or products to the organization's clients.

Double-Entry Accounting is today's accounting method, which requires that for every amount added to one account an equal amount must be taken away from one or more other accounts.

Long-Range Financial Plans is a document prepared by every organization to cover the next 5 to 10 years in terms of goals and dollars.

Variance is a general term to describe the difference between a budgeted number (or planned cost) and an actual result. There are many kinds of variances.

Revenue refers to incoming cash or cash equivalents received during a specific span of time.

Assets are those holdings of the organization that have a dollar value.

Resources are commodities of the organization that have value.

Expenditures are those resources used by the organization to provide service. This may include compensation for employees or providers of goods or services.

Liabilities are the dollar amounts owed to other organizations.

Budget Work Sheet is a tool used by managers to prepare their budget.

■ MANAGING FINANCIAL RESOURCES

The preparation of a department's budget is actually one of the last steps in handling organizational finances. It is part of the interrelated activities that fall within the scope of **financial management.** This major department in health care institutions coordinates financial operations throughout the entire organization or network. It does so through the establishment of a financial structure and management of the resultant system. The usual objectives of the office of financial management are as follows:

- To ensure that the organization has an efficient and effective financial management structure that supports strategic objectives, including those of individual operating units
- To establish a uniform set of internal financial controls across the entire organization
- To provide appropriate financial information to make timely decisions

These objectives can only be met with the cooperation of all managers who plan and evaluate budgeted resources. To illustrate the financial concepts presented in this chapter please read the Lobsterville case study on page 334, which illustrates how financial concepts impact and interact with health care delivery.

■ FINANCIAL STRUCTURE

The creation of a **financial structure** enables managers to know what is expected of them and in so doing to judge the organization's viability in today's competitive environment. A **financial management system** is a plan that uses and maximizes the economics of the organization. This plan consists of:

1. Centralized policies (those control policies that apply to all departments),
2. Decentralized financial operations (each department has separate operating costs), and
3. Establishment of interrelated responsibilities of those who play a part in financial management (Fig. 16-1).

The actual financial system that results from the financial management plan balances assets (those holdings of the organization that are of value) and

Budget types

Zero based   or   Flexible based

Figure 16-1. The different types of variance to the budget.

revenues with **expenditures** and **liabilities**. Financial data are integrated into the day-to-day operations, and subsequent reporting on financial conditions keeps the system functioning. The usual means of incorporating financial data is through the **budget**, or the planning document, used by a department and organization that forecasts both receipts and expenditures:

- The Financial Plan
    Positive (assets and resources)
        Balances
            Negative (losses)

▓ THE BUDGETING PROCESS

Budgeting is an important part of every organization's planning and control function. It requires that the manager:

- Review the financial performance during the prior budgeting time frame, month, quarter, or year, and
- Formulate a new budget or financial plan for the coming period in relation to the organization's goals and financial projections.

The **budgeting process** can be filled with anxiety and uncertainty. Anxiety exists because the prior budget must be assessed, and variances (the difference between the budget numbers and the actual results) must be fully understood and explained to upper management. Uncertainty exists because translations of long-term goals and projections into detailed dollar estimates raise questions that are difficult, if not impossible, to answer precisely; yet, the process must go forward. Nevertheless, budgeting can be an exciting and challenging activity for the nurse manager to focus on the overall plan of the organization.

Fundamental to the budgeting process is careful design and direction. This is accomplished through a general policy statement as well as through clear goals and reciprocal financial projections, which follow.

A Policy Statement

A general policy statement makes clear that (1) budgeting is an important part of the organization's planning and control process, (2) uniform standards and definitions are used across the organization in carrying out the budgeting process, and (3) all managers are expected to provide the necessary data within a specific time frame. This policy statement is general in nature, widely publicized, and should be changed rarely or not at all.

Goals and Financial Projections

Specific goals and financial projections are prepared on a regular, set schedule (e.g., every 12 months for publication in a formal document). Goals and projections contain operating (that which affects day-to-day activities) and capital (that which affects major or unusual expenditures) plans. They convey a general sense of where the organization is headed and enough specifics so that goals can be integrated with the capital and operating budget.

These statements and projections demand the attention of administrators and managers who must use them when doing their own budgeting tasks. These statements must be detailed enough to provide each department or division manager with the hard numbers needed to begin the budgeting process.

■ RELATED BUDGETING CONCEPTS

Budgeting is a complex process and requires specific knowledge and skill. The following section describes related concepts that are necessary to complete a budget. These concepts include: (1) accounting, (2) long-range financial plans, and (3) budget terms. Accounting methods provide an accurate record of expenditures and drive the budgeting process. Long-range financial plans focus the budget. Budget terms are offered to define the jargon that is used in the budgeting process. The reader may select appropriate sections to review.

Accounting

Accounting is the activity that records and reports all financial transactions and thus generates the data for the budget. There are different types of accounting methods. This section will discuss standard accounting, cost accounting, and a method that is used by both types of accounting activities, double-entry accounting. **Standard accounting**, or general accounting, consists of activities that formulate reports of financial performance on a monthly, quarterly, or yearly basis. These reports can be prepared in many formats, but the most common formats fall into one of three categories:

Accounting Reports
1. Income statements
2. Balance sheets
3. Cash-flow statements

Category One: Income Statements. Income statements (also known as profit or loss statements) record receipts and expenditures. These statements disclose whether the organization or department made or lost money in the time period in question (month, quarter, or year). The income statement has two important sections. In the revenue section, the organization records all its receipts (or expected receipts due) from its normal operating activities. These would typically include such things as income from patient services. The expenses section records (1) the expenses directly incurred in caring for patients (labor, material, utilities, etc.); (2) the prorated portion of the cost of buildings and equipment used by the enterprise; and (3) the overhead expenses incurred in running the organization (administrators' salaries, interest expense on debts, etc.).

Category Two: The Balance Sheet. The balance sheet (also known as the position statement) records where the organization stands financially at any given point in time. These are usually prepared at the end of a period, month, quarter, or year. The balance sheet reports two types of **resources**: those owned by the organization and those owed to others. Those that are owed to others are further divided into those that are owed to others as a matter of debt and those that are owed to the owners of the organization.

The balance sheet is divided into two sections. **Assets** is the section for the organizations' owned resources: cash, buildings, equipment, inventory, etc. In this section, assets are generally ranked by the speed with which they could be converted into cash. Cash is presented first, money due from others for services already rendered is second, inventory ready to be sold is third, and so on.

Liabilities and owners equity is the section where resources owed to others are shown. In the liabilities portion, debts are shown, such as amounts due to suppliers for goods and services already received, and amounts due to bankers for loans received. Liabilities are generally ranked by urgency. Those that will have to be paid quickly are ranked first. Owner's equity is the difference between assets and liabilities. This difference is normally a positive amount and represents what the owners would receive if all the organization's assets were sold and all its debts paid.

Category Three: Cash-Flow Statements. The third form of accounting format is a cash-flow statement, which records the sources and uses of cash for a period. This statement is used to determine if the organization improved (or hurt) its cash position over a specific time period. This report is different from an income statement in that it measures the organization's ability to pay its bills. An organization can be profitable while at the same time be weak from a cash position. For example, the organization's cash may have been used to buy too many nonliquid items, such as buildings or equipment.

Cost Accounting

Another type of accounting is **cost accounting**. Cost accounting activities produce reports that tell managers how much it is costing to provide specific services. These reports are published on a monthly, quarterly, or yearly basis and contain details about the various elements of cost: labor, material, and overhead. There are two ways to approach cost accounting. Standard costing is used in an organization where all services or products fall into a manageable number of groups and where the costs to produce each item in that group are identical or so close to identical that the differences are not meaningful. The current prospective payment system uses standard costing concepts.

Actual costing (also known as job costing) is used in an organization where each product, patient, or client is unique and will have its own unique requirements. This is the actual cost system that is used by today's acute care organizations.

Cost accounting also takes into consideration the change in value through depreciation and amortization. Depreciation is the expense item that shows the drop in the value of a major asset from time period to time period. A related term is amortization, which is the drop in the value of a major, nonphysical asset from period to period. Items that are depreciated are buildings, equipment, additions, improvements, furniture, etc. Items that are amortized are copyrights, patents, legal fees associated with organizing the organization, etc. Although both depreciation and amortization are expense items on the income statement, they do not require any expenditure of cash and do not weaken the organization's cash position. An organization with depreciation and amortization may show losses on its income statement while actually improving its cash position.

Double-entry Accounting

Double-entry accounting is the system used by today's accountants to record all financial transactions. This system requires that for every amount added to one account, an equal amount must be taken away from one or more other accounts. The system works because some accounts are expected to have negative balances (called credit balances), while other accounts are normally expected to have positive balances (called debit balances). Assets and expense items normally have debit (positive) balance accounts, while revenue, liabilities, and shareholder equity items normally have credit (negative) balance accounts (Table 16-1).

Consider the following example: If the organization increases its bank debt, two things must happen. The liability account for bank debt would increase, and the asset account, cash, would also increase. The double entry must add to (debit) cash and subtract from (credit) bank debt. On paper the result would be that the asset account, called cash, would increase, and the liability account, called bank debt, would also increase.

Long-range Financial Plans

A long-range financial plan is a document prepared by every organization to cover the next 5 to 10 years. This plan shows how the long-range vision for the organization will take shape in terms of dollars and cents. This kind of a document is also known as a *projection*. Typically, a goal/financial projection document will begin with a statement about the steps to be taken in the next 5 to 10 years to improve the organization. For example, the administrator of a medical clinic might include discussions about (1) building new buildings, (2) adding a wing to modernize or increase the efficacy of certain types of care, or (3) eliminating or scaling back on underused services (e.g., obstetrics/gynecology [ob/gyn] in a clinic that serves an aging population).

The second part of the document explores the capital side of the items mentioned above. *Capital expenditure plans* set forth the costs for what has been planned. Where will the money come from for the new building or new wing, and when will it be finished? What disruptions will occur to the existing staff and departments? What will be necessary to accompany the improvements? Also included would be a discussion about which departments or divisions might be relocated to (or allowed to expand into) the space being vacated by the underused department.

The third part of the document discusses the *operating budget* of the overall clinic. An operating plan sets forth the changes that are anticipated in the organization as the long-range plan is implemented. This plan contains general and long-term language. An example of such a plan follows.

> The new building will increase our patient capacity by approximately 30%. This will necessitate the addition of 3 to 5 examining rooms, an "in-clinic" X-ray facility and blood-testing machinery. Additional staff will be necessary to implement this plan.

Following the long-term discussion, a more specific, detailed discussion of the expected impact over the next 18 months would be provided:

> The clinic will be adding new examining rooms in February and November of next year. Construction disruptions will be adversely affecting two of the existing examining rooms so appointment scheduling during that period will have to be stretched out and patients seen over a twelve-hour, rather than the usual eight-hour, day. Staffing and budgeting decisions should be made with these scheduling problems in mind.

Budget Terms

The *operating budget* is a planning document used by a department, a division, or the entire organization that forecasts both receipts and expenditures. The budget must be done often enough and in detail to allow the nurse manager to effectively address any differences that develop between the budget's numbers and the actual results. Budgets are generally prepared in one of two ways. *Zero-based budgets* are prepared as though all items of expense in the department, division, or organization are out and must be rejustified to be reincluded in the coming budget. This form of budgeting is time-consuming. A supporting rationale must be composed for each assumption, each planned expenditure, and each planned revenue (Fig. 16-1).

Flexible-based budgeting builds off the budget used in the prior period and is mostly a series of adjustments and refinements to the prior budget. Most budgeting falls into this category, mostly because zero-based budgeting is so time consuming, can result in major changes in direction or emphasis, and can therefore require a great deal of coordination between and among interacting departments and divisions.

TABLE 16-1. LOBSTERVILLE CLINIC'S STATEMENTS FOR DECEMBER 25 AND DECEMBER 31 WITH DOUBLE-ENTRY ACCOUNTING ENTRIES FOR THE WEEK SHOWN

	Dec 25, 1996		Activity for Week		Dec 31, 1996	
	DR+	CR−	DR+	CR−	DR+	CR−
BALANCE SHEET:						
Assets:						
Cash in clinic's account	2913				2913	
Due from patients	4577		50[1]	100[4]	4627	
Inventories	2588				2488	
Land	60000				60000	
Equipment	20000				20000	
less: depreciation	0			2000[3]	−2000	
Buildings + improvements	220000				220000	
less: depreciation	0			7333[3]	−7333	
Goodwill (amt paid for practice)	140000				140000	
less: amortization	0			14000[3]	−14000	
Liabilities						
Due to suppliers		1879		4000[6]		5879
Due to doctors		11923		3577[5]		15500
Due to nurses		2884		866[6]		3750
Due to other employees		641		192[5]		833
Due to St. Johns		673		6500[2]		7173
Equity						
St. Johns initial capital		422000				422000
Profit & Loss for year		10078				−28440
PROFIT AND LOSS STATEMENT:						
Revenues:						
Patient fees year to date		394338		50[1]		394388

Expenses			
Doctors	182423	3577[5]	186000
Nurses	54134	866[5]	55000
Other employees	9808	192[5]	10000
Supplies	52500	100[4]	52600
Maintenance	24000		24000
Utilities and office supplies	7155		7155
Rent for trailers	51000	4000[6]	55000
Uncompensated & emergency	3240	6500[2]	9740
Cash Flow (year to date)	10078		−5107
Cash Flow (during 12/25–12/31 period)		−15185	
Depreciation	0	9333[3]	9333
Amortization	0	14000[3]	14000
Profit and Loss (year to date)	10078		−28440
Profit and Loss (during 12/25–12/31 period)		−38518	

Notes:

[1]The clinics revenues are credited with $50, the usual St. John's HMO/PPO reimbursement for an expectant mother visit. (Thirty-three patients from Lobsterville visited the St. John's ER during the week. St. John's billed the insurance carriers, the patients HMO/PPO, or these patients directly.)

[2]The clinic was charged with $6500 emergency expense for delivering the doctors and equipment during the storm.

[3]Depreciation for year is charged on Dec. 31. This amount is 1/30 of the value of the building & improvements ($220,000) and 1/10 of the value of the equipment ($20,000). Also Goodwill is being amortized at the rate of 1/10 per year. (Goodwill is a term used when money is paid for a non-tangible asset, in this case the doctor's practice.)

[4]The shot given to the expectant mother came from the clinics drug supply. It was charged a standard $100 per dose.

[5]The doctors, nurses, and other employees of the clinic are paid on the first day of each month for the prior month's work. The liabilities section of the Dec. 25th balance sheet show the money due employees from Dec. 1 to Dec. 25. The expense section shows the amount of accrued payroll liabilities for period Dec. 25 to Dec. 31.

[6]The $4000 rent bill for the trailers for December is received on Dec. 31.

Another term, **variance**, describes the difference between a budgeted number (or planned number) and an actual result. Some variances are positive (better than expected); some are negative (not as good as expected). All variances, both positive and negative, should be analyzed and understood. Managers are expected to classify variances as controllable and noncontrollable, simply meaning that the person responsible for the department or division had the power (or did not have the power) to control a specific variance. Although variances are classified as controllable or noncontrollable, studies of specific variances have shown that most have elements that are controllable and elements that are noncontrollable.

A more useful way to classify variances is as mix variances, volume variances, cost variances, and price variances. These classifications allow the variances to be divided into component parts and quantified by category. Each of these will be addressed below:

- A *mix variance* is a variance or part of a variance that is attributable to a change in the mix of work that the department or division experienced. For instance, a division, whose budget for the year was devised with the expectation that most patients would be middle-aged to older patients recovering from elective gastrointestinal (GI) surgery would experience a super mix variance if suddenly it became a step-down unit for patients from a cardiac intensive care unit (ICU). The occupancy rates might be the same, but the budget numbers on staffing and supplies would never match the actual.
- A *volume variance* occurs when the utilization rate is higher or lower than expected. If a budget is built around a utilization rate, even a small variation from that rate will create a variance.
- A *cost variance* occurs when the cost of the key inputs to the process begin to change. If labor rates go up in the organization, a cost variance will result.
- A *price variance* occurs when the price paid for the product or service offered is different than that used in the budget.

The managerial structure needed to support a budgeting effort is substantial. Top-level decisions must be made and reinforced. Computer systems must be revised to support two parallel sets of numbers, budgeted numbers, and actual accounting results so that side-by-side comparison reports can be generated. The timing of the budgeting cycle and the accounting cycle must be compatible and appropriate so that those individuals who watch over the system make sure the budget and accounting systems are coordinated. Managers must be educated to the process so that the accounting and budgeting data flow accurately and quickly into the computers.

A small group of knowledgeable health facility planners must be involved to help the administrators prepare the goal statement with financial projections. The health planners cannot provide the vision that can only come from the organization's leaders, but they can see to it that the overall document is internally consistent and realistic.

■ PREPARATION OF THE BUDGET

The temptation for the hard-pressed department head is to put budgeting on the back burner and then rush something out the door at the last minute. This temptation should be resisted. The budgeting process, if carried out thoroughly, demonstrates the seriousness the nurse manager exhibits in controlling finances. It gives familiarity with the dollar realities in the nurse manager's area and will inevitably trigger a series of "what if" questions. Those questions are the essential ingredients of change, and change can lead to greater productivity. Below are the several steps each manager must follow to properly prepare a budget.

Step One: Review Past Performance

Past financial performance must be reviewed and understood. This involves several steps. Placing the budgeted numbers next to the actual numbers for a given time period (month, quarter, or year) and identifying any and all significant variances is the first step. The meaning of the variance is interpreted as significant under different conditions. If the budgeted number is small, variations of less than 10% are generally not considered significant. If the budgeted number is large, variations of 2% or 3% may be considered significant.

The interpretation of the variances is facilitated by determining the degree of control held by the nurse manager. Each item in the budget should be identified as "beyond my control," "partly under my control," or "under my control." "Revenue per patient" and "number of patients treated" are items beyond the nurse manager's control. However, "overtime expended" items might be classified as under the nurse manager's control.

Each significant variance, whether under the manager's control or not, should be looked into, commented on, and explained. Usually the reason for a variance is a function of either a volume, mix, price, or cost variance. These generic terms can be understood with a few examples.

- If the budget had been prepared on the basis of an 80% average occupancy rate on a unit and the actual occupancy rate was 65%, there would be a volume variance of significant proportions.
- If several additional beds increased the unit's capacity as well as the need for professional staff, registered nurse (RN) budget numbers would be below actual. In this case, the total nursing-cost budget number would be below actual and both a combination mix and cost variance would exist; different and higher cost inputs had to go into providing the service.
- If a higher percentage of older and sicker, uninsured patients were admitted, the variance on the revenue side would be both a mix variance (greater acuity) and a price variance (full payment was not recovered).

Step Two: Review the Organization's Goals and Projections

The organization's goals and financial projections should be studied thoroughly. The manager has to assume that the administrators and the health planners have a good grasp on future plans for the organization. Items in the major report that affect an individual department should be highlighted. An example of this is as follows:

> This division is going to lose 4 beds from February to November and then gain 12 additional beds after that. A gerontologist and clinical specialist in gerontology have been added to the staff. This division will then admit older and sicker patients. If the shortage of nurses continues, nursing service will have to consider alternative staffing patterns to deal with this situation.

Step Three: Review the Variance

Once the goal statement is finished, it, together with the actual versus budget analysis done earlier, should be reviewed with higher level management. The departmental goals proposed should be carefully considered; the variances, their causes, and proposed corrective actions should also be reviewed. Once the final statement for the department is in place, the new budgeting process can begin in earnest.

Step Four: Actual Preparation of the Budget

The actual preparation of a new budget can be done at several degrees of depth. Types of budgets were discussed earlier, but for review, different types of budgets serve different departments more appropriately. Zero-based budgets are used when prior assumptions are rejected and all items are questioned anew. Less rigorous budgeting or flexible budgeting uses the prior year's operation as the model for the coming year, and changes are made as needed to fit new realities. Most budgeting is flexible budgeting in which the prior year becomes the model for the current year.

To complete the budget, a **budget worksheet** is essential, which includes a condensed version of the department's goal statement. The actual worksheet is composed of columns. These columns should include one with historic information with the old budget and a column for actual numbers with comments explaining the variances. Another column should display revenue and cost, both direct and indirect. The items that are fully controllable within the department should be highlighted.

The manager should be able to enter an estimate of the budget numbers they see growing out of the process. Next to each number should be a notation on the source of the number. Some organizations provide these budgetary worksheets with guidelines that explain what each line and column should contain. Table 16-2 offers an example of a budgetary worksheet for a medical clinic that is growing and changing.

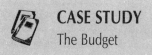

CASE STUDY
The Budget

Brenda Smith has been a head nurse on Division 6 West for three years. She has been a competent and thoughtful manager. She has been wanting to expand her role and spoke to her director of nursing about her thoughts. Brenda explained that she needed to know more about the organization's plans so that she could feel she was keeping pace.

The director, Mr. Brown, suggested that Brenda think about the financial component of her division. He suggested that she consider becoming involved with the creation of the budget for her division rather than allowing financial management to dictate the budget for 6 West.

TABLE 16-2. LOBSTERVILLE CLINIC BUDGET AMOUNTS FOR 1996 WITH ACTUAL AMOUNTS, VARIANCES AND ANALYSIS SHOWN TO THE RIGHT

	Budgeted	Actual	Difference or Variance	Type of Variance	Cause
REVENUE:					
Children patients					
% St. John's HMO/PPO payment ***	3.8%	6.3% *	–2.5%		Insignificant variance
Number of visits	675	496	179	– volume	St. John's letter directing injured athletes to go to St. John's ER
Average $ per visit	168	169 *	–1		Insignificant variance
Total $	113400	83824			
Adult patients					
% St. John's HMO/PPO payment ***	2.0%	1.9%	0.1%		Insignificant variance
Number of visits	1250	1274 *	–24		Insignificant variance
Average $ per visit	119	116	3	– price	Private payers refused to pay for things formerly covered
Total $	148750	147784			
Pregnant women patients					
% St. John's HMO/PPO payment ***	6.5%	77.4%	–70.9%	– mix	Catholic Facility added patient load at lower payment rates
Number of visits	184	775	–591	+ volume	Catholic Facility added patient load increasing dollars to clinic
Average $ per visit	59	52	7	– price	Catholic Facility added patient load at lower payment rates
Total $	10856	40300			
Older patients					
% St. John's HMO/PPO payment ***	3.0%	75.0%	–71.9%	– mix	Catholic Facility added patient load at lower payment rates
Number of visits	800	2401	–1601	+ volume	Catholic Facility added patient load increasing dollars to clinic
Average $ per visit	59	51	8	–price	Catholic Facility added patient load at lower payment rates
Total $	47200	122480			
Total Dollars	320206	394388	74182		

EXPENSE:

	Planned		(+ or −)	
Doctor #1	75000	75000	0	
Doctor #2	75000	75000	0	
Nurse/midwife	35000	35000	0	
Part time receptionist 6 hrs/day +$9/hr	12000	10000	2000 + cost	Receptionist quits and is replaced by less costly person
Extra help (part-time resident mid-year)**	0	18000	−18000 − volume	Catholic Facility added patient load
Extra help (part-time resident mid-year)**	0	18000	−18000 − volume	Catholic Facility added patient load
Extra help (full-time geriatric nurse practitioner added mid-year)**	0	20000	−20000 − volume	Catholic Facility added patient load
Total Personnel Costs:	197000	251000	−54000	
Other Ordinary Costs:				
Rent	24000	55000	−31000 − volume	Trailers needed to handle increased patient arrivals
Utilities/phone	6000	6300*	−300	Insignificant variance
Office supplies	800	855*	−55	Insignificant variance
Supplies & testing agents:				
Urine testing	7500	9000*	−1500	Insignificant variance
Bandaging	6500	2000	4500 + mix	Transfer of sports injuries to ER says on splints and bandages
Syringe	14000	17000	−3000 − volume	Catholic Facility added patient load
"In clinic" blood testing	12000	19000	−7000 − volume	Catholic Facility added patient load
Other	4200	5600*	−1400	Insignificant variance
Maintenance	15000	24000*	−9000	Insignificant variance
Total Other Costs:	90000	138755	−48755	
Uncompensated care	3200	3240*	−40	Insignificant variance
Emergency	0	6500	−6500 − cost	Emergency with mother in early labor
Expense Total	290200	399495	−109295	
Toward clinic's depreciation and St. John's overhead costs (+ or −)	30006	−5107	35113	

* Variance on this item is too small to deserve investigation

** Not represented in the original budget but was needed to provide needed care

*** St. John's HMO/PPO reimbursement rates are generally 20% less than private payers

Brenda considered this possibility and felt that this would enhance her ability to plan for and control the division. However, she also considered that new technical knowledge had to be gained if she were to feel confident with this task. She devised a plan and a timetable that included what she needed to know.

She gave herself one year and scheduled meetings with financial management directors. She asked for and received previous budgets for Division 6 West.

- What information and new knowledge does she need?
- In what real way will this new responsibility enhance productivity on the division?

(Author's Note: The illustrative examples in this chapter are all drawn from the financial experiences of a single hypothetical medical clinic. The reader will need to read this case to fully understand the discussion of capital expenditures on page 336, as well as general ledger and budget information in Table 16-1 and Table 16-2).

CASE STUDY
The Lobsterville Clinic: A Study in Financial Resource Management

Location and Economics of Lobsterville

The Lobsterville Clinic is located in the small community of Lobsterville (pop 3,250), situated at the end of a long, thin, sandy peninsula, 40 miles long, that parallels the seacoast. Lobsterville is 2.5 miles from downtown New Providence, the nearest major seaport city, but, by car, Lobsterville is ninety miles from New Providence. Lobsterville is an economically depressed community with a small fishing fleet and some small businesses, who cater to the tourist trade, causing an economic surge every summer. The town would never have grown to 3,250 except for the fact that from 1940 to 1990, the Navy ran a mine-sweeping training facility in Lobsterville. This training facility, had been used to conduct six-week training classes, which all sailors and officers who served on destroyers had to attend. The only things remaining on the training base were two large housing facilities, each with 400 small efficiency apartments. These apartments had been used by the sailors when they came to Lobsterville for their training.

To enhance transportation, the state and federal governments finished construction of a suspension bridge, which connected New Providence to Lobsterville. This bridge was very high to allow the largest ocean-going vessels to pass under the bridge on their way into New Providence harbor. The bridge was not intended to serve only Lobsterville but was built to provide easier access to New Providence from the north. The road from Lobsterville going north was also being improved to handle the additional traffic.

Establishment of The Medical Clinic

Long-range Planning
Financial Management

The planning department at St. John's of New Providence projected that with the new bridge, medical care in Lobsterville would no longer be within the orbit of the hospital in Oceanside, a town located 40 miles to the north, but would soon come within the orbit of New Providence, which has eight major hospitals and two medical colleges, including one that was affiliated with St. John's. St. John's was well-connected to the large Catholic population in New Providence and in fact had a HMO/PPO contract with the Archdiocese of New Providence, under which St. John's provided all health care for the employees of the Archdiocese, its parish employees, and all people residing in Catholic charitable institutions.

Thus, in late 1995, St. John's Hospital of New Providence created the Lobsterville Clinic by buying the medical practices of two doctors, an internist and a pediatrician, who were operating a joint partnership practice out of a small aging building with a gravel parking lot situated in the center of a ten-acre lot. Their office consisted of a waiting room, four examining rooms, a small lab, a unisex rest room, a coffee room, and a file room. The doctors employed an RN, who was also a certified nurse midwife, and 2 part-time receptionists. Among her other duties, the nurse midwife also served as the part-time bookkeeper/administrator for the clinic.

In the past, these two doctors had staff and admitting privileges at the Oceanside hospital. As part of the buy-out, these two doctors were given staff and admitting privileges at St. John's, they were promised the clinic would not be closed or relocated for at least five years, and they were given employment contracts with the new clinic. The hospital paid $100,000 for the building, $60,000 for the land, $20,000 for the equipment and fixtures, and $140,000 for the practice. The financial department of St. John's managed the contract, and the total package came to be $320,000.

Formation of the Capital Budget

Financial Management Structure
Accounting
Assessment of Assets, Resources, and Expenditures

In December, the planning department at St. John's assigned an administrator to the new Lobsterville Clinic to set up the first capital budget and operating budget for the facility. The administrator met the nurse midwife to design the clinic's first budget. After reviewing the assets and resources, they were faced with an unexpected problem. The location of the Lobsterville Clinic was 6 miles from the main hospital. Within a twelve-mile radius of the clinic were 500,000 people, but in the narrow 3-mile radius, there were only 3,500 people. Ideally, the clinic should be relocated to the other side of the bridge, but there was the five-year nonrelocation clause, and there was the uncertainty about what future growth might occur in Lobsterville as a result of the new bridge. The administrator and the nurse midwife decided on a "steady-state" budget, keeping the same staff in place, and planning only minor physical improvements to the facilities, including a new large examining room that had the air, water, and power hookups to accommodate more sophisticated diagnostic equipment and two new bathrooms (a male and female), to replace the old unisex facility. The budgeting process reflected these small improvements.

Expenditures

In January, the Lobsterville Clinic, under the ownership of St. John's, began to see patients with its former staff (two doctors, nurse midwife, and two part-time receptionists). The administrator's operating budget for the clinic is shown in Table 16-2 (to the left of the vertical line). The capital budget for the new rest rooms was $120,000, including the costs for the trailer to keep the clinic open during construction.

Also, in January, again in response to the new bridge, the Archdiocese of New Providence decided to purchase the two apartment buildings from the Navy. The Archdiocese needed a place to put 650 indigent elderly who were under the care of Catholic Charities, and another facility for 120 poor pregnant women who needed housing during their pregnancy. The archdiocese' current facilities were old and were scheduled to be closed for code violations as soon as the acceptable alternative facilities could be found.

Events that Produce Variance

Revenue and Expenditures
Revenue

In March, patients began arriving at the new Archdiocesan facility, and they begin coming to the Lobsterville Clinic for care. By May, the geriatric patient flow had increased from four per day to 20 per day, and the expectant mother patient flow increased from two per day to 16 per day. Needless to say, the clinic was totally unequipped for these additional patient visits.

Additional Expenditures

The main hospital arranged for two additional trailers to be parked next to the existing trailer and be converted into examining rooms. A gerontological nurse practitioner was assigned to the Lobsterville Clinic full-time, a gerontologist resident was scheduled to be in Lobsterville three days per week, and an ob-gyn resident was scheduled three days per week.

The facilities were poor, but patients were being examined, blood and urine samples were taken, and morale was generally high. In November, the contractor finished the new rest rooms and large examining room. The administrator met with the nurse midwife to discuss the budget and future of the Lobsterville Clinic. The town of Lobsterville was beginning to experience a boom. Several contractors were planning new subdivisions, but building permits were not being issued because the community was not sure where the necessary fresh water would come from. The meeting ended with a decision to maintain the clinic as is with a combination of trailers and permanent structure until the town of Lobsterville found a source for additional fresh water. The operation budget was kept on a steady state (using a budget worksheet), although both the nurse midwife and administrator agreed that things were more likely to change than remain steady.

Events That Lead to Unusual Expenditures

To unwind after a hectic year, the clinic decided to schedule no appointments during the last week of December. Everyone was encouraged to get a good vacation. However, the nurse midwife was forced to stay in Lobsterville, her husband was the fire chief, and so she remained on call.

The clinic's phone was forwarded to the main hospital, patients would be seen if needed at the hospital's emergency room, and the St. John's ER was told that if someone there needed access to the clinic, they were to call the nurse midwife in Lobsterville and she would help them.

On December 29th, an expectant mother at the Catholic Charities facility went into early labor (she was in her sixth month), as very high winds raged and the new suspension bridge was declared impassable. Catholic Charities in Lobsterville called the clinic, the call was picked up at the main hospital, and the emergency room dispatched an ambulance to get the woman. In ten minutes, the ambulance driver radioed that he was at the bridge, but the police had blocked all traffic. The dispatcher told the driver to go the old way to Lobsterville via the ninety miles of road through Oceanside. Then the dispatcher called the nurse midwife in Lobsterville and explained the situation.

The nurse midwife rushed to the Catholic Charities facility to make a preliminary examination of the woman and called St. John's and asked to speak to the ob-gyn resident on duty. The nurse told the resident that the woman had not progressed very far in labor and could still be transported the short distance to the clinic where there are medicines that might control her labor. She also explained that the new room at the clinic had hook-ups needed for neonatal equipment. If this equipment could be delivered to the clinic, the clinic would have a good chance of saving the baby if it was delivered. Calls were also made to the neonatal unit and St. John's maintenance department, which would be responsible for dismantling the equipment and packaging it for transport to Lobsterville.

The decision was made to move the woman to the Lobsterville Clinic and send the equipment and an ob-gyn resident and pediatrician from St. John's via the old road to Lobsterville. The Lobsterville fire department was called to move the woman. At the clinic, the nurse midwife administered the medicine, but she also began a course of soothing hypnosis. This process involved giving the patient repeated suggestions that the baby really wanted to remain with the mother for the time being. The hypnosis was meant to mobilize the mother's system toward keeping, rather than separating from, the infant.

Radio/telephone contact was established with the truck bringing the doctors and equipment. Their progress was slow. Traffic accidents and water-covered roads were problems. What was supposed to be a two-hour trip was turning into a three- or four-hour trip. The winds remained high, but the well-built windowless room was quiet, and the expectant mother remained very calm in the care of the nurse midwife. Gradually, the contractions slowed and then stopped.

The equipment from Lobsterville arrived, but the decision to remove it from the truck was never made. The doctors and the nurse midwife discussed the episode in the hall as the expectant mother slept in the examining room. The doctors shook their heads as the course of hypnotic suggestion was explained.

The patient was not transferred to St. John's.

Cost Accounting

Double-entry Accounting

When the year-end financial reports arrived the nurse midwife noticed that all the extra expenses incurred on the 29th were being charged to the Lobsterville Clinic. What was going to be a positive cash-flow year became a losing year. She thought to herself, at least the premature baby was not delivered in the middle of that storm.

■ SUMMARY

This chapter has discussed the management of financial resources with special attention to the budgetary process. The major department in an organization that handles finances is the office of financial management. However, managers may be called upon to give input into decisions about finances as well as to manage a budgeted amount of money for specific divisions or departments.

It is with this responsibility in mind that a discussion concerning the budgetary process was offered. The major financial management office dictates to what degree the individual managers engage in financial management, which may include preparation of a budget.

The activity of preparing a budget requires some fundamental orientation to related budgetary concepts. Accounting is important to the process. There are different types of reports and formats, but today double-entry accounting is the most useful. Long-range financial plans for the organization dictate to what degree financial resources will be allocated for the present and the distant future. Budgetary terms are also fundamental to understanding what is involved with budgeting. Finally, the actual steps necessary to complete a budget are provided.

The manager's role may vary in relation to finances, but knowledge of the process is critical to the planning and control functions of the manager. The more information available to the manager, the better the decisions and the better the input into the long-range plans for the organization.

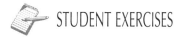

STUDENT EXERCISES

1. What do you think the nurse manager's role should be concerning the finances of the organization?

2. What is a budget? Develop a personal budget for yourself for the next week. Is this a difficult task?

3. Do some double-entry accounting of the money you began the week with and how you spent your funds. Was your spending what you anticipated?

4. On your next clinical rotation, observe the pattern of staff, use of drugs and equipment, and anything that is unusual. Determine a simple budget for the division. Use a category for salaries, drugs and equipment, and housekeeping expenses. Then observe to see if there will be a deviation from your plan. For instance, observe if extra patients are admitted, if a disaster occurs, or if too few staff require the use of nurses from an outside float pool.

■ SUGGESTED READINGS

Ehrat K, "The Cost-quality Balance: An Analysis of Quality, Effectiveness, Efficiency, and Cost", *J Nurs Admin*, 17:5, 1987, p. 6–13.

Finkler SA, Budgeting Concepts for Nurse Managers, Philadelphia, WB Saunders, 1992.

Finkler SA, Knickman JR, Hanson KL, "Improving the Financial Visibility of Primary Care Health Centers," *Hospital and Health Services Administration*, 39:1, 1994, p. 117–131.

Gabrielson R, Lund C, "Enhancing the Financial and Operational Performance of the Nursing Department," *J Nurs Admin.*, 15:11, 1985, p. 28–32.

Holder W, Williams J, "Better Cost Control with Flexible Budget and Variance Analysis." In Schied E (editor), *Maintaining Cost Effectiveness*, Chicago: Nursing Resources, 1979.

Wellever A, "Variance Analysis: A Tool for Cost Control." *J Nurs Admin.*, 12:7&8, 1982, p. 23–26.

West DJ, "Involving Physicians in Cost Reduction Strategies," *Healthcare Financial Management*, 48:4, 1994, p. 46–47.

Wilburn D, "Budget Response to Volume Variability," *Nursing Management*, 23:2, 1992, p. 42–44.

INDEX

A

Accountability, 8, 180, 181
Accounting, 318, 321–323. *See also*
    Budgeting
Accreditation, 194
Active listening, 52–53
ADA (Americans with Disabilities Act),
    254
Administrative management, 126–129.
    See also Management; Nursing
    management
Advanced practice nurses (APNs), 11
Affirmative action, 100, 109, 252, 253
Age Discrimination Act, 254
Agency for Health Care Policy and
    Research (AHCPR), 197, 202
Aggressive communication, 46, 54
AHCPR (Agency for Health Care
    Policy and Research), 197, 202
AIDS, 99
Ambulatory care, 4, 9
American Hospital Association, 113
American Nurses' Association (ANA),
    107, 166, 197, 258, 260
Americans with Disabilities Act (ADA),
    254
ANA. *See* American Nurses' Association
Analysis, 74–76

Answerability, 194
APNs (advanced practice nurses), 11
Argyris, Chris, 131, 156
Assertive communication, 46, 54
Assets, 318, 322
Assignment of work, 181
Associate nursing, 170, 171
Authority, 136–137, 146, 180, 181
Autocratic decision-making style, 22,
    25–26, 80
Autonomy, 100, 104, 113

B

Balance sheets, 322–323
Bargaining, 92
Baylor plan, 300–301
Behavioral school, 22, 25
Behavioral science, 130–131
Behavioral/situational framework, 4, 16
Behavior theory and motivation theory,
    212
Beneficence, 100, 104, 200
Benefits, 218, 144–145
Bennett Amendment of 1972, 201
Bennis, Warren, 131
Bill of Rights documents, 113
Boards of nursing, 199

Brainstorming, 84
Budget, 318
Budgeting, 317–340
  policy statement for, 321
  process of, 318, 320–321, 329–331
Budget work sheet, 318
Bureaucratic model of organization, 129–130
Burnout, 106

C

Capital expenditure plans, 324
Capitation, 4, 9
Career ladder, 228, 242–244
Case management, 154, 163, 171–173
Case method, 154, 168
Case mix, 294, 295
Cash-flow statements, 323
Centralized authority, 136
Central tendency errors, 246
Certification, 194, 197–198
Certified nurse midwives (CNMS), 11
Certified registered nurse anesthetists (CRNAs), 11
Change agents, 14, 268, 280–281
Change management, 267–290
  evaluation of, 284–285
  in nursing, 270–273
  process of, 273–277
  resistance to, 281–284
  stages of, 277–280
  theoretical perspective of, 269–270
Chaos theory, 124, 134
Children, 11, 12
Citizen's Committee for Employment Rights, 261
Civil Rights Act of 1964, 253, 255
Classical theory of organization, 125–130
Climate
  for communication, 46, 48, 51
  internal, 74

and motivation, 210, 215–219
for nursing practice, 195–196
Clinical ladder, 228, 242–244
Clinical nurse specialists (CNSs), 11
Clinical nursing, 12
Clinton, Bill, 6, 11–12, 261
Clinton, Hillary, 6
CNMs (certified nurse midwives), 11
CNSs (clinical nurse specialists), 11
Code for Nurses, 101–104, 106, 107, 111, 112
"Code for Nurses with Interpretive Statements," 113
Coercive power, 135
Collective bargaining, 252, 257–260
Combination plan, 301
Communication, 46–60
  blocks to, 55–56
  climate for, 46, 48, 51
  with difficult people, 57–60
  with health team, 56–60
  process of, 46, 47–49
  in time management, 306
Communication networks, 60, 61
Competition, managed, 4, 9, 14, 144
Computer technology, 216, 267
Conflict, 74, 86–94
  basis of, 87–93
  examples of, 89–91
  management of, 91–94
  nature of, 86–87
Confrontation, 92
Connection power, 136
Connective leadership, 23, 34–35
Consensus, 80–81
Consequentialism, 103
Contingency design, 124
Contingency model of leadership, 22, 29–30
Contingency structure, 142–143
Contracts in managed care, 8–9
Controlling, 154, 165
Coordinating, 154, 165
Corporate planning groups, 6

Cost accounting, 318, 323–324. *See also* Budgeting
Cost centers, 124
Costs of health care, 6, 144, 183
Covy, Stephen, 131
Creativity, 74
Crisis control, 306, 310–311
Criteria, 194
Critical care, 12
CRNAs (certified registered nurse anesthetists), 11

D

Daily planning, 310
Death and dying, 106, 113
Decentralized authority, 136, 180, 183
Decision, 74
Decision making, 74–86
    impact of, 79–80
    in nursing, 77–79
    process of, 74, 81–86
    styles of, 22, 25–26
    systems of, 80–81
Decoding, 48–49
Delegation, 138, 179–190
    barriers to, 187–189
    guidelines for, 186–187
    purpose of, 183–184
    in time management, 307
Delphi technique, 84
Deming, W. Edwards, 201
Democratic decision-making style, 22, 25–26, 80
Deontology theories, 100, 103–104
Descriptive methodology, 294, 296
Diagnosis related groups (DRGs), 4, 5–6, 201
Directing, 154, 164–165
Disabilities, people with, 254
Disciplinary action, 229, 239–240
Discrimination, 235, 252. *See also* Ethnic groups; Minorities

Dissatisfiers, 210, 212–213
Division of work, 124
Dock, Lavina, 14
Double-entry accounting, 318, 324, 326–327. *See also* Budgeting
Downsizing, 159, 267
DRGs. *See* Diagnosis related groups
Due process, 239

E

EEOC (Equal Employment Opportunity Commission), 252, 253, 255
EEO (Equal Employment Opportunity laws), 252, 253
Effectiveness, 306, 307, 311
Efficiency, 306, 307, 311
Elderly, 11
Empirical-rational strategy, 268, 269
Employer-employee relationships, 108–110
Encoding, 47–49
Epidemiology, 7–8
Equal Employment Opportunity Commission (EEOC), 252, 253, 255
Equal Employment Opportunity (EEO) laws, 252, 253
Equal employment regulations, 240
Equitable treatment, 108–109
Ethical issues, 13, 99–120
    barriers in, 105–106
    in health care rationing, 200
    in nursing practice, 106–108
Ethical principles, 104–105
Ethical theories, 103–104
Ethics, 100
Ethics committees, 100, 107–108
"Ethics in Nursing: Position Statements and Guidelines," 113
Ethnic groups, 109. *See also* Discrimination; Minorities

Evaluation. *See* Performance appraisal system

Evaluation of groups, 67

Evaluation interview, 229, 238–241

Excellence approach to management, 157–158

Expectancy theory, 210, 214–215

Expenditures, 318

Expert panel method, 294, 298

Expert power, 135

Extrinsic motivation, 156

F

Family and Medical Leave Act (FMLA) of 1993, 261–262

Fayol, Henri, 126

Fee for service, 5, 14

Field theory, 281–282

Financial management, 317. *See also* Budgeting

Financial management system, 318, 319–320. *See also* Budgeting

Financial projections, 321, 324–325, 330. *See also* Budgeting

Financial structure, 318, 319–320. *See also* Budgeting

Flat/horizontal organizational structures, 141–142, 163

Flexible-based budgeting, 325

FMLA (Family and Medical Leave Act of 1993), 261–262

Forced association, 84

Formal groups, 61–62

Fringe benefits. *See* Benefits

Functional nursing, 154, 168

Future for health care, 13–14

G

Gender roles, 106

General systems/social systems theory of organization, 131–134

Gene therapy, 106

Goal prioritizing in time management, 307–308

Goal setting, 211

Goals and financial projections, 321, 324–325, 330. *See also* Budgeting

Goodrich, Annie Warbuton, 14

Governmental regulations, 200–202

Great Depression, 130, 217

Greater social system, 146

Great man theory, 22

Grievance, 229, 240

Group dynamics, 46, 61–67

Group evaluation, 67

Guessing error, 246

"Guidelines on the Termination of Life-Sustaining Treatment and the Care of the Dying," 113

Gullick, Lyndall, 126

H

Habit, 312

Halo effect, 246

Hastings Center, 113

Hawthorne Studies, 130, 131

Health care

characteristics of, 10–13

costs of, 6

dynamics of, 4, 10–13

forecast for, 13–14

integrated system of, 5, 143–148

rationing of, 200

reform in, 5–7

See also Mental health care; Preventive care; Primary care

Health maintenance organizations (HMOs), 5, 144

Herzberg, Frederick, 131, 156

Hierarchy of needs, 211–212

HIV, 99

HMOs (health maintenance organizations), 5, 144

Home care, 113
Horizontal/flat organizational structure, 141–142, 163
Hospitalization
  and DRGs, 5–6
  and managed care, 9, 12
  and Medicare reimbursement, 201
Hostile environment harassment, 255
Hygiene factors, 121

I

Idea generation, 84
Ideation, 47, 49
"I" messages, 54
Immigrants, 12
Immunizations, 12
Incident report, 194
Income statements, 322
Indicator, 194
Industrial engineering, 294, 297
Informal groups, 61–62
Information in managed care, 8
Information power, 136
Institute of Medicine (IOM), 202
Institutional ethics committees. See Ethics committees
Institutional loyalty, 109–110
Instrumentality, 210
Insurance industry, 6, 7
Integrated health care system, 5, 143–148
Intentionally disinviting and inviting, 210
Interactional phenomena, 134–138
Interdependence in managed care, 8
Internal climate, 74
Interview, evaluation. See Evaluation interview
Intrauterine diagnosis, 106
Intrinsic motivation, 156
IOM (Institute of Medicine), 202

J

JCAHO (Joint Commission on Accreditation of Healthcare Organizations), 197, 201
Job security, 108
Job sharing, 301
Johnson, Lyndon, 253
Joint Commission on Accreditation of Healthcare Organizations (JCAHO), 197, 201
Judeo-Christian doctrine, 105
Justice, 100, 105, 200

L

Labor-management laws, 167, 257–261
Laissez-faire decision-making style, 22, 25–26
Lambertson, Eleanor, 168
Lateral communication, 46
Leader Behavior Description Questionnaire (LBDQ), 28
Leadership
  definition of, 4, 23–25
  and groups, 63–67
  heritage of, 14–17
  and management, 16–17
  styles of, 22, 25–26
  theories of, 21–43
Leadership behaviors, 22, 26–35
Legal constraints, 253
Legal issues, 105–106, 198–200, 235, 251–265
Legislation. See Governmental regulations, 200–201
Legitimate power, 135
Liabilities, 318, 322. See also Budgeting
Liability, 194
Licensed practical nurses (LPNs), 168, 259
Licensure, 198
Life-cycle theory, 22, 30

Life-sustaining treatment, 113. *See also* Death and dying
Likert, Renes, 156, 157
Line authority, 136–137
Litigation, 253
Long-range financial plans, 318, 321, 324–325. *See also* Budgeting
Lorenz, Edward, 134
Loyalty to institution, 109–110
LPNs (licensed practical nurses), 168, 259

M

McGregor, Douglas, 131, 156
Macromotivation, 210, 218–219
Magaziner, Ira, 7
Maintenance functions in groups, 65
Malpractice, 194
Managed care, 4, 7–10
Managed care organizations, 9. *See also* HMOs; PPOs
Managed competition, 4, 9, 14, 144
Management
    administrative, 126–129
    definition of, 4, 154
    and leadership, 16–17
    levels of, 155–156
    scientific, 126
    See also Nursing management; Organization and management theory
Management Assessment Guide, 175–176
Management by objectives, 229
Management engineering, 294, 297–298
Management science, 156–158
Management theory. *See* Organization and management theory
Maslow's hierarchy of needs, 211–212
Matrix organizations, 142, 230
Medicare, 5, 197, 201
Mental health care, 7
Meritor Savings Bank v. Vinson, 255

Message, 46, 47–48
Micromotivation, 210, 218–219
Minorities, 12. *See also* Discrimination; Ethnic groups
Mission statements, 233
Modern theory of organization, 130–138
Modular nursing, 154, 163, 171
Monitoring performance, 227–250
Monitoring standards, 194
Mooney, James D., 126
Morality, 100
Mothers, 11, 12
Motivation, 156, 209–225
    and behavior theory, 212
    and personality type, 212–214
    problems in, 219–221
    theories of, 211–215
Moving, 268, 279, 281

N

National Health Planning and Resource Development Act of 1974, 201
National Labor Relations Act (Wagner Act) of 1935 (NLRA), 130, 258–260
National Labor Relations Board (NLRB), 258–260
National Labor Relations Board v. Health Care Retirement Corporation of America, 259
National League for Nursing (NLN), 15
Needs theorists, 211–212
Negligence, 194
New theory of leadership, 22, 32–33
Nightingale, Florence, 168
NLN (National League for Nursing), 15
NLRA. *See* National Labor Relations Act (Wagner Act) of 1935
Nondiscrimination. *See* Discrimination
Nonintervention in change, 268, 277
Nonmaleficence, 100, 104

Nonverbal behavior, 46, 48, 52
Normative-reeducative strategy, 268, 270
NPs (nurse practitioners), 11
NRLB (National Labor Relations Board), 258–260
Nurse-patient relationship, 112–115
Nurse practitioners (NPs), 11
Nurse's Bill of Rights, 54
Nursing
    climate for practice, 195–196
    clinical and career ladders, 242–243
    Code for, 101–104, 106–107, 111, 112, 113
    conflicts in, 89–91
    decision making in, 77–79
    ethical issues in, 106–108
    organizational chart for, 140
    systems of care, 154, 167–174
    See also Nursing management; Standards
Nursing homes, 113
Nursing management, 153–177
    assessment guide for, 175–176
    controlling, 165
    coordinating, 165
    directing, 164–165
    evolution of, 159
    objectives of, 149–160
    organizing, 163
    planning, 161–162
    policies in, 166–167
    and risk management, 195, 202–205
    in staff planning, 163–164, 301–302
    transition to, 173–174
    See also Administrative management; Management; Nursing; Standards
Nutting, M. Adelaide, 14

O

Objectives of organizations, 233
Omnibus Budget Reconciliation Act of 1986, 202

Operating budgets, 325
Organizational chart, 124, 138–139
Organization and management theory, 123–151
    classical theory, 125–130
    link between, 147–148
    modern theory, 130–138
Organizations, 124
    concepts about, 138–143
    learnings about, 124, 134
    models of, 145–146
    philosophy, mission, and objectives of, 233
    structures of, 138–142
Organizing, 124, 134–135, 154, 163
Organ transplants, 99
Outcomes management, 194, 201, 202
Outcome standards, 197–198

P

Palmer, Sophia F., 14
Part-time work, 301
Passive communication, 46, 55
Paternalism, 104
Patient-nurse relationship, 112–115
Patient's Bill of Rights, 113–115
Patient's Choice of Treatment Options, 113
Patient Self-Determination Act, 101, 104
Peer Assistance Programs, 111
Peer relationships, 110–111
Performance appraisal system, 229
    criteria for, 230–232
    elements of, 233–237
    obstacles in, 245–246
    participation in, 232
    process of, 237–241
    purpose of, 229–230, 234
    and rewards, 241–245
Performance monitoring, 227–250
Performance standards, 194, 198. *See also* Standards

Perkins, Francis, 168
PERM complex, 271–273
Personality type and motivation, 212–214
Peters, Thomas J., 131, 157
Philosophy of organizations, 233
Planned change, 268, 276
Planning, 154, 161–162
  daily, 310
  in time management, 307
Policy statement in budgeting, 321
Position descriptions, 231
Power, 74, 88, 124, 135–136
Power-coercive strategy, 268, 269
PPOs (preferred provider organizations), 5, 144
Practice guidelines, 194, 197, 198
Prediction of outcomes, 74, 76–77
Preferred provider organizations (PPOs), 5, 144
Pregnancy Discrimination Act, 254
Premises, 74, 77
Prenatal care, 12
Prepaid medical groups, 9
President's Task Force on National Health Care Reform, 6, 11–12
Preventive health care, 7, 10, 12.
  See also Health care
Primary care, 4, 7, 144
  in managed care, 8, 9, 10
  and primary nursing, 170
  See also Health care
Primary groups, 61
Primary nursing, 154, 163, 169–171
Problem analysis in time management, 311
Problem distortion, 246
Problem identification, 274
Problems, 194
Process model of conflict management, 93–94
Process model of leadership, 23, 35–39
Process standards, 197
Professional growth, 184

Professional standards review organizations (PSROs), 201
Public health, 7–8
Purkey's Intentional Model, 220

Q

Quality, 195, 196–197
Quality assurance, 201
Quality management, 195, 201
Quid pro quo, 255

R

Radical change, 268, 276–277
Rater temperament effect, 246
Rationing of health care, 200
Reagan, Ronald, 261
Recency effect, 246
Referant power, 136
Reform in health care, 5–7
Refreezing, 268, 279–280
Registered nurses (RNs), 168, 258, 260
Registration, 195
Reiley, Alan C., 126
Reliability, 229, 235
Resource management
  budgeting, 317–340
  of staff, 293–304
  of time, 305–315
Resources, 294
Resources in budgeting, 318
Response, 48–49
Responsibility, 138, 179, 181
Revenue, 318
Revolutionary eras, 215
Reward power, 135
Rewards, 241–245
Risk management, 195, 202–205
Risk taking, 268
RNs (registered nurses), 168, 258, 260
Robb, Isabel Hampton, 14

S

Satisfiers, 211, 213
Scalar chain, 180, 182–183
Scheduling patterns, 294, 299. *See also*
    Work schedules
Scientific knowledge, 13
Scientific management, 126. *See also*
    Management; Nursing
    management
Secondary groups, 61
Second wavers, 217, 232
Self-actualization, 156
Self-interrogation checklist, 84
Self-management, 306, 308
Sexual harassment, 109, 252–253,
    254–256
Shalala, Donna, 7
Single-parent families, 12
Situational theory, 22, 29, 30–32
Smoothing, 92
Social Security Act Amendment of
    1983, 201
Social Security Amendments of 1983, 5
Social system, 124
Social systems theory of organization,
    131–134
Span of control, 124, 127–128
Specialists, 10–11
Staff authority, 136–137
Staffing, 154, 163–164, 294
Staff management, 293–304
    methodologies of, 296–298
    role of management, 301–302
    See also Work schedules
Staff plan, 294–296
Standard accounting, 318. *See also*
    Budgeting
Standards, 165–166, 193–207, 230–232.
    See also Performance standards
Standards of Nursing Practice, 195,
    196–197, 199, 217
Standards of Patient/Client Care, 195
State boards of nursing, 199

Status, 138
Stewart, Isabel Maitland, 14
Stress, 306, 307
Strikes, 253, 260–261
Structure, 124
Structure standards, 195, 197
Style of leadership, 22, 25–26
Substance abuse, 106, 111
Sunflower effect, 246
Systems of nursing care delivery, 154,
    167–174

T

Taft-Hartley Amendment, 248
Tailoring, 231
Tall/vertical organizational structures,
    141, 163
Task analysis in time management, 311
Task functions in groups, 64
Taylor, Frederick W., 126
Teaching Improvement Projects
    System (TIPS), 91–92
Team nursing, 154, 163, 168–169
Technology, 13
Ten-hour shifts, 300
Terminal patients. *See* Death and dying
Theory X and Y, 156, 213-214
Think tanks, 84
Third-party payers, 202
Third wavers, 217, 232
Time analysis, 309–310
Time control, 311
Time evaluation, 311
Time management, 305–315
    barriers to, 312
    strategies of, 308–311
Time savings, 184
Time styles, 305, 308
TIPS (Teaching Improvement Projects
    System), 91–92
Total care, 170
Traditional eight-hour shifts, 300

Trait approach, 22, 24
Transactional leadership, 23
Transformational leadership, 23, 33–34
Transmission, 48–49
Tsunami (tidal wave), 217
Twelve-hour shifts, 300
Two-factor theory, 212–213

U

Unfair employment practices, 235
Unfreezing, 268, 278
Unilateral action, 92–93
Unions, 130, 252, 257–260
Unity of command, 124, 127
Unity of direction, 124, 127
Utilitarianism, 200

V

Valence, 211
Validity, 229, 235
Values, 100
Variances, 318, 328, 330
Vertical/tall organizational structure,
     141, 163

W

Wagner Act of 1935 (National Labor
     Relations Act), 130, 258–260
Wald, Lillian, 14

Wallenda factor, 33
Waterman, Robert H., Jr., 131, 157
Whistle-blowing, 100, 110
Work assignment, 181
Work expansion, 312
Work load, 294, 295
Work sampling, 297
Work schedules, 242, 299–301. *See also*
     Scheduling patterns

X

X characteristics, 211. *See also* Theory X
     and Y
X chart, 282

Y

Y characteristics, 211. *See also* Theory X
     and Y
York, James, 134
"You" messages, 54

Z

Zero-based budgets, 325
Zone of indifference, 129